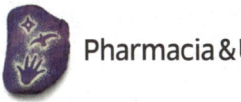

Movement Disorders in Clinical Practice

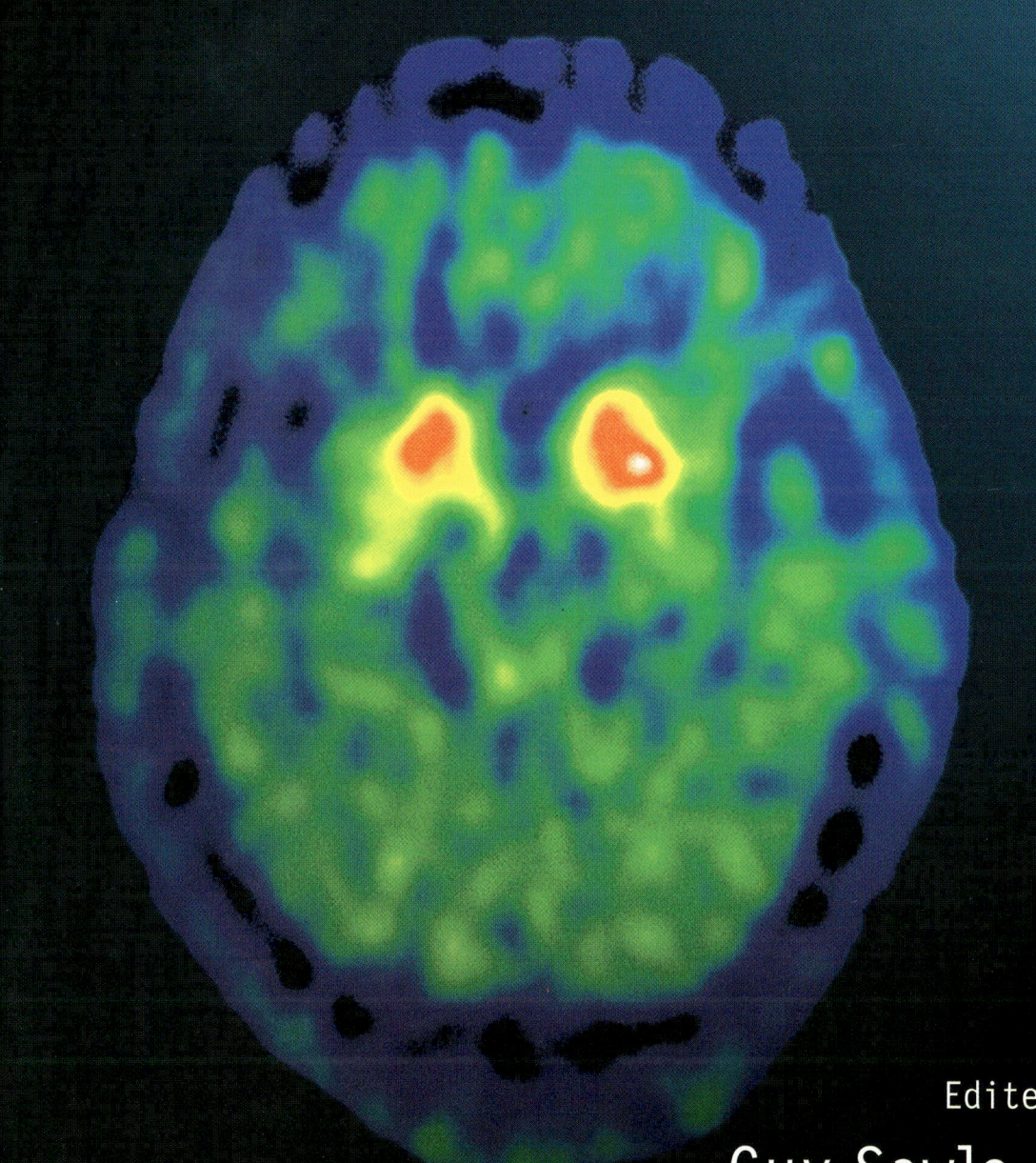

Edited by

Guy Sawle DM FRCP

*Reader in Clinical Neurology and Consultant Neurologist,
University Hospital, Nottingham, UK*

**ISIS
MEDICAL
MEDIA**

© 1999 by Isis Medical Media Ltd.
59 St Aldates
Oxford OX1 1ST, UK

First published 1999

British Library Cataloguing in Publication Data.
A catalogue record for this title is available
from the British Library.

ISBN 1 899066 60 8

Sawle, G. V. (Guy)
Movement Disorders in Clinical Practice
Guy V. Sawle (ed)

Always refer to the manufacturer's Prescribing
Information before prescribing drugs cited in this book.

Design and Illustration
Lee Smith & Paul Wilkinson of InPerspective Ltd.

Indexer
Laurence Errington

Isis Medical Media staff
Publisher: Jonathan Gregory
Senior Editorial Controller: Sarah Carlson
Production & Editorial Manager: Julia Savory

Printed by
KHL Printing Co PTE Ltd, Singapore

Distributed in the USA by
Books International, Inc., P.O. Box 605,
Herndon, VA 20172, USA

Distributed in the rest of the world by
Plymbridge Distributors Ltd., Estover Road,
Plymouth PL6 7PY, UK

Contents

Contributors

Stewart G. Boyd
Consultant Clinical Neurophysiologist, Great Ormond Street Hospital for Children NHS Trust, Great Ormond Street, London, WC1N 3BG, UK

Peter Brown
Consultant Neurologist, MRC Human Movement and Balance Unit, The Institute of Neurology, National Hospital for Neurology and Neurosurgery, Queen's Square, London WC1N 3BG, UK

Lucinda Carr
Consultant Paediatric Neurologist, Great Ormond Street Hospital for Children NHS Trust, Great Ormond Street, London, WC1N 3BG, UK

Cynthia L. Comella
Associate Professor, Rush Presbyterian St. Luke's Medical Centre, 1725 West Harrison, Chicago, IL 60612, USA

J. Helen Cross
Consultant Paediatric Neurologist, Great Ormond Street Hospital for Children NHS Trust, Great Ormond Street, London, WC1N 3BG, UK

Thomas B. Freeman
Professor, Departments of Neurosurgery, Pharmacology and Experimental Therapeutics, University of South Florida, 4 Columbia Drive, Suite 730, Tampa, FL 33606, USA

Robert A. Hauser
Associate Professor of Neurology, Pharmacology and Experimental Therapeutics; Director, Parkinson's Disease and Movement Disorders Center, University of South Florida, 4 Columbia Drive, Suite 410, Tampa, FL 33606, USA

Graham Lennox
Consultant Neurologist, Department of Neurology, Addenbrookes Hospital, Hills Road, Cambridge CB2 2QQ, UK

Guy V. Sawle
Reader and Consultant Neurologist, Division of Clinical Neurology, University Hospital, Queen's Medical Centre, Nottingham NG7 2UH, UK

Foreword

Abnormal movement disorders represent a common and at times bewildering area of clinical neurology. Many patients defy definite categorisation and phenomenology continues to dominate the subject. Even at post-mortem, disorders as disabling and severe as generalised torsion dystonia or the Lance–Adams syndrome are found to have no detectable histopathological lesion. In spite of this uncertainty and relative insubstantiality, the morbid impact on quality of life is considerable.

Jean Martin Charcot and his colleagues at the Sâlpetrière Hospital in Paris were the first to try to dissect and categorise scrupulously these chaotic dyskinetic patterns. A department of medical photography under the direction of Monsieur Londe was opened in order to capture abnormal movements for subsequent publication and case discussions. Charcot and his colleagues also sketched many of the grotesque and handicapping maladies seen on the wards and Paul Richer sculpted a wonderfully evocative statuette of a patient with paralysis agitans. Even today the study of movement disorders remains a visual act.

Despite these early efforts the semiology of abnormal movement disorders remained confused and confusing with the same disorder often being described in the literature under several different medical names. Even the concept of a relatively well-defined disorder like Parkinson's disease changed with the wind as preconceptions came and went and knowledge accrued. In the last fifteen years or so there have been modest gains; molecular genetics has started to make inroads into classification of biochemical and degenerative neurological disorders and more refined methods of imaging the brain have facilitated diagnoses. The arrival of the camcorder has further aided uniformity in clinical description, and video workshops at international meetings and the pioneering work of the Movement Disorder Society with its accompanying video journal have also improved diagnoses. Many patients with movement disorder can now be diagnosed accurately from a written clinical description and accompanying video clip by specialists in the field.

Guy Sawle is to be congratulated on providing a detailed but readable text, liberally embellished with photographic material. The accompanying CD-ROM text places this book as one of the first in what will be a further educational leap forward in assisting the clinician to recognise the often complex and heterogeneous disorders which present with abnormal movement. I wish this book the success it undoubtedly deserves.

Dr Andrew J. Lees
London, 1999

Acknowledgements

My heartfelt thanks go to all of my movement disorder patients, particularly those I have diagnosed and treated slowly or wrongly, and those who have generously allowed me to include them in this book and CD.

I am also grateful to those friends, colleagues and strangers who have supplied illustrations to fill some of the gaps in my own collection. Additional video images have been supplied by Peter Bain, Peter Brown, Robert Hauser, Adrian Wills, Professor P. Polak and Professor A. Benabid. I thank Karen Anderton, Stephen Butterworth, Miles Humberstone and Graham Lennox for their help videoing patients in Nottingham.

I thank Jonathan Gregory, Julia Savory, Sarah Carlson and their colleagues at Isis Medical Media for their encouragement and support, and for seeing this project through. I am grateful to Sean Morrow and his colleagues at Bereza Associates for programming the CD.

My co-authors have been an enormous help and I have oftentimes wished I had enlisted help with more of the chapters. When asked to write a chapter for a book such as this there is a danger in writing too soon, else by the time of publication one's contribution may be out of date. Several of my co-authors took no such risks, and the chapter on tics should be completely up to date at the time of publication.

This book is dedicated to my wife Fiona (who, like me, has been astonished by how much time it has taken) and my children Chloe, Oliver and Tristan who view this ground-breaking book/CD product as a rather ordinary format.

Guy Sawle
Nottingham, 1999

About the CD-ROM

The video clips in this book are mostly my own, taken using a digital video camera in the course of normal outpatient clinics. For each patient shown, I have included a brief clinical history. Also included on the CD are a number of still images (such as brain scans of the patients illustrated) which are not in the book. Hyperlinks direct you to other video clips of related interest.

The principal technical objective has been to show clear images in real time without motion artefact. This is possible with current compression techniques. In order to optimise image quality most of the clips have been kept short; where necessary these can be replayed using the 'loop' button. The image size can be zoomed to 4x normal by pixel replication; this is best used when the images are being viewed at a distance.

Most of the clips have an audio track which is used to convey the ambient noise including the road outside and groaning patients in adjacent rooms as well as any conversations taking place during recording. The clinic rooms are sometimes untidy and cluttered with relatives or medical students. Nevertheless, I hope that these video clips will provide a useful illustration of a broad range of movement disorders.

The CD-ROM runs from the desktop and does not need to be installed onto the host hard drive. Further instructions are found on the CD disc located at the back of this book.

chapter 1

Introduction

Guy Sawle

Movement disorders are common. They are varied. Many are treatable. But faced with a patient who has involuntary movements or a failure of normal movement it may be difficult to make a diagnosis and this may preclude effective treatment.

How do we make diagnoses in neurology? In truth, we diagnose many of the patients we see by pattern recognition. This makes it particularly difficult to diagnose a condition if we have not seen it before.

A particular difficulty in movement disorder diagnosis is that many of the commonest conditions are either of unknown aetiology, have no known pathology, have no known genetic basis, or are inaccessible to conventional investigations. Most movement disorders cannot presently be diagnosed by a brain scan, blood test, or any other kind of investigation. Clinical skills are therefore of supreme importance.

One way to pick up the relevant clinical skills is to work as an 'apprentice' to an (acknowledged or unsung) expert in the field. But not all of those with a neurological interest will be able or sufficiently eager to follow this approach. All wise clinicians turn, at some stage, to the written word.

Faced with a patient with an unrecognized skin condition, one sensible way forward would be to compare the patient's skin with the illustrations in a contemporary dermatological text, many of which are brimming with helpful photographs. But still photographs are much less helpful for movement disorders which lend themselves to the use of video recording, hence the widespread use of video records in movement disorders research and teaching, and the video supplement to the journal of the Movement Disorder Society.

So the intention in writing this book has been to produce a combined text and video product, to enable the reader to see real-time images of as many of the conditions described as possible.

Diagnosing movement disorders: a short overview of movement disorder phenomenology

On the assumption that few readers will be entertained by more than a brief introduction and most will skip straight to the subject chapters, the following overview is intentionally short.

Taking the history

Even though an abnormality of movement may be obvious as soon as a patient enters the room, a careful clinical history is still essential. In particular, a detailed drug history and family history are necessary. Patients may have drug-induced movement disorders as a result of over-the-counter medicines, drugs they were prescribed weeks earlier, illicit drugs, and drugs used to treat gastrointestinal or vestibular disorders, as well as the more 'obvious' psychiatric agents.

Also enquire carefully about the family history. The condition may have low penetrance and very different phenomenology in different family members. Furthermore, previous generations may have been misdiagnosed, so be wary about taking a grandparent's diagnosis of 'Parkinson's disease' at face value. Occasionally, other family members have undiagnosed symptoms or signs; this hardly justifies an exploratory visit to the family home, but some patients bring a relative along who has an undiagnosed head tremor or similar which may unlock the diagnosis.

Examination

Some patients have other neurological symptoms or signs (such as concurrent epilepsy, or extensor plantar responses) or even non-neurological signs (such as hepatomegaly or skin changes) and these must of course be discovered and explored in the conventional way.

Turning now to the movement disorder itself, in the broadest terms, affected patients are either moving too

CLASSIFYING MOVEMENT DISORDERS

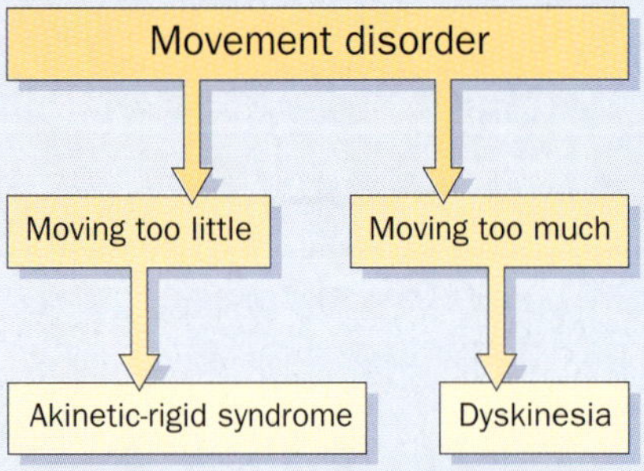

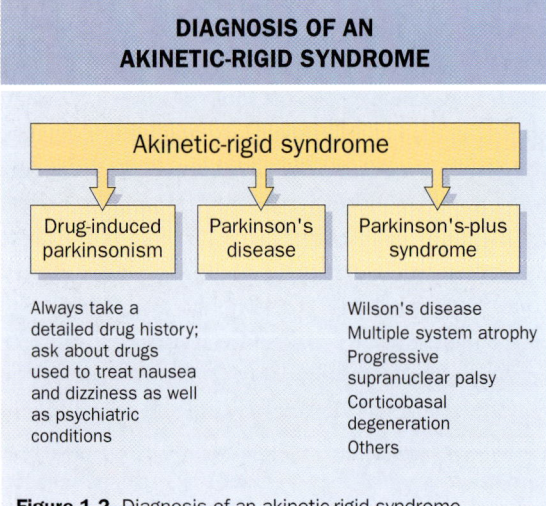

Figure 1.1. Classifying movement disorders.

DIAGNOSIS OF AN AKINETIC-RIGID SYNDROME

Always take a detailed drug history; ask about drugs used to treat nausea and dizziness as well as psychiatric conditions

Wilson's disease
Multiple system atrophy
Progressive supranuclear palsy
Corticobasal degeneration
Others

Figure 1.2. Diagnosis of an akinetic-rigid syndrome.

DIAGNOSIS OF DYSKINESIAS

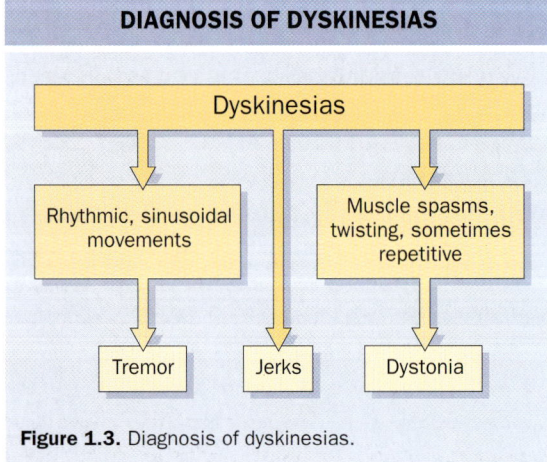

Figure 1.3. Diagnosis of dyskinesias.

much, or too little. Patients who are moving too little are often slow and stiff, and they are said to have an akinetic-rigid syndrome (Fig. 1.1).

Patients with an akinetic-rigid syndrome either have Parkinson's disease, drug (usually neuroleptic)-induced parkinsonism, or something more complicated. Patients with Parkinson's disease may have tremor, but not all do. Those who have an akinetic-rigid syndrome with symptoms in life which are incompatible with the diagnosis of Parkinson's disease are said to have a Parkinson's plus syndrome, common examples of which are multiple system atrophy and progressive supranuclear palsy (Fig. 1.2; CDs 1.1, 1.2).

If the problem is not one of moving too little, then it is often a problem of moving too much, or at least in an abnormal way. These conditions are together called the dyskinesias. When faced with a patient with involuntary movements and searching for the right diagnostic label, it is wise to begin by describing the movements as dyskinetic, since this word embraces so many conditions and does not run the risk of making an incorrect diagnosis by being too specific too soon (Fig. 1.3).

Of the dyskinesias, patients with tremor are fairly easy to recognize. They have rhythmical and approximately sinusoidal movements. Tremors may be specific to certain activities or limited to certain body parts (CDs 1.3, 1.4, 1.5).

Next are the various kinds of 'jerking' movements. These break up into chorea, myoclonus, and tics. Of these, the easiest to separate out are the tics. These are the only kind of involuntary movements which most affected patients are able to stop fairly easily, by an act of will. Furthermore the movements are generally similar to normal 'fragments' of facial expression, such as nose-wrinkling, eyebrow raising, etc. (CD 1.6). Some patients also have vocal tics, which are more commonly sniffs or throat clearing than swearing.

If patients cannot suppress their jerks, they probably have chorea or myoclonus. Chorea is Greek for 'dance', and patients with chorea have jerky, restless, purposeless movements which give a fidgety appearance (CD 1.7). The movements typically flit from one body part to another; you never know which body part will jerk next. Patients may try and hide choreic movements by continuing the movement into an apparently purposeful action,

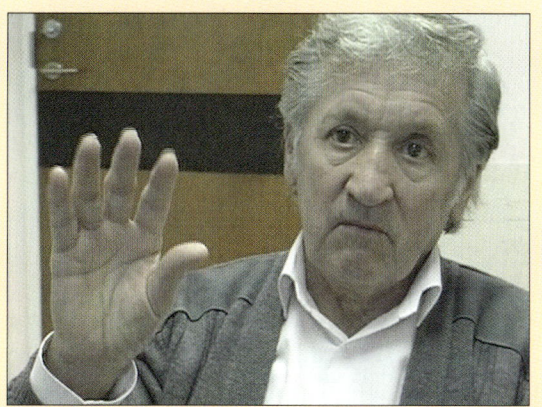

CD **1.1.** Parkinson's disease.

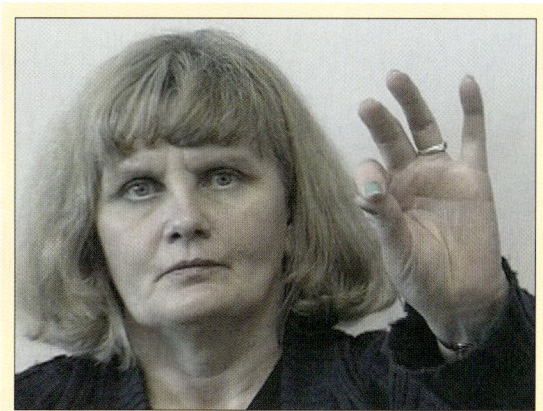

CD **1.2.** Multiple system atrophy.

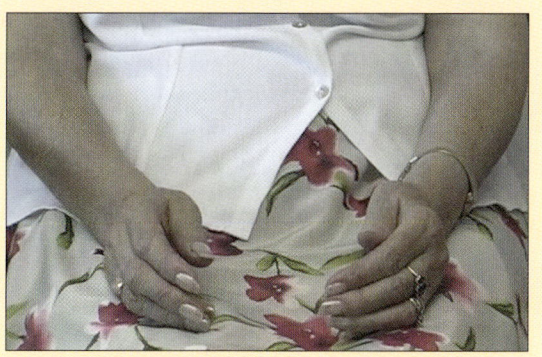

CD **1.3.** Rest tremor.

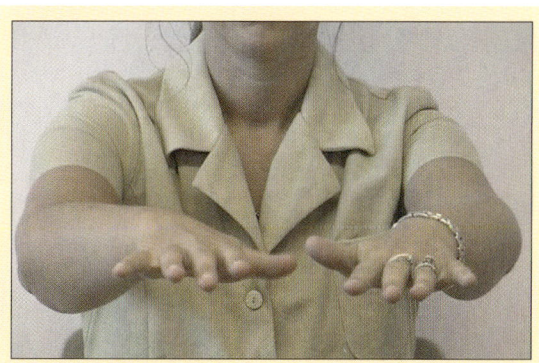

CD **1.4.** Postural tremor.

CD **1.5.** Neck and voice tremor.

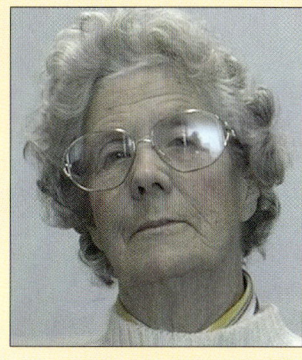

CD **1.6.** Gilles de la Tourette syndrome.

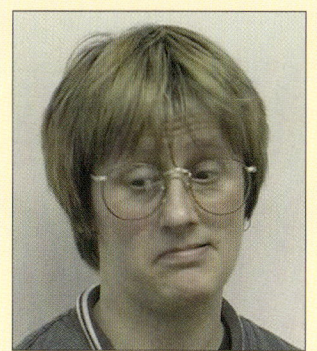

such as adjusting their clothing or hair (CD 1.8). Ballism refers to very large amplitude jerking movements, a kind of severe proximal chorea. It is almost always unilateral and referred to as hemiballism (Fig. 1.4; CD 1.9).

Patients with myoclonus have brief shock-like jerks or lapses in muscle tone (negative myoclonus). Myoclonic jerks are sometimes generalized but may be focal (CD 1.10). They may occur only during action. The clinical differentiation between chorea and myoclonus can be one of the most difficult in movement disorder phenomenology, particularly when the jerks are infrequent.

Patients whose dyskinesias are not simply jerking movements may have dystonia. This refers to muscle

DIAGNOSING 'JERKS'

Jerking movements

Can be voluntarily suppressed → Tics

'Dance-like' Unpredictable → Chorea

Fast 'Shock-like' → Myoclonus

Figure 1.4. Diagnosing jerks.

spasms which often have a twisting component and are typically repetitive (CDs 1.11, 1.12). There is usually simultaneous contraction of agonist and antagonist muscles. Some patients with dystonia have tremor as well, and many have superimposed muscle jerks which are considered to be part of the dystonia. In a patient with a mixture of spasms, twisting, tremor and jerks, the movements may all be due to the dystonia. As with tremor and myoclonus, the movements of dystonia may be action-specific (CD 1.13).

The term 'athetosis' has been largely dropped from usage, except in the context of cerebral palsy. Most other patients whose movements would hitherto have been called athetoid are now recognized to have one of the forms of dystonia.

Conditions which do not fit comfortably into any of the above are those comprising severe (usually axial) rigidity, such as the stiff person syndrome, a miscellaneous group of dyskinesias including belly dancer's dyskinesia, the condition called painful legs and moving toes, and hemifacial spasm. Once encountered, most of these conditions are easily recognized the second time around (CDs 1.14, 1.15, 1.16).

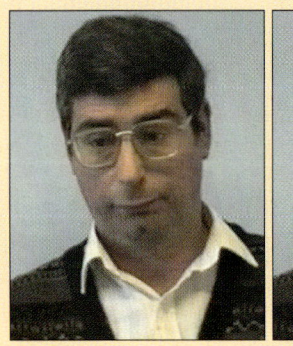 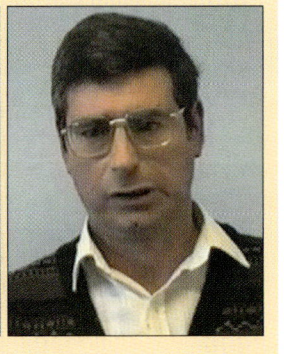

CD **1.7.** Facial chorea.

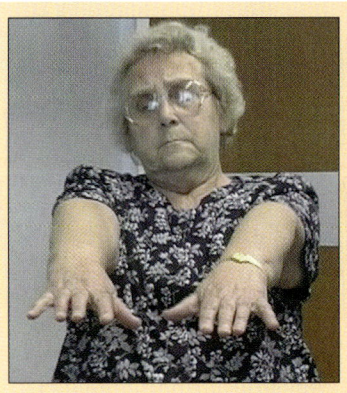

CD **1.8.** Limb chorea.

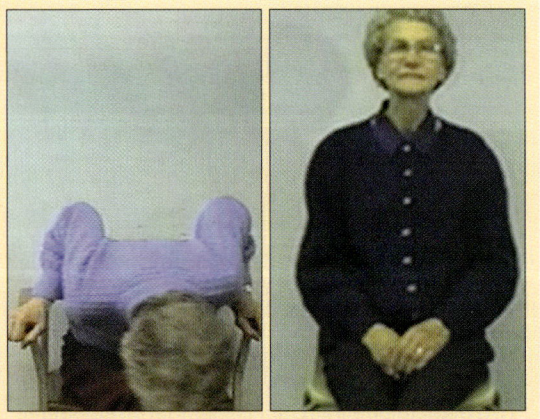

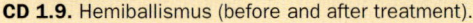

CD **1.9.** Hemiballismus (before and after treatment).

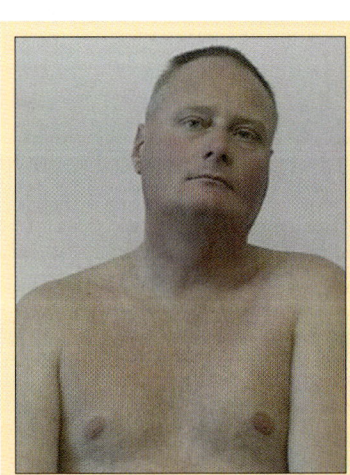

CD **1.10.** Segmental myoclonus affecting left pectoralis muscle.

Finally with regard to phenomenology, it is important to recognize that many patients have a mixture of the various types of movement described above. So patients may have dystonia plus myoclonus, or an akinetic-rigid syndrome plus myoclonus. Or the symptoms of their condition may change with time, starting with chorea but later showing evidence of an akinetic-rigid syndrome and dystonia.

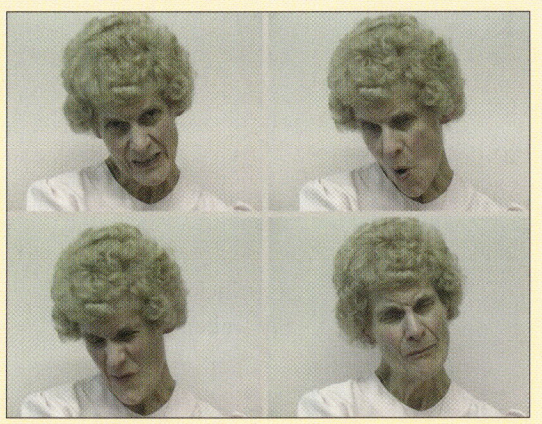

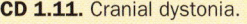
CD 1.11. Cranial dystonia.

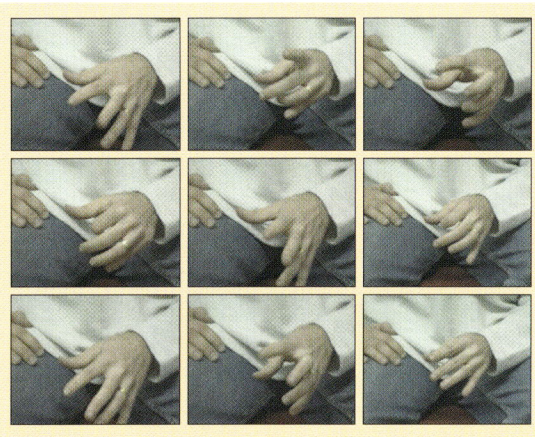
CD 1.12. Arm dystonia.

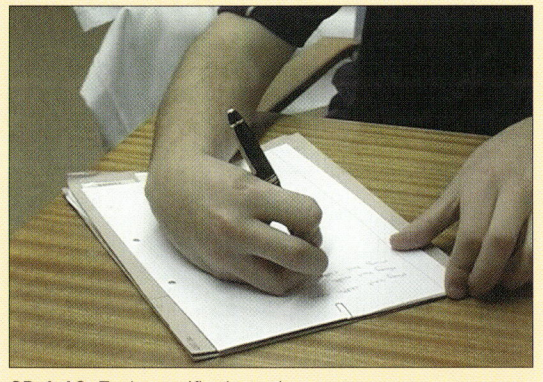
CD 1.13. Task-specific dystonia.

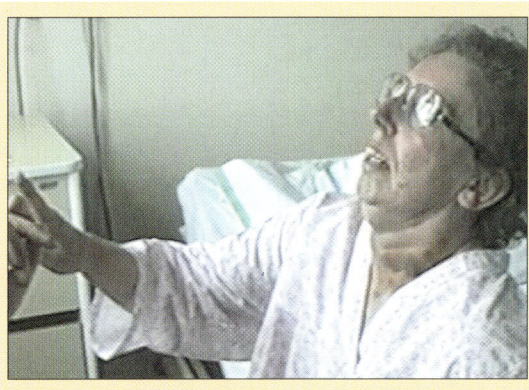
CD 1.14. Stiff person syndrome.

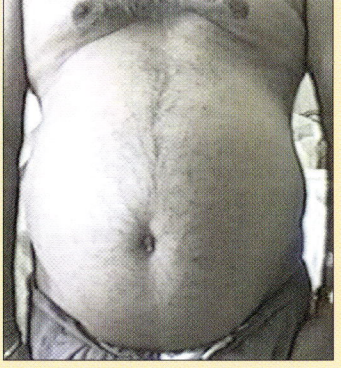
CD 1.15. Belly dancer's dyskinesia.

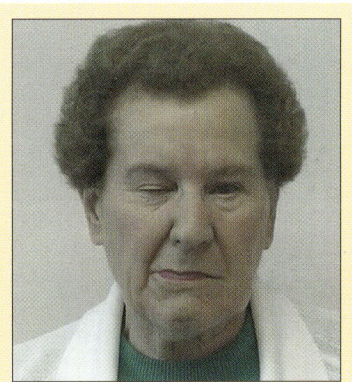
CD 1.16. Hemifacial spasm.

Organization of this book

The movement disorders in this book are grouped mainly into the above categories. Special chapters deal with movement disorders presenting in childhood or induced by exposure to drugs. The small collection of disorders which occur during sleep form another chapter and a miscellaneous chapter completes the overview of organic disorders. Psychogenic movement disorders (chiefly a warning against making the diagnosis too lightly) are discussed separately. Therapy is considered together with each condition, except in the case of Parkinson's disease, where a special chapter is included to discuss neurosurgical treatment.

chapter 2

Parkinsonism: *Parkinson's disease*

Guy Sawle

History

Recognition of the condition and beginning of levodopa therapy

Born in 1755, James Parkinson was 62 years of age when he wrote of 'the shaking palsy'.[1] In this essay he described six patients he had observed in the course of his work as a general practitioner in Shoreditch, two of whom he had met quite casually in the street, and one of whom he seems only to have seen at a distance. Parkinson noted the slow and relentless progression of a disease characterized by a tremor most obvious at rest, with festinant gait, flexed posture, dysarthria, dysphagia, insomnia and constipation.

Charcot some 40 years later noted that tremor was not always present and furthermore that strength was actually normal. It was he who proposed that this condition be referred to as 'Parkinson's disease'. The suggestion that the substantia nigra was abnormal in Parkinson's disease dates back to 1893, although the classic description is that of Trétiakoff in 1919. Hassler, writing in 1938, gave a detailed account of the microscopic anatomy of the substantia nigra, and showed that the pathology of Parkinson's disease is most striking within the ventrolateral cell groups of the pars compacta.[2] In 1957, Carlsson and colleagues demonstrated that levodopa reversed the effects of reserpine in mice and rabbits. Three years later Ehringer and Hornykiewicz reported low dopamine levels in the striata of patients with parkinsonism. In 1961 Birkmeyer and Hornykiewicz and (independently) Barbeau and colleagues each showed an improvement in parkinsonian symptoms after administration of levodopa. Subsequently Cotzias and colleagues used rather larger doses of (oral) levodopa and in 1967 they showed that a therapeutic effect could be obtained.

What is Parkinson's disease?

A clinical, or a pathological condition?

At the present time it is generally acknowledged that around a quarter of all patients diagnosed in life by neurologists who profess a special interest in Parkinson's disease will turn out to have some other pathology at postmortem. This is despite regular follow-up and 'weeding out' of patients thought initially to have Parkinson's disease but in whom the doctors subsequently suspect a different underlying condition. So we cannot make an accurate purely clinical definition of Parkinson's disease.

Can the pathologists help us here? The pathological features of Parkinson's disease seem robust enough to the uninitiated clinician; cell loss in the substantia nigra with Lewy bodies in some of the surviving neurons (and a host of other pathological features).[3] Yet there are well described cases where all of the classical pathological findings have been present at postmortem, yet the patients have had absolutely no symptoms during life.

We are left, therefore, with a compromise. Parkinson's disease is best defined (for the moment) as a condition where typical clinical features are present in life and a particular pathology is found at postmortem. So diagnosis in life can, in truth, only be provisional.

Parkinson's disease versus parkinsonism

Parkinsonism is that constellation of clinical features which are characteristic of Parkinson's disease but which may also form the clinical core of other conditions. Specifically, parkinsonism refers to the combination of bradykinesia and rigidity. Rest tremor is a common but not invariable accompaniment in Parkinson's disease and it is typically absent in some of the other causes of an akinetic-rigid syndrome.

Clinical diagnosis of Parkinson's disease

Because of the known difficulty in making a clinical diagnosis of Parkinson's disease, various sets of clinical criteria have been put forward. One in popular clinical trial use is the set devised by the United Kingdom

● **Table 2.1.** UK Parkinson's Disease Society Brain Bank clinical diagnostic criteria

STEP 1. Diagnosis of Parkinsonian syndrome.

BRADYKINESIA (slowness of initiation of voluntary movement with progressive reduction in speed and amplitude of repetitive actions).

And at least one of the following:

a. muscular rigidity

b. 4–6 Hz rest tremor

c. postural instability not caused by primary visual, vestibular, cerebellar or proprioceptive dysfunction

STEP 2. Exclusion criteria for Parkinson's disease.

History of repeated strokes with stepwise progression of parkinsonian features

History of repeated head injury

History of definite encephalitis

Oculogyric crises

Neuroleptic treatment at onset of symptoms

More than one affected relative

Sustained remission

Strictly unilateral features after 3 years

Supranuclear gaze palsy

Cerebellar signs

Early severe autonomic involvement

Early severe dementia with disturbances of memory, language and praxis

Babinski sign

Presence of a cerebral tumour or communicating hydrocephalus on CT scan

Negative response to large doses of levodopa (if malabsorption excluded)

MPTP exposure

STEP 3. Supportive prospective positive criteria for Parkinson's disease. Three or more required for diagnosis of definite Parkinson's disease

Unilateral onset

Rest tremor present

Progressive disorder

Persistent asymmetry affecting the side of onset most

Excellent response (70–100%) to levodopa

Severe levodopa-induced chorea

Levodopa response for 5 years or more

Clinical course of 10 years or more

Parkinson's Disease Society Brain Bank[4] (Table 2.1). This involves three steps. First is the diagnosis of a parkinsonian syndrome (defined as bradykinesia and at least one of either muscular rigidity, 4–6 Hz rest tremor, or postural instability not caused by primary visual, vestibular, cerebellar or proprioceptive dysfunction). The second step is a checklist of exclusion criteria such as a history of definite encephalitis or the presence of cerebellar signs. The third step is to look for supportive prospective criteria for Parkinson's disease such as unilateral onset and levodopa response for 5 years or more. When three or more of the supportive criteria are present the *clinical* diagnosis is said to be 'definite Parkinson's disease'.

An alternative set of clinical criteria proposes that patients be classified as having 'possible', 'probable', or 'definite' idiopathic parkinsonism depending on the presence of various combinations of resting tremor, rigidity, bradykinesia and impairment of postural reflexes,[4] subject again to various exclusion criteria. In this case, a variety of 'supportive' laboratory features are mentioned including fluorodopa positron emission tomography (PET) scans and electrophysiological measurements.

Bradykinesia

This is the absolute centrepiece of the clinical diagnosis of parkinsonism and it refers to *slowness of initiation of voluntary movement with progressive reduction in speed and amplitude of repetitive actions.* We must bear this carefully in mind if we are to differentiate between the kind of slowness so characteristic of Parkinson's disease and the slowness seen in other patients, where the underlying cause may be anything from depression to arthritis. Patients with Parkinson's disease have a special difficulty in sustaining repetitive self-initiated movement. In the hand this is best seen when the patient is asked to repetitively open and close the thumb and index finger (I mime the act to my patients and suggest they open and close their thumb and finger 'like a crocodile') (CD 2.1). Patients with Parkinson's disease are often able to make two or three full-amplitude movements like this even though they may start off slowly. What then happens is that successive movements become slower and smaller and movement may even grind to a halt. Patients may be able to re-start of their own accord, only for the movements to peter out again. One catch for the unwary is that this test may be more difficult to interpret in patients who have a lot of tremor; they may unwittingly 'cheat' by synchronizing the requested thumb and finger movements with their tremor frequency, the net result of which can be fairly substantial movements sufficient to make it harder to spot the underlying bradykinesia (CD 2.2). Few patients are as dextrous with their toes as they are with their fingers and in the lower limb the best sitting test is repetitive foot tapping using the toe or heel. Again, the characteristic pattern seen in bradykinesia is a slowing and decrementing amplitude of movement (CD 2.3).

Rigidity

The increased tone of Parkinson's disease is commonly referred to as either 'lead pipe' rigidity, or 'cog-wheel' rigidity. The former is a reminder that the increased tone is constant throughout the range of movement, and that it is similarly felt in passive movements both of flexion and extension — this is similar to the (entirely unfamiliar but easily imagined) resistance to movement encountered in bending a pipe made of lead. Cogwheel rigidity refers to the additional 'ratchety' feel of superimposed tremor. Tone should be assessed at each of the four limbs and also in the trunk, with the patient as relaxed as possible. Arm tone can be tested standing, sitting, or lying. Leg tone is best tested on the bed. Trunkal tone is best tested with the patient standing, holding them by the shoulders and rotating them gently from side to side. It is unusual for patients with Parkinson's disease to have higher tone in trunkal muscles than in the limbs, whereas the converse is true for patients with some other akinetic-rigid syndromes (particularly progressive supranuclear palsy). When rigidity is not obvious, it may be brought out by asking the patient to move the contralateral limb (CD 2.4).

Rest tremor

The misinterpretation of postural tremor as rest tremor is probably the commonest reason for false-positive diagnoses of Parkinson's disease. It is easy to forget how unrestful it is for patients to consult a doctor. True rest tremor means tremor *at rest* and when in doubt this may be most easily enquired about by history ('do you have tremor when you are relaxed at home watching your favourite television programme?') or when the patient has been given time to relax during the consultation and is then either sitting or lying quietly for a minute or two. The classical rest tremor of Parkinson's disease is said to be in the 4–6 Hz frequency range although I have never found my own efforts to check tremor timing against my wristwatch to be very helpful (or easy). Rest tremor is the first clinical symptom in about three-quarters of

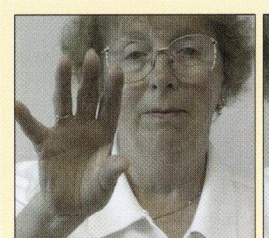
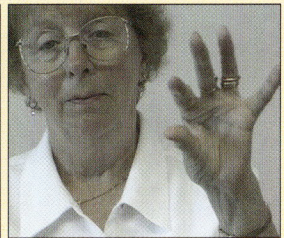

CD 2.1. Upper limb bradykinesia.

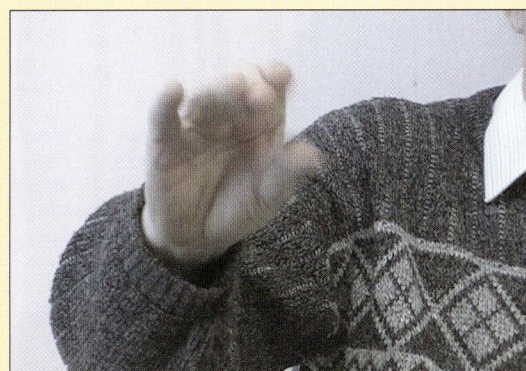

CD 2.2. Assessing bradykinesia in the presence of severe tremor.

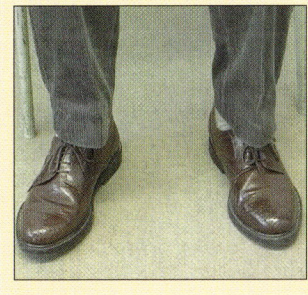

CD 2.3. Lower limb bradykinesia.

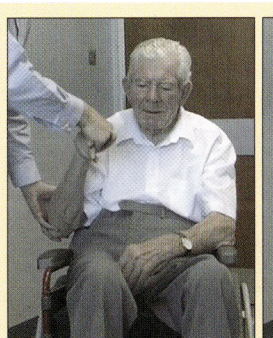
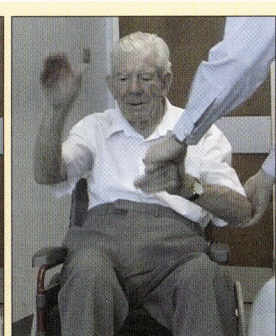

CD 2.4. Test rigidity in Parkinson's disease.

patients. It usually begins in a single extremity, and it may remain localized to one hand or even a single finger for months and sometimes for years. Resting tremor in a limb classically stops when the limb is moved. At the same time, there may be an *increase* in tremor in other parts of the body which are still at rest. In the same way, resting tremor in the hands often increases during walking (even though the arms are not truly at rest).

Patients with Parkinson's disease may also have a postural tremor at a slightly faster frequency. Some patients develop a postural tremor before they develop either a resting tremor or any other cardinal features of parkinsonism and diagnosis at this early stage can be particularly difficult as most patients with a pure postural tremor have some other condition (such as essential tremor or dystonia). Tremor of the head (which is really of the neck) almost never occurs in Parkinson's disease, whereas chin tremor is seen very much more often (CD 2.5).

Loss of postural reflexes

A feature of advancing Parkinson's disease which cannot easily be explained by bradykinesia, rigidity or tremor, is the impairment and eventual loss of postural reflexes. Other causes of postural instability include visual, proprioceptive and cerebellar deficits and these must be identified and/or excluded. The loss of postural reflex control heralds the onset of falls and defines progression to 'stage III' of the Hoehn and Yahr rating scale (Table 2.2). To test postural reflexes it is best to stand behind the patient and (after an appropriate warning) give them a gentle tug backwards. If postural reflex control is normal, efforts to pull a patient over in this way will be met with by a resolute refusal to fall. If the reflexes are impaired, the subject will totter a little, but regain control and remain standing. If the patient's postural reflexes are severely impaired they will fall over unless you catch them.

Other clinical signs in Parkinson's disease

Patients with Parkinson's disease commonly have a reduction in facial expression and it is important not to misinterpret this sign alone as evidence of depression or mental slowness.

Many patients notice a change in their handwriting. The usual complaint is that writing has become small and more difficult to read (Fig. 2.1). Where a patient has had cause to keep samples of their handwriting over years (entries on cheque-book stubs, for example), changes may be seen (in retrospect) going back for months or years before the first recorded cardinal sign such as rest tremor.

● **Table 2.2.** Modified Hoehn and Yahr staging

Stage 0	No signs of disease
Stage 1	Unilateral disease
Stage 1.5	Unilateral plus axial involvement
Stage 2	Bilateral disease, without impairment of balance
Stage 2.5	Mild bilateral disease, with recovery on pull test
Stage 3	Mild to moderate bilateral disease; some postural instability; physically independent
Stage 4	Severe disability; still able to walk or stand unassisted
Stage 5	Wheelchair bound or bedridden unless aided

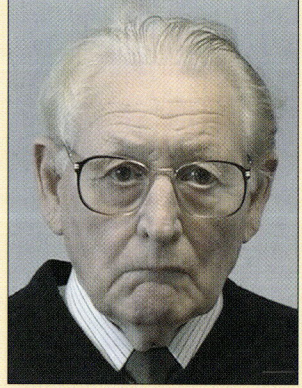

CD 2.5. Chin tremor.

MICROGRAPHIA

Mary had a little Lamb and didn't know what to do

Figure 2.1. Micrographia. Handwriting becomes progressively smaller.

Patients rarely report any difficulty with eye movements. Nevertheless, careful examination may show slowed and hypometric saccadic movements and rather jerky smooth pursuit movements. Although patients may have some loss of upgaze (also seen in healthy elderly patients), they do not lose downgaze.

The glabellar tap sign, also known as Myerson's sign (persistence of the blink response on repetitive tapping between the eyebrows) is not particularly helpful as a diagnostic clinical sign, as it may be seen in normal people.

Few doctors ask their patients about their sense of smell. A small number of parkinsonian patients notice a reduction in olfactory function. Careful testing using scratch-and-sniff testing cards may reveal impaired olfactory perception. The abnormality occurs quite early on in the disease, and has even been suggested as a possible presymptomatic marker.

Changes in skin texture have been noted; a 'greasy' complexion is not uncommon.

In fairly advanced disease, patients may be plagued by drooling of saliva, which is mainly due to defects in the oral, pharyngeal and oesophageal phases of swallowing.

Asymmetry

It is common for patients with Parkinson's disease to present with unilateral symptoms and signs; in fact an absolutely symmetrical presentation is rather unusual. Most patients remain more severely affected one side than the other and when symptoms on the worst affected side are severe enough to warrant treatment, this of course has the effect of further masking the development of signs on the less affected side. Positron emission tomography using fluorodopa as tracer generally shows asymmetrical bilateral involvement even when symptoms and signs are exclusively unilateral (Fig. 2.2). Likewise single photon emission computed tomography (SPECT) scans using [I-123] β-CIT as tracer (to image dopamine transporter sites) also show bilateral involvement in hemiparkinsonian patients.[5]

Gait disorders in Parkinson's disease (CD 2.6)

In the early stages of Parkinson's disease there may be little more to see than a unilateral reduction in arm swing, but as the disease progresses patients tend to adopt a slightly stooped posture. Stride length shortens

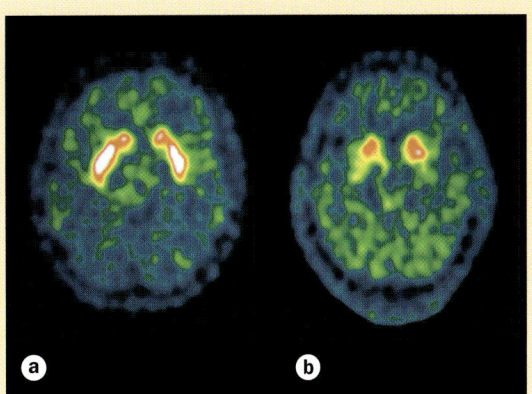

Figure 2.2. Striatal fluorodopa uptake in control (a) and Parkinson's disease (b) brain. Patient scan shows bilateral reduction in putamen uptake.

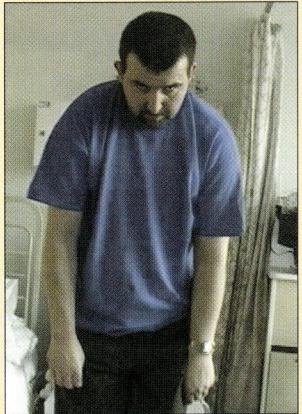

CD 2.6. Loss of arm swing.

and patients may have particular difficulty in stepping out; it is said that some patients find it easier to walk up stairs than they do on the flat and this is almost certainly because the stairs act as an external cue for each pace. Similar 'assistance' with walking has been reported from other visual cues such as walking along a disused railway line (these lines are never in very helpful places) or auditory cues, such as listening to marching music on a personal stereo.

Cognitive function in Parkinson's disease

James Parkinson noted that the intellect was unaffected in the shaking palsy. Slowly, doctors came to realize that this was not strictly true, but even though careful psychometric testing showed mild deficits in certain cognitive tasks, the overall message as passed on to patients was that 'broadly speaking', Parkinson's disease did not affect their intellect.

Such a stance can no longer be reasonably maintained since it is now appreciated that dementia occurs in around a quarter of parkinsonian patients and a similar pathology is identified at postmortem as one of the commonest causes of dementia, even in the absence of any evidence of parkinsonism during life.

In an effort to distinguish the slow thinking (bradyphrenia) and visuospatial and perceptual deficits identified in parkinsonian patients from the cognitive profile of other known dementing illnesses such as Alzheimer's disease, the phrase *subcortical dementia* was coined. This served to explain why some 'cortical' functions such as language were spared. The notion was that the dementia of Parkinson's disease was due principally to a disruption of subcortical connections. This was a useful concept, particularly as it took into account the observation that the pathology of Parkinson's disease was subcortical.

When newer histopathological methods such as ubiquitin staining showed that the cortical pathology was so much greater in Parkinson's disease than had hitherto been appreciated (see below), then the concept of subcortical dementia fell somewhat by the wayside.

Dementia with Lewy bodies accounts for 15–25% of elderly demented patients. The central feature of dementia with Lewy bodies is a progressive disabling mental impairment progressing to dementia. Attentional impairments and disproportionate problem-solving and visuospatial difficulties are often early and prominent. Fluctuation in cognitive function, persistent well-formed visual hallucinations, and spontaneous motor features of parkinsonism are core features and help distinguish between dementia with Lewy bodies, and Alzheimer's disease.[6] Similar clinical features arise in a proportion of patients who initially present with a parkinsonian syndrome, whilst other parkinsonian patients remain mentally sharp throughout their disease. The precise relationship between these two ends of a possibly continuous disease spectrum remains presently unclear.

The pathology of Parkinson's disease

The brain in Parkinson's disease appears macroscopically normal, except for the loss of pigment in the substantia nigra (Fig. 2.3) and locus coeruleus. Together with neuronal cell loss and the presence of Lewy bodies in surviving neurons of the pigmented brainstem nuclei, there is uptake of neuromelanin into macrophages and astrocytes.

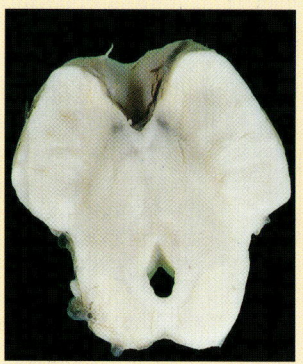

Figure 2.3. Section through midbrain to show abnormal pallor of the substantia nigra. This macroscopic appearance correlates with loss of neuromelanin-containing cells. (Courtesy of J. Lowe.)

There are two types of Lewy body, the classical type which is found in the brainstem, and the type which is found in the cortex. The classical Lewy body is a rounded 8–30 μm diameter intraneuronal inclusion body with an eosinophilic colour, a hyaline core, and a pale peripheral halo. Ultrastructurally they have a dense osmiophilic core composed of granular and vesicular material and a concentric rim of radiating to haphazardly arranged 8–10 nm diameter fibrils. These bodies are found in the substantia nigra, the locus coeruleus, dorsal vagal motor nucleus, thalamus, hypothalamus, and the substantia innominata. A single neuron may contain more than one Lewy body (Fig. 2.4).

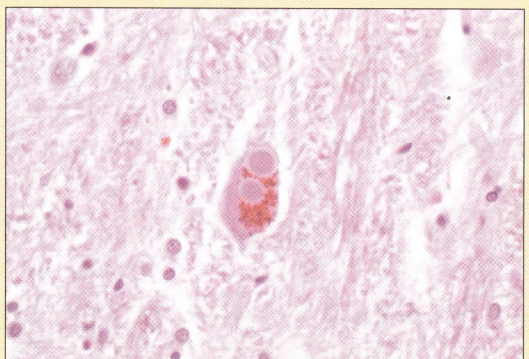

Figure 2.4. A pigmented neuron from the substantia nigra containing two classical Lewy bodies (H&E stain). (Courtesy of J. Lowe.)

The cortical Lewy bodies are mostly found in neurons within layers V and VI of the temporal, insular and cingulate regions. They are found in all patients with Parkinson's disease, but are more numerous in patients who have 'dementia with Lewy bodies' (formerly Lewy body dementia). Unlike their cousins in the brainstem, cortical Lewy bodies have no obvious halo and they are more variable in shape (Fig. 2.5). Ultrastructurally they have comparatively loosely-arranged fibrils and granular material, but no distinct core.

Lewy bodies may also be seen in a variety of extracerebral sites, including sympathetic and parasympathetic neurons and in the enteric nervous system.

Brainstem and cortical Lewy bodies both contain ubiquitin (a heat shock/cell stress protein present also in some other inclusions) (Fig. 2.6). The normal function of ubiquitin is believed to include targeting proteins for breakdown.

Ubiquitin staining makes Lewy bodies more easily visible, particularly in the cortex (Fig. 2.7). Lewy bodies have also more recently been shown to contain alpha-synuclein[7] (Fig. 2.8). Point mutations in the gene for alpha-synuclein have been shown to be responsible for Lewy body parkinsonism in some families.[8,9]

A third kind of inclusion, pale bodies, are also seen in the substantia nigra and locus coeruleus. These granular rounded bodies may be precursors of Lewy bodies.

Subdivisions of the substantia nigra

Microscopically the substantia nigra can be divided into a series of cell tiers. The nigral cell loss which occurs with normal ageing is greatest in the dorsal tier. In Parkinson's disease the converse is true, with the greatest cell loss in the ventral, then the intermediate, then the dorsal tier[10] (Fig. 2.9).[11]

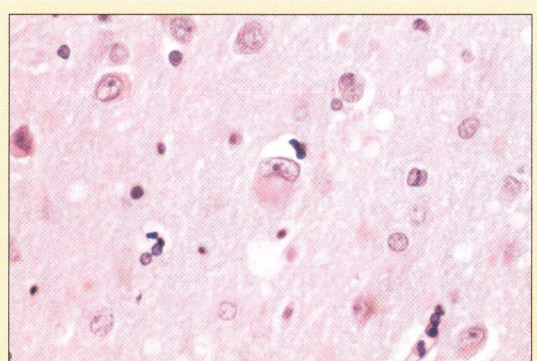

Figure 2.5. A cortical Lewy body presented in a small neuron from layer VI in the temporal neocortex (H&E stain). (Courtesy of J. Lowe.)

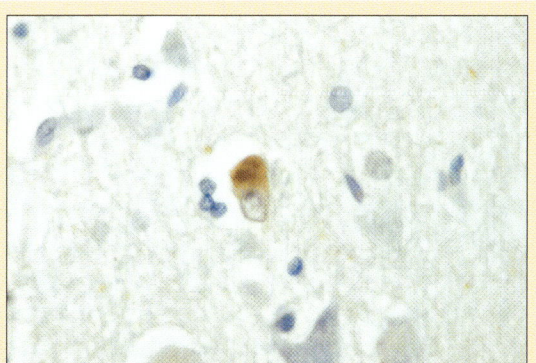

Figure 2.6. Cortical Lewy body (anti-ubiquitin stain). (Courtesy of J. Lowe.)

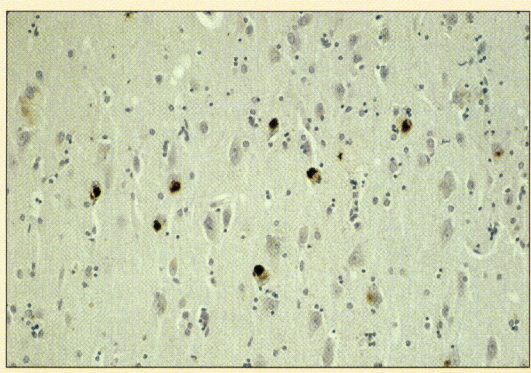

Figure 2.7. A low magnification view showing a high density of cortical Lewy bodies (anti-ubiquitin stain). (Courtesy of J. Lowe.)

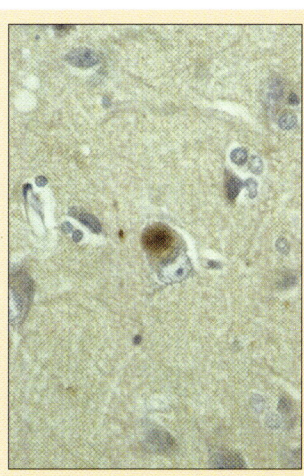

Figure 2.8. Cortical Lewy body (anti-α-synuclein stain). (Courtesy of J. Lowe.)

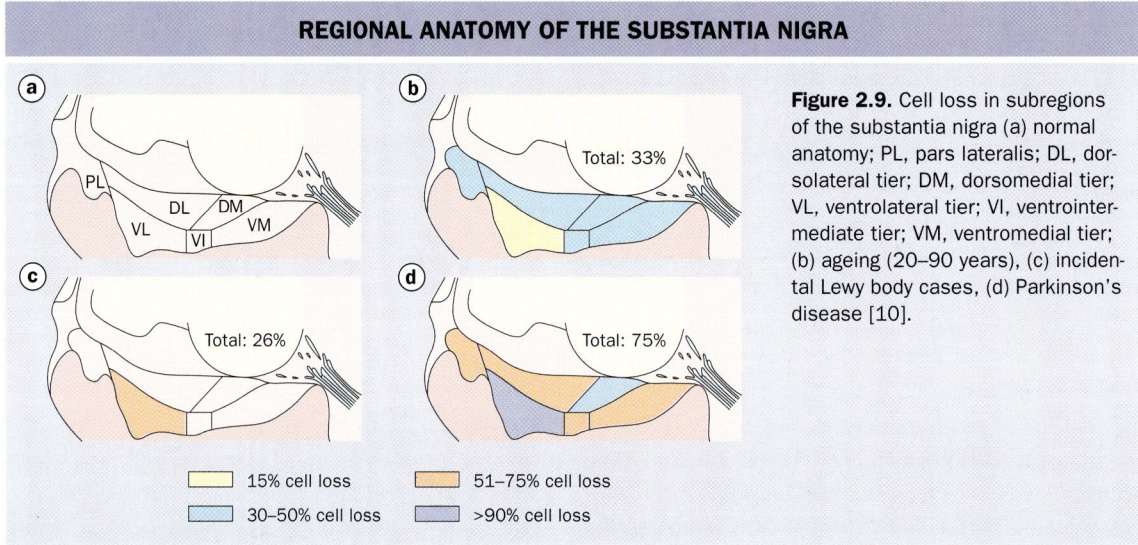

REGIONAL ANATOMY OF THE SUBSTANTIA NIGRA

Figure 2.9. Cell loss in subregions of the substantia nigra (a) normal anatomy; PL, pars lateralis; DL, dorsolateral tier; DM, dorsomedial tier; VL, ventrolateral tier; VI, ventrointermediate tier; VM, ventromedial tier; (b) ageing (20–90 years), (c) incidental Lewy body cases, (d) Parkinson's disease [10].

The loss of nigral dopamine from the striatum follows a corresponding pattern, with the most severe loss being in the putamen, particularly the dorsal putamen, and lesser loss in the caudate, except for its most dorsal part.[12]

Incidental Lewy bodies

Lewy bodies are also found at postmortem in individuals who have had no recognized neurological symptoms in life. The frequency of these so-called incidental Lewy bodies increases with age, rising from 3.8% in those dying at age 50–59 to 12.8% in those dying over the age of 80[3,13] (Fig. 2.10).[3] Because Parkinson's disease

is not usually manifest before the nigral cell loss exceeds 20–50%, those who die with incidental Lewy bodies are widely assumed to have preclinical Parkinson's disease. The implication of this is that if they had survived longer, many would ultimately have developed clinical evidence of parkinsonism.

With regard to nigral subdivisions, the least affected incidental Lewy body subjects have cell loss with Lewy bodies only in the ventrolateral tier. Subjects with moderate or severe (but still subclinical) pathological changes, show Lewy bodies and cell loss also in the dorsal tier (Fig. 2.9).[11]

Specificity of Lewy bodies

Although Lewy bodies are required for a pathological diagnosis of Parkinson's disease, they are *not* specific to that condition, having also been described in a number of other neurological conditions, some of which are clinically similar to Parkinson's disease. The list of clinically and neuropathologically diagnosed conditions in which Lewy bodies have so far (rightly or wrongly) been described includes multiple system atrophy, progressive supranuclear palsy, corticobasal degeneration, motor neuron disease, Hallervorden–Spatz disease, neuroaxonal dystrophy, ataxia telangiectasia, subacute sclerosing panencephalitis, sporadic and familial Alzheimer's disease, Down's syndrome, cranial dystonia and in the postpartum period (Table 2.3).[14] Since Lewy bodies are known to occur in patients who have no obvious neurological disease in life, it is possible that they might also

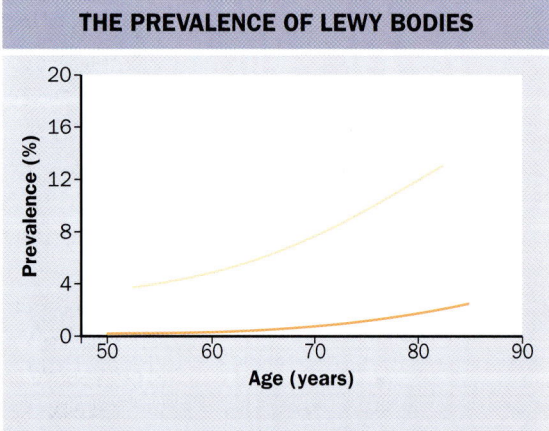

THE PREVALENCE OF LEWY BODIES

Figure 2.10. Relative frequency of incidental Lewy body disease (pathological data) and idiopathic Parkinson's disease (clinical prevalence data) with age. (———) Incidental Lewy bodies. (———) Parkinson's disease.

occur as an incidental finding in patients who have a wide variety of other illnesses, simply as a chance finding. This is a possible explanation for some of the above reported associations.

Some patients who have the typical changes of established Parkinson's disease at postmortem have been documented to have other phenotypes in life, including dementia without parkinsonism and a levodopa unresponsive parkinsonism.[15,16]

Lastly, Lewy bodies are found in some types of motor neuron disease, in which they may be restricted to motor nuclei of cranial nerves and anterior horn cells, but in this instance they do not occur in the dopaminergic system; so they are not absolutely specific for the neurons which are affected in Parkinson's disease.[17]

Aetiology

Several major hypotheses vie for primacy in the causation of Parkinson's disease. The genetic hypothesis has had a rocky ride but has gained important ground recently with the identification of strong evidence for a single gene responsible for causing parkinsonism in a large kindred spread across Italy and the USA. The 'environmental' hypothesis had been kept alive for years, much fuelled by the 1-methyl-4-phenyl-1,2,3,6-tetrahydropyridine (MPTP) story. Oxidative stress and xenobiotic metabolism have each held our

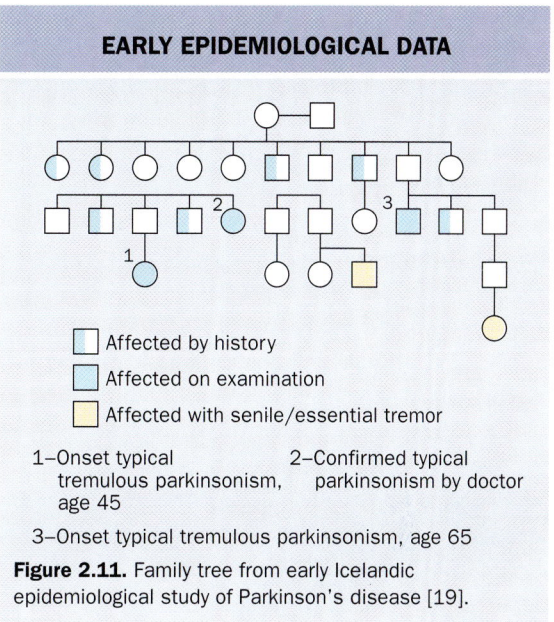

EARLY EPIDEMIOLOGICAL DATA

☐ Affected by history
☐ Affected on examination
☐ Affected with senile/essential tremor

1–Onset typical tremulous parkinsonism, age 45

2–Confirmed typical parkinsonism by doctor

3–Onset typical tremulous parkinsonism, age 65

Figure 2.11. Family tree from early Icelandic epidemiological study of Parkinson's disease [19].

attention at major international conferences. The winner? Probably the answer will prove to be a combination of several of the above.

Parkinson's disease: a genetic disorder?

Most patients with Parkinson's disease do not have similarly affected first-degree relatives. But quite a few patients report that someone or other in their extended family has or did have Parkinson's disease, and there are occasional families in whom the condition appears to obey the rules for an autosomal dominant condition. How do we tally these findings?

Taken at face value, the observation that many patients have one or more (usually distant) affected relatives does suggest some sort of genetic aetiology. Certainly this was the conclusion reached in some early epidemiological studies[18,19] (Fig. 2.11).[19] More information came from twin studies.[20] Whilst several pairs of identical twins concordant for Parkinson's disease have been reported,[21–23] in a larger study of 62 twin pairs, *no* difference was found between the clinical concordance in monozygotic and dizygotic twins. Furthermore, the frequency of Parkinson's disease in the monozygotic co-twins of index cases with Parkinson's disease was no higher than in the general population (though a later reappraisal of the data concluded that these findings did not exclude the

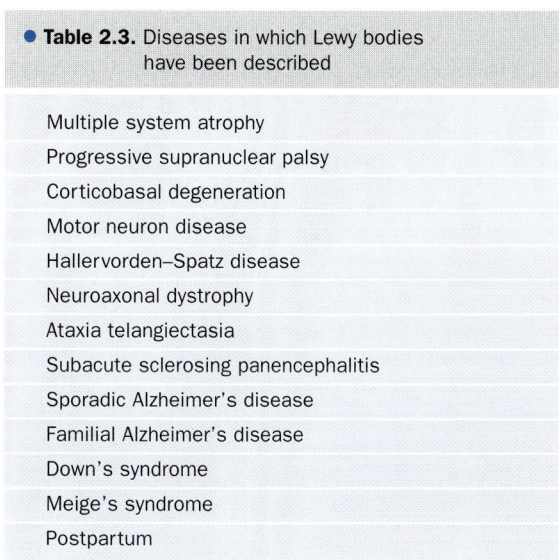

Table 2.3. Diseases in which Lewy bodies have been described

Multiple system atrophy

Progressive supranuclear palsy

Corticobasal degeneration

Motor neuron disease

Hallervorden–Spatz disease

Neuroaxonal dystrophy

Ataxia telangiectasia

Subacute sclerosing panencephalitis

Sporadic Alzheimer's disease

Familial Alzheimer's disease

Down's syndrome

Meige's syndrome

Postpartum

possibility of a genetic contribution).[24] So despite some protestations, the concept of Parkinson's disease as an inheritable disease rather fell by the wayside and the apparent clustering of parkinsonian symptoms in families was explained away on the basis of misdiagnosis (older relatives who are dead or at least unavailable for examination may in reality have had essential tremor or some other condition rather than Parkinson's disease) or clustering by chance.

Even bearing these possible confounding errors in mind, still many physicians were struck by the number of Parkinson's disease patients who reported other affected family members. Rigorous studies have followed. Many families exist in which two or more members are affected and in which the clinical features are indistinguishable from those observed in sporadic Parkinson's disease patients.[25] In such families clinical data suggest autosomal dominant inheritance with low penetrance. In a questionnaire study (with clinical examination of a subset of cases) the susceptibility to Parkinson's disease was found to be increased in the first-degree relatives both of patients with 'familial' Parkinson's disease and those who (prior to the study) were believed to have sporadic disease.[26]

More rarely, there exist families in which penetrance is high.[27–30] In some such families, autopsy data confirm the typical pathological changes of Parkinson's disease with Lewy bodies[27,31] (Fig. 2.12).[31] Following the discovery that trinucleotide repeat genes were responsible for Huntington's disease and a variety of other disorders, kindreds with familial parkinsonism have been scrutinized for evidence of anticipation (earlier age of onset in successive generations). This pattern of age-at-onset has been identified in a small number of families,[30,32] but has not been confirmed in others, in some of whom apparent anticipation was found to be due to age-ascertainment bias.[33,34] Efforts to identify CAG or other trinucleotide repeat genes in these families have been thus far unrewarding.[35,36]

PET scan studies have shown that some clinically normal subjects have impaired fluorodopa uptake, at a level intermediate between normal control values and the values seen in affected family members[37,38] (Fig. 2.13),[37] suggesting that the penetrance for nigrostriatal dopaminergic dysfunction in familial clusters of parkinsonism may be higher than the prevalence estimated from clinical examination alone.

An important positive finding in the genetics of Parkinson's disease was the discovery in a large Italian kindred of genetic markers on chromosome 4q21–q23 which are linked to the parkinsonian phenotype.[39] This region contains more than 30 genes. Further study led to the discovery of a point mutation in the alpha-synuclein gene in the same family as well as in three apparently unrelated Greek families.[8] Another point mutation in the same alpha-synuclein gene has been reported in a family with Parkinson's disease of German descent.[9]

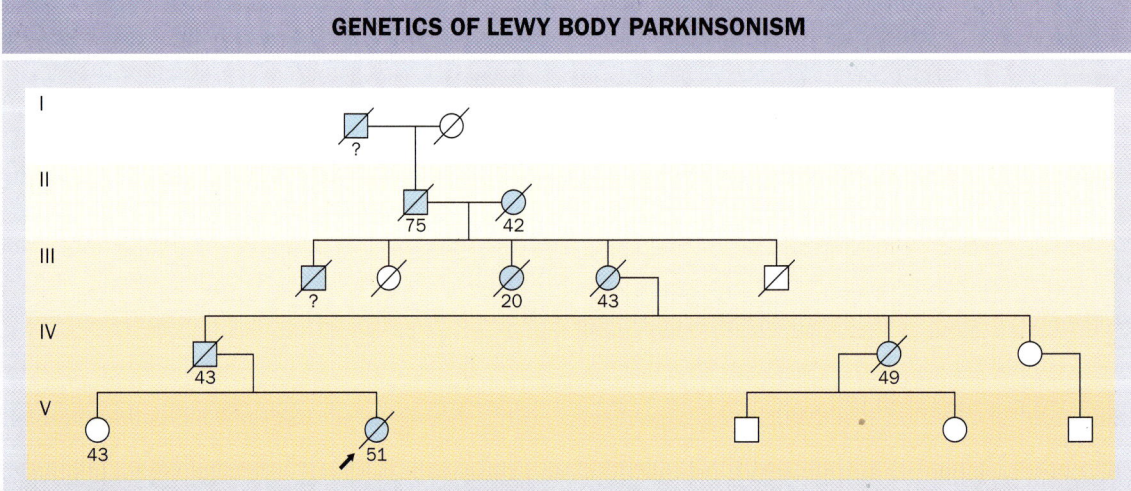

GENETICS OF LEWY BODY PARKINSONISM

Figure 2.12. Pedigree of family with autosomal dominant Lewy body parkinsonism. Arrow represents propositus. Numbers below symbols represent age at death [31].

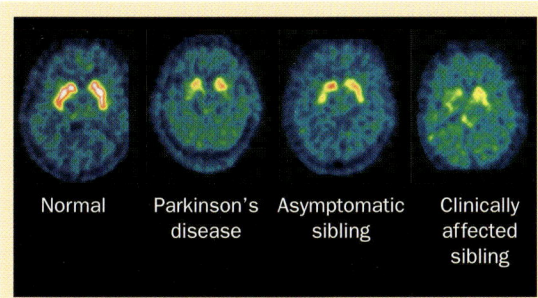

Figure 2.13. Fluorodopa PET scan in familial parkinsonism. Note subclinical changes in clinically unaffected family member.

Alpha-synuclein has been shown to be present in Lewy bodies (Fig. 2.8);[7] hopefully the discovery of these genetic causes for Lewy body parkinsonism will lead to an improved understanding of the aetiology of Parkinson's disease in other patients.

MPTP: a clue to an environmental, or a genetic aetiology?

One of the major landmarks in Parkinson's disease research has been the recognition of a Parkinson's disease look-alike condition induced by the toxin MPTP. The details of the 'MPTP story' are well known. Briefly, a group of drug addicts in the USA injected a bad batch of synthetic narcotic and some of them became severely ill with a Parkinson's disease-like illness within weeks.[40] It transpired that the chemist who had made the offending drug had unwittingly synthesized MPTP. This proved to be a potent and specific nigral toxin. An autopsy of one such affected patient showed prominent cell loss in the substantia nigra with a single eosinophilic inclusion similar to a Lewy body.[41]

There have been a series of off-shoots from this initially serendipitous discovery. Firstly, it has prompted further searching for a more widespread toxin that might lead to Parkinson's disease in the generality of affected patients. Secondly, observation of the manner in which the drug is toxic has been a stimulus to research into mitochondrial function in Parkinson's disease. Thirdly, the MPTP model (using rodent or primate species) has become a standard and powerful tool in the laboratory investigation of parkinsonism.

Although MPTP parkinsonism is similar to human Parkinson's disease, there are a small number of important differences. The onset is typically rapid over a few weeks, whereas in Parkinson's disease the onset is insidious over months or even years. Next, there is little evidence of the subsequent slow progression typical of Parkinson's disease. MPTP parkinsonism appears to require intravenous injection of the toxin, whereas such a route of exposure cannot explain the sporadic disease. Also whereas MPTP parkinsonism (due to a known environmental risk factor) caused a cluster of cases, similar clustering of Parkinson's disease cases seems not to occur. Lastly, the pathological findings although similar to sporadic Parkinson's disease were not indistinguishable from it.[41]

The mechanism of toxicity is that MPTP is first oxidized by glial monoamine oxidase-B (MAOB) to 1-methyl-4-phenylpyridinium (MPP^+)[42] (Fig. 2.14). Animals pretreated with MAOB inhibitors and then given MPTP may be spared from toxicity.[43] MPP^+ is then taken up by the dopamine reuptake pathway and it is further concentrated in mitochondria, where it is a specific inhibitor of complex I. Quite how MPP^+ inhibits complex I is not fully understood, but it binds close to the binding site of rotenone (another complex I inhibitor), it binds loosely, and its inhibition of complex I can be prevented by free radical scavengers.

So it can be seen that the MPTP story provides firm evidence of an environmental cause of parkinsonism in a tiny minority of patients, and it provides a clue to the possible relevance of mitochondrial function in the mechanism of nigral cell death. Might Parkinson's disease be another mitochondrial disease?

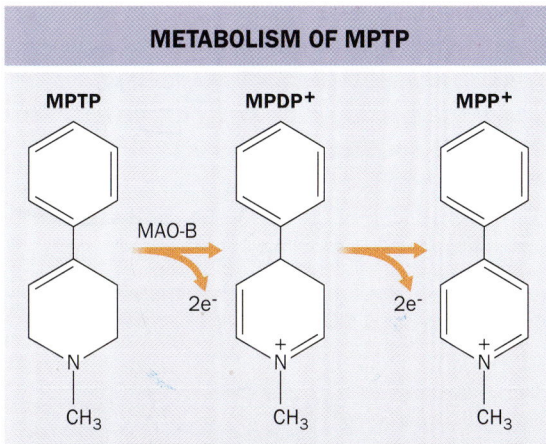

Figure 2.14. In the striatum, MPTP is converted into its toxic metabolite MPP^+ via an enzymatic oxidation catalysed by monoamine oxidase-B (MAO-B).

Mitochondrial genetics and function in Parkinson's disease

In an era where mitochondrial genetics have been found to explain a variety of neurological disorders including some myopathies and some kinds of ataxia and myoclonus, evidence of a mitochondrial gene defect has, naturally, been sought in Parkinson's disease. No such gene defect has been confirmed to date. This is not particularly surprising, since mitochondrial inheritance occurs from mother to child (of either sex), whereas in those large kindreds that have been studied both clinically and genetically, no such mode of transmission has been apparent. It is important to remember, however, that complex I is encoded by both mitochondrial and nuclear DNA.

Turning to mitochondrial function, various laboratories have measured postmortem nigral mitochondrial respiratory chain activities. Nigral tissue homogenates contain both glial cells and neurons, and in Parkinson's disease the neurons are outnumbered by the glia. So the reported 30% decrease in (citrate synthase corrected) complex I activity may reflect both glial and nigral changes.[44] Mitochondrial function in parkinsonian frontal cortex, cerebellum and tegmentum is normal. It is not yet agreed whether there are significant changes in striatal mitochondrial function.

Mitochondrial function in muscle has been reported both as normal and abnormal. The extent to which the different results from different laboratories reflect differences in patient and control selection, tissue storage, and assay methods is not known. Muscle power is normal in Parkinson's disease, and patients do not have either a resting or an exercise-induced lactic acidosis.[45]

Platelet complex I activity was first reported to be 55% reduced.[46] Subsequent studies using different methodologies have shown less severe reductions[47] or normal function[48] and whether any reduction is real remains controversial. Certainly, the results are not presently robust enough and the overlap with normal results is too great to allow such a test to be used for diagnostic purposes in clinical practice.

The cause of complex I deficiency in Parkinson's disease is of interest. Since studies in multiple system atrophy do not show a nigral complex I deficit,[49] the abnormal activity in parkinsonian brain cannot simply be a non-specific consequence of nigral cell degeneration. The possibilities are that either the complex I deficit is secondary to whatever is causing the nigral damage (such as oxidative stress) or that it is itself a cause of nigral damage, perhaps arising as a primary genetic defect (even though evidence of exclusive maternal transmission is not apparent). Alternatively an entirely different (even unknown) biochemical deficit could precipitate a sequence of events ending with complex I deficiency and free radical formation.[44]

Oxidative stress

Free radicals contain one or more unpaired electrons; examples are superoxide anions and hydroxyl radicals. Such species are formed in all respiring cells. They are highly reactive and may cause cellular damage via non-selective oxidation of proteins, DNA, lipids and fatty acids.

In order to prevent this potential damage, respiring cells employ a series of 'scavenging' systems which destroy free radicals. These systems include superoxide dismutase (SOD) which metabolizes superoxide anions to hydrogen peroxide and molecular oxygen (Fig. 2.15). SOD exists in several isoenzymes, including copper-zinc (Cu-Zn SOD) which is cytosolic and manganese (Mn SOD) which is mitochondrial. Increases in one or other of these isoenzymes in parkinsonian substantia nigra have been reported.[50,51] Increased SOD activity leads to more hydrogen peroxide formation. Where iron is present this leads in turn via the Fenton reaction to an increase in hydroxyl radicals (Fig. 2.16), which themselves increase lipid peroxidation.

Iron is believed to accumulate in the nigra in Parkinson's disease,[52] in association with melanin-containing zona compacta nigral neurons.[53] The reason for this accumulation of iron is unknown. Iron acts as a catalyst to the so-called Haber–Weiss reaction, leading to further production of hydroxyl radicals from hydrogen peroxide (Fig. 2.17).

Dopamine has also been implicated in oxidative stress, and this underlies one of the theoretical reasons for avoiding levodopa therapy where possible (in case the resulting increase in nigral dopamine causes disease progression). Once taken back into the neuron (after neurotransmission), non-vesicular dopamine may be oxidized by monoamine oxidase, with the formation of hydrogen peroxide.

Glutathione is a natural antioxidant which scavenges hydroxyl radicals. Its reduced form (GSH) is lower in Parkinson's disease;[54] this may be a secondary change, but is indicative of oxidative stress.

Other substances known to scavenge hydroxyl radicals include vitamin E, uric acid, ascorbate, ubiquinone and salicylate.

The extent to which impaired mitochondrial function leads to oxidative stress, or vice versa, remains controversial.

Evidence for an environmental cause

Although the environmental hypothesis gained a significant boost from the MPTP story it was by no means new at the time. Epidemiological observations over a number of years had already given rise to theories of an environmental cause.

The Chamorro people of the Pacific island of Guam suffer a particular neurodegenerative condition referred to as the amyotrophic lateral sclerosis-parkinsonism-dementia complex (ALS-PDC). This is obviously not the same as Parkinson's disease, but a component of the disorder is a slowly progressive parkinsonism and if an environmental cause could be shown to operate in the genesis of ALS-PDC, might not the same be true also for Parkinson's disease? The incidence of ALS-PDC has been reducing in recent decades. An analysis of the incidence data between 1944 and 1985 suggests that the critical age of exposure to an (unknown) environmental factor was probably during childhood.[55]

$$2O_2^- + 2H^+ \longrightarrow H_2O_2 + O_2$$

Figure 2.15. Action of superoxide dismutase.

$$H_2O_2 + Fe^{2+} \longrightarrow HO\bullet + OH^- + Fe^{3+}$$

Figure 2.16. The Fenton reaction.

$$O_2^- + H_2O_2 \longrightarrow HO\bullet + OH^- + O_2$$

Figure 2.17. The Haber–Weiss reaction.

Racial factors have been examined and most authors have reported Parkinson's disease to be more common in Caucasians than in other ethnic groups. Also, Parkinson's disease appears to be slightly more common in men than in women. Community-based prevalence studies have generally shown Parkinson's disease to be more common in areas where industrialization is relatively long-standing.[56]

One risk factor which has been identified in several studies is 'rural living'.[57,58] This means living in a community with a small population. In one study of 150 case-control pairs, rural living was reported by 105 patients and 83 controls. The greatest difference was seen in the first decade of life and was independent of age of onset. Although drinking well water was more common in patients than controls, the difference was no longer significant when controlled for rural living.[58] No particular association with chemical exposure use was found, despite the known mitochondrial toxicity of rotenone (a commonly used pesticide) and the chemical similarity between paraquat (a herbicide) and MPP+. Other case-control studies have found an association with prior herbicide and pesticide exposure.[26,59,60]

Whilst it is generally assumed that environmental associations with disease reflect uneven exposure to causative agents, the opposite may be true. That is to say there may be a *protective* factor which is unevenly distributed and to which some people have greater exposure than others. In the context of Parkinson's disease, this possibility has been considered most closely in dietary studies where some foodstuffs (such as vitamin E, for example) could act by influencing free radical formation. Studies of prior legume consumption (a dietary variable selected for high vitamin E content) suggest that Parkinson's disease is subsequently less common in those with a higher intake; but the data do not allow any conclusions about the likely benefit or otherwise of taking vitamin E supplements.[61]

Disease progression and treatment complications

Wearing-off

Early in the course of Parkinson's disease, drug treatment results in a smooth motor response; patients are equally mobile throughout the day. With disease progression, however, a variety of motor fluctuations usually emerge, the first of which is typically so-called 'wearing off'. This is akin to recurrence of pain after analgesia wears off. Quite often this effect can be ameliorated by treatment with longer-acting drugs, or by more frequent dosing with shorter-acting agents.

On–off fluctuations

After several years of comparatively predictable motor response to drug treatment, many patients begin to notice marked variability in their motor performance with precipitous swings from being 'on' (i.e. with good treatment effect) to 'off' (akin to untreated parkinsonism). These so-called on–off attacks may occur in a chaotic pattern with no two consecutive days the same. The degree to which these fluctuations reflect either neuronal loss (with consequent loss of dopamine storage capacity), receptor instability (with sudden changes in dopamine receptor sensitivity) or variability in transport between gut, blood and brain remains the subject of considerable debate. Likewise, we do not know for sure whether the development of on–off fluctuations is a consequence of advancing disease severity or prolonged levodopa treatment.

Freezing

This refers to sudden gait failure. A patient is walking along and suddenly becomes unable to move any further, as if suddenly turned to ice. It is a common sign in late Parkinson's disease and is rarely helped much by dopaminergic medication. Although there have in the past been claims of benefit from treatment with L-threodops, the usefulness of such treatment has not been widely confirmed.

Dyskinesias

'Dyskinesia' is a useful word to describe a vast range of involuntary or impaired movement. When describing involuntary movements it is often wisest to start off with a relatively non-committal word, and dyskinesia is ideal. But when used in the context of Parkinson's disease, dyskinesia is usually reserved for use in describing drug-induced (usually levodopa or dopamine agonist) involuntary movements. These dyskinesias are generally fluid, restless, fidgety movements which are quite different from the signs of untreated parkinsonism.

Peak-dose dyskinesias

Most easily understood are the dyskinesias which occur in patients at the peak of their plasma (and presumed brain) drug levels (CD 2.7). This is akin to side-effects of other drugs, such as tinnitus in aspirin toxicity or ataxia with anticonvulsant overdose. In early Parkinson's disease, the dose of levodopa (or agonist) required to provide symptomatic benefit is initially very much less than the dose required to produce dyskinesia; but as the disease progresses, these two doses come closer together (akin to a narrowing of the therapeutic index) so that the dose at which dyskinesias begin is barely (if at all) higher than the dose required to switch a patient 'on' (Fig. 2.18).[62]

Diphasic dyskinesias

Whether or not patients suffer peak-dose dyskinesias, they may also develop similar dyskinetic movements which occur as they are changing from being 'off' to being 'on', or vice versa. So a patient starts 'off', takes a levodopa (or agonist) tablet and then becomes dyskinetic *prior to* switching on. Later, as the plasma (and presumably brain) drug level falls, the patient may become dyskinetic again during the transition from 'on' to 'off'.

Off-period dystonia

Some patients suffer dystonic posturing, usually in the foot. This is typically most troublesome on waking in the morning (Fig. 2.19).

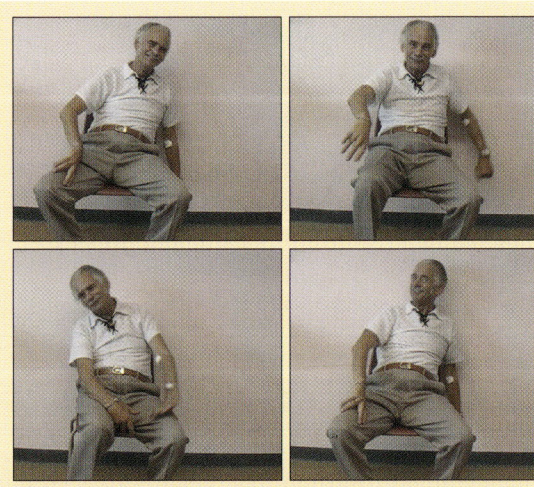

CD 2.7. Peak-dose dyskinesia in Parkinson's disease.

INDUCING LEVODOPA DYSKINESIA

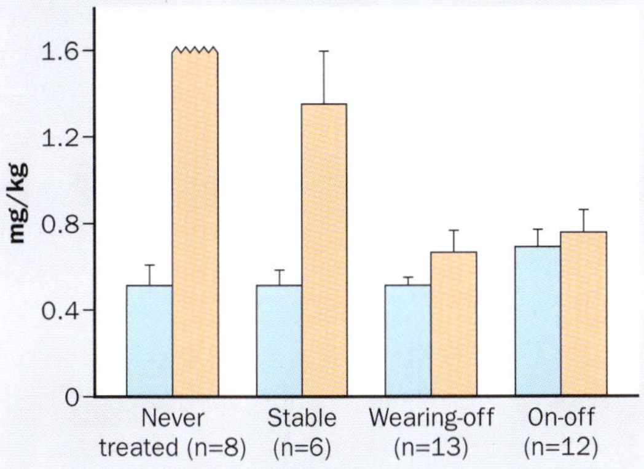

Figure 2.18. Threshold dose of levodopa required to turn on (green) or induce dyskinesia (orange) in patients with Parkinson's disease at various stages of the disease [62].

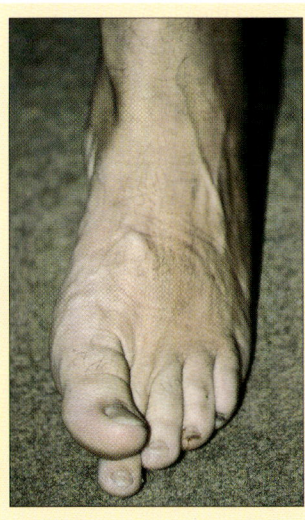

Figure 2.19. 'Off' period dystonia in Parkinson's disease.

Non-motor fluctuations

Whilst the most obvious on–off changes are a fluctuation in motor performance, patients also report a variety of other symptoms which come and go together with their ability to move and which are presumably a further reflection of their dopamine status.[63] Such phenomena have been categorized as sensory (reported by 24% of 130 fluctuating patients), autonomic (44%), and cognitive/psychiatric (32%).[64] Sensory complaints include a feeling of breathlessness without any overt signs of dyspnoea and limb dysaesthesia. Autonomic symptoms include abdominal pain, sweating, nausea, belching and urinary frequency. Cognitive/psychiatric complaints include anxiety, panic and depression. Many patients report that they feel as if they are a different person when they are 'on' and 'off'; as a doctor it can be helpful to meet 'both patients', in order to better understand their disabilities and frustrations.

Drugs used in treating Parkinson's disease

There can be few other neurological conditions which afford the treating physician an opportunity for logical treatment schedules with such detail and complexity as are possible for Parkinson's disease. Patients are very often treated with a combination of agents having complementary effects.

Levodopa

Despite the panoply of other available agents, levodopa remains the single most effective agent in the symptomatic treatment of Parkinson's disease. Perhaps this is hardly surprising, since its metabolism by brain aromatic amino acid decarboxylase yields dopamine, the very chemical which is deficient in Parkinson's disease. Levodopa is almost never given without a peripheral decarboxylase inhibitor (either benserazide in Madopar or carbidopa in Sinemet) to block peripheral dopamine formation.

Levodopa (as Madopar or Sinemet) is available in a variety of preparations designed for very rapid absorption (Madopar dispersible, or regular Sinemet dissolved in water), for 'normal' absorption, or for slow absorption (Madopar CR and Sinemet CR). Sinemet and Madopar are broadly comparable; many physicians choose and stick to one or the other for simplicity.

Most patients tolerate the introduction of levodopa without side-effects. Some, however, notice nausea and occasionally patients vomit.

Anticholinergics

A variety of anticholinergic drugs (benzhexol, procyclidine and others) have been used in the treatment of Parkinson's disease. Anticholinergics have more effect on tremor and rigidity than they do on bradykinesia.

The reason these drugs work at all is most likely because they block intrastriatal cholinergic transmission. The particular disadvantage of these drugs (and the reason that many neurologists avoid them in all but their youngest parkinsonian patients, and even in young patients use them for a short while only) is their side-effect profile. Confusion and urinary retention are both common side-effects especially in elderly patients.

Amantadine

Developed as an antiviral agent, amantadine was long ago recognized to have some benefit in Parkinson's disease patients. It is a weak *N*-methyl-D-aspartate (NMDA) antagonist, and this is presumed to be the basis of its antiparkinsonian activity. The dose is usually 100–200 mg daily, best taken before 4 p.m. because it can cause insomnia.

Selegiline (Eldepryl)

Selegiline is an inhibitor of monoamine oxidase type B (MAOB). There are two strings to the logic of using selegiline for the treatment of Parkinson's disease. Firstly, MAOB is responsible (along with catechol-*O*-methyl transferase) for the intrastriatal catabolism of dopamine after its release in the course of neurotransmission. So blocking brain MAOB acts to potentiate the effect of both endogenous dopamine and any dopamine formed in the brain as a consequence of levodopa administration. As might be expected, selegiline has therefore been shown to prolong the efficacy of single doses of levodopa and it also has a small symptomatic treatment in its own right. Although it does not have the cheese-effect (characteristic of MAOA inhibition) it also has a small antidepressant effect which is usually no disadvantage.

The second reason for prescribing selegiline is tied in closely with the MPTP story. Since MPTP is not itself a neurotoxin, but rather it depends upon toxification by MAOB to MPP$^+$ (which is a powerful nigral toxin), it has been suggested that if Parkinson's disease is caused by the toxic effect of an environmental substance, then perhaps MAOB is necessary for toxification of that agent too. So selegiline could be a neuroprotective agent, not just a drug with symptomatic effect. When given to patients with mild Parkinson's disease, selegiline definitely delays the need for further treatment with, for example, levodopa.[65] In part this effect is due to the mild symptomatic effect of the selegiline. There may also be a neuroprotective effect although the size of any such effect remains unclear at this time.

At the time of writing, the selegiline story has been further complicated by the emergence of data demonstrating an increase in the mortality rate in a British cohort of parkinsonian patients prescribed selegiline together with levodopa in comparison to a group of patients given levodopa alone.[66] The significance of this observation is still uncertain.

Dopamine agonists

The curious thing about levodopa as drug treatment for Parkinson's disease, is that it must be decarboxylated and then stored in and released by the remaining nigrostriatal neurons; and these are the very cells which are dying off. In part, it may be that the various response fluctuations which characterize the later stages of the disease are the consequence of this smaller and dwindling population of surviving (and presumably sick) neurons struggling to cope with such a demand. It seems logical, therefore, to avoid this problem altogether by using a dopamine agonist which has its effect directly on the postsynaptic dopamine receptor.

The number of identified subtypes of dopamine receptor has increased considerably in recent years. Within the striatum the dominant groups of dopamine receptors are the D1-like and the D2-like groups. The D1 group receive excitatory input from the nigrostriatal projection and form an integral part of the 'direct' corticostriatothalamic feedback loop. The D2 group receive inhibitory input from the nigrostriatal projection and their host neurons form part of the indirect corticostriatothalamic loop. The currently available dopamine agonists provide either selective (D2 only) or less selective (D1 and D2) stimulation; though it has yet to be proven that either approach has an overwhelming advantage over the other (Table 2.4).

Bromocriptine

This is the dopamine agonist which has been in consistent clinical use for the longest. It is a D2 agonist with D1 antagonist activity at very low (nanomolar) concentration and D1 agonist activity at rather higher (micromolar) concentration. The half-life of bromocriptine is around 7 hours. It has been used extensively as add-on therapy, in patients already on levodopa, and as *de novo* treatment. There has also been a vogue for starting patients on the combination of levodopa and bromocriptine together, from the start of treatment.

When patients tolerate and derive satisfactory clinical benefit from bromocriptine monotherapy, they suffer fewer of the long-term complications of levodopa therapy.[67] Unfortunately, however, only around one-third of patients started on bromocriptine as monotherapy are able to continue on that single drug for more than 2 years, because it either causes unacceptable side-effects, gives insufficient early clinical benefit, or else patients deteriorate and the lost ground cannot be regained by increasing the bromocriptine dose.

Lisuride

Lisuride has mainly D2 agonist activity with slight D1 antagonist activity. It also has central serotonin agonist activity. The duration of clinical effect is around 2–4 hours. Lisuride stands apart from other orally active dopamine agonists for being easily water soluble. This allows its use as an oral solution. It can also be given by intravenous infusion. 1 mg of lisuride is approximately equivalent to 15 mg bromocriptine.[68] It has been shown to be an effective adjunct to levodopa in patients with advanced disease.[69] Continuous subcutaneous or intravenous infusions of lisuride may benefit severely fluctuating patients.[70,71] After prolonged administration (mean 21 months), recurrence of dyskinesias, an increase in 'off' periods, psychosis, and the technical inconvenience of the pump reduce the usefulness of this approach.[72] When used as *de novo* monotherapy, the same effect is noted as with bromocriptine, that is that those (minority of) patients who tolerate and derive sufficient clinical benefit from lisuride fare better than those treated from the start with levodopa.[73] Combination *de novo* lisuride plus levodopa treatment has been advocated.[74]

Pergolide

Pergolide has strong agonist activity at D2 receptors and D3 receptors, with weak agonist activity at D1 sites. The duration of action is longer than either bromocriptine or lisuride, but it is still usually necessary to give pergolide two or three times a day. It is effective as an adjunct to levodopa treatment[75–77] and is also active as a *de novo* agent.[78] Just as with other agonists, a significant proportion of patients cannot tolerate the side-effects which include nausea and vomiting, somnolence and psychiatric disturbance.[76] 1 mg of pergolide is approximately equivalent to 10 mg bromocriptine.

Ropinirole

Active only at the D2 receptor, ropinirole is a non-ergoline dopamine agonist. In patients with fluctuations on levodopa, addition of ropinirole has been shown to reduce the frequency of 'off' periods.[79] Side-effects are similar to those in patients treated with other agonists. Ropinirole has been shown to be effective in the treatment of *de novo* patients.[80] As with other agonists, fewer *de novo* patients derive sufficient symptomatic response to ropinirole than to levodopa.[81]

Cabergoline

This agent is an ergoline derivative which is specific for the D2 receptors. It has a particularly long plasma half-life (65 hours), so it can be given once a day. It has been shown to be an effective adjunct when used together with levodopa in patients who are either undertreated or who are already noticing motor fluctuations.[82–86] Dose limiting side-effects are similar to those reported with other agonists, including nausea and vomiting, visual hallucinations, orthostatic hypotension and dyskinesias. Peripheral oedema has also been reported.[87] In a double-blind comparison with bromocriptine, a mean dose of 3.2 mg cabergoline gave generally similar benefit to a mean dose of 22 mg bromocriptine.[88] In one recent study 60% of *de novo* patients were able to manage 1 year on monotherapy.[87]

● **Table 2.4.** Comparison of dopamine agonists (principal site of action shown in bold)		
Drug name	**Receptor specificity**	**Half-life (hours)**
Bromocriptine	D1 antagonist/ agonist (see text) **D2**	7
Lisuride	D1 partial antagonist **D2**	2–4
Pergolide	D1 **D2** **D3**	15–42
Ropinirole	**D2**	6
Cabergoline	**D2**	65
Pramipexole	**D2, D3**	13
Apomorphine	**D1, D2**	0.5

Pramipexole

This agent is an agonist at D2 and D3 receptors. It has been shown to be effective as an adjunct to levodopa in patients with motor fluctuations.[89] In a *de novo* study, pramipexole led to a significantly greater improvement in the 'activities of daily living' section of the UPDRS than placebo over 9 weeks.[90]

Apomorphine

Unlike the above agonists, apomorphine is inactive when taken orally because of extensive first-pass metabolism in the liver. It is usually therefore delivered by subcutaneous injection (Fig. 2.20), although nasal,[91,92] rectal[93] and sublingual[94] delivery systems have also been used. It is active at D1 and D2 receptors. The half-life of apomorphine is the shortest of the agonists, with typical clinical effect lasting between 0.5 and 1 hour after a single subcutaneous injection. Balanced against this short duration of action is a similarly rapid time to onset of clinical effect; patients generally notice benefit within about 5 minutes of injection, so apomorphine has found a particular niche role for patients who need a rapid and reliable onset of clinical effect and can cope with a brief duration of benefit.

Apomorphine is not a new agent, having first been used many years ago.[95,96] When used alone it is very liable to cause extreme nausea and vomiting; it has therefore enjoyed a renaissance since the advent of the peripherally active dopamine antagonist, domperidone. It is common practice to begin patients on domperidone for 2 or 3 days before starting apomorphine therapy. Once a patient has become accustomed to apomorphine it is then normally possible to slowly withdraw the domperidone without severe nausea or vomiting. Apomorphine causes somewhat less psychiatric side-effects than most of the other available dopamine agonists.

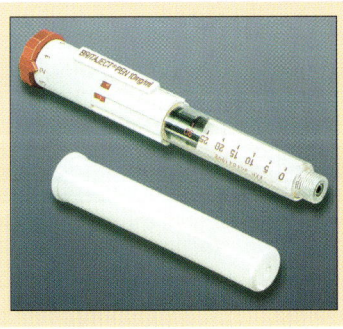

Figure 2.20. Apomorphine penject system. (Courtesy of Britannia Pharmaceuticals Ltd.)

Fluctuating patients have been shown to increase 'on' time using subcutaneous apomorphine via a penject system.[97] The quality of the response obtained after apomorphine is virtually indistinguishable from the 'on' effect of levodopa.[98] The motor response to apomorphine is similar after repeated injections both acutely[99] and in the longer term.[97,100] Apomorphine can also be given by continuous subcutaneous injection using a mini pump system.[101,102] Whether given by continuous infusion or by intermittent injection, some patients experience local tissue reactions at the site of needle entry,[103] although these are rarely a serious problem. Patients vary in the extent to which they rely on apomorphine as the backbone of their parkinsonian therapy. Some use it by continuous infusion without any levodopa or other agonist treatment. Others take levodopa or a different agonist as their primary treatment and use frequent apomorphine boosts at regular strategic times during the day. Still others use apomorphine intermittently when they experience a dose failure and some simply keep a dose of apomorphine available for very occasional use. Having a preloaded syringe at hand can provide a considerable boost to self-confidence for a patient who suffers severe and unpredictable 'off' periods.

Apomorphine has also been used as a 'test' for drug responsiveness in parkinsonian syndromes.[104] The attraction of this approach is that the response to an injection of apomorphine is fairly short, and can be observed directly. The clinical response to a single dose of levodopa is similar but the time course more variable and as a diagnostic test a levodopa challenge is more time consuming.

In untreated parkinsonian patients, an apomorphine test has predictive value, in that *most* patients who will subsequently respond to levodopa will respond to a test dose of apomorphine. But a subgroup of patients respond to chronic (several weeks of) treatment with levodopa after negative apomorphine testing and so even if a *de novo* patient has a negative apomorphine test, most clinicians would still give a trial of longer-term dopaminergic treatment.

In patients on long-term treatment with levodopa or an agonist who report lack of drug efficacy, an apomorphine test can provide an indication of their current agonist responsiveness. This can be helpful in patients who lose their initial levodopa or agonist response after a period of initially successful treatment.

COMT inhibitors

The peripheral metabolism of levodopa to dopamine via aromatic amino acid decarboxylase (AAAD) is well known and almost all patients receiving levodopa take it together with an AAAD blocker (carbidopa in Sinemet and benserazide in Madopar). This still leaves another enzyme in the peripheral blood, catechol-O-methyl transferase (COMT) which also metabolizes levodopa, this time to the inactive product 3-*O*-methyl-dopa. The effect of this metabolism is a decrease in the amount of levodopa available for uptake into dopaminergic neurons and decarboxylation to dopamine.

This same enzyme, COMT, is also present in brain where together with MAOB, it is responsible for the breakdown of dopamine, after release in the context of neurotransmission, to homovallinic acid. So peripheral COMT inhibition offers the potential for increasing the uptake and duration of levodopa, and central COMT inhibition may additionally reduce central dopamine catabolism.

Entacapone

Active only in the periphery, entacapone has been shown to extend the clinical effect of a single dose of levodopa. Positron emission tomography studies using fluorodopa as tracer have shown increased striatal uptake of tracer after entacapone premedication[105,106] (Fig. 2.21). Clinical single-dose studies have shown a prolongation of the antiparkinsonian effect of levodopa,[107] and pharmacokinetic studies have shown an increase in the half-life of levodopa with an increased duration of action over a period of weeks.[108]

Tolcapone

This agent inhibits the action of COMT both centrally and in the periphery. After a single dose, tolcapone has been shown to prolong the antiparkinsonian response to levodopa.[99] Tolcapone has been shown to reduce 'off' time in fluctuating patients when given together with levodopa/carbidopa.[109]

Practicalities of drug treatment

This is a rapidly evolving field. Nevertheless, there are some general principles of treatment which are widely agreed and there are areas of controversy where experts agree to differ. There are several common problems, particularly in the management of fluctuations and dyskinesias, where most practising clinicians would agree that there are no easy answers. The surgical treatment of Parkinson's disease is considered in Chapter 4.

When to begin symptomatic treatment?

Patients with Parkinson's disease have a progressive and disabling disease. Effective drug treatment should be given when the symptoms and signs of the disorder are sufficient to cause disability of practical importance to the patient. Doctors have previously been advised to defer symptomatic treatment for as long as possible, in an effort to defer long-term treatment complications. Whilst the avoidance or at least the delay of on–off fluctuations and drug induced dyskinesias remains an important goal in treating Parkinson's disease, simply delaying all effective symptomatic treatment is probably an ineffective means to that end. Patients with MPTP-induced parkinsonism developed capricious dyskinesia and response fluctuations almost immediately they were treated with levodopa, suggesting that these symptoms were evidence of the depth of their dopamine deficiency, rather than the length of their levodopa exposure.

When to start neuroprotective treatment?

An effective neuroprotective treatment, if free from important side-effects, should be started as early as possible in the clinical course of the illness. At the present time, however, although there is almost universal agreement that early treatment with selegiline delays the

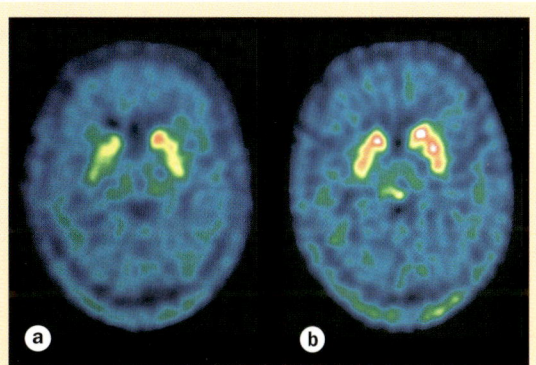

Figure 2.21. Fluorodopa uptake in Parkinson's disease after premedication with carbidopa alone (a) *versus* carbidopa plus entacapone (b).

subsequent need to add another (more symptomatically effective) drug treatment,[65,110,111] the balance of the protective and symptomatic components of this effect is disputed. Furthermore, concern over the long-term safety of selegiline in treating early Parkinson's disease has been raised by the finding in a British study of an increase in mortality amongst patients randomized to levodopa plus selegiline in comparison to those given levodopa alone.[66] At the present time, physicians are divided on whether or not they prescribe selegiline as a neuroprotective agent.

The drug of choice in symptomatic treatment

The single most reliable and clinically effective drug in the symptomatic treatment of Parkinson's disease is levodopa. So 'all other things being equal', levodopa is the drug to use when a reliable symptomatic effect is required. So why don't we *always* use levodopa first and what do we use in its place? The reason for not using levodopa first in all patients is that long-term levodopa treatment is associated with a host of response fluctuations and dyskinesias as given above. And there is a nagging doubt that in part these complications are the consequence of the levodopa treatment itself, even though some lines of evidence (such as the experience of the MPTP affected patients referred to above) argue against this hypothesis. So doctors have been eager to explore other drug treatments which might be used to delay or avoid the need for treatment with levodopa.

The incentive to avoid early levodopa treatment is greater in younger patients since they have the longest potential period of disease ahead and since they also tend to develop dyskinesias earlier than patients who are older at clinical disease onset. In younger patients, therefore, drugs having only a modest symptomatic effect (such as anticholinergics and amantadine) are commonly used (Fig. 2.22). When these agents no longer suffice, either levodopa or dopamine agonists are prescribed.

Prescribing anticholinergics and amantadine

Both of these agents have definite symptomatic effect, although neither are as effective as levodopa or dopamine agonists, and very few patients derive adequate long-term benefit from these drugs alone. They can both be useful, however, particularly in patients who are mildly affected, in whom symptomatic treatment is desirable, and yet in whom there is

a wish to delay the prescription of levodopa or agonists.

Once very popular as initial symptomatic treatment, cholinergic drugs are used less now, particularly because they can lead to such unpleasant side-effects in older patients. For this reason many neurologists regard them as suitable only for younger patients (below 40, or at least below 50). When they are started in this age bracket it is sensible to reduce and stop them at the point of later introducing levodopa or an agonist, hopefully before side-effects become a major problem.

Rarely, anticholinergics are appropriate in older patients with severe tremor in whom other medications (including levodopa and dopamine agonists) have been ineffective.

Levodopa versus dopamine agonists

This is one of the issues in Parkinson's disease treatment where experts agree to differ. The arguments in favour of dopamine agonist treatment centre around observations that patients treated with agonists accumulate fewer response fluctuations and dyskinesias than those treated with levodopa. On the other hand, when patients are randomized to receive either levodopa or an agonist,

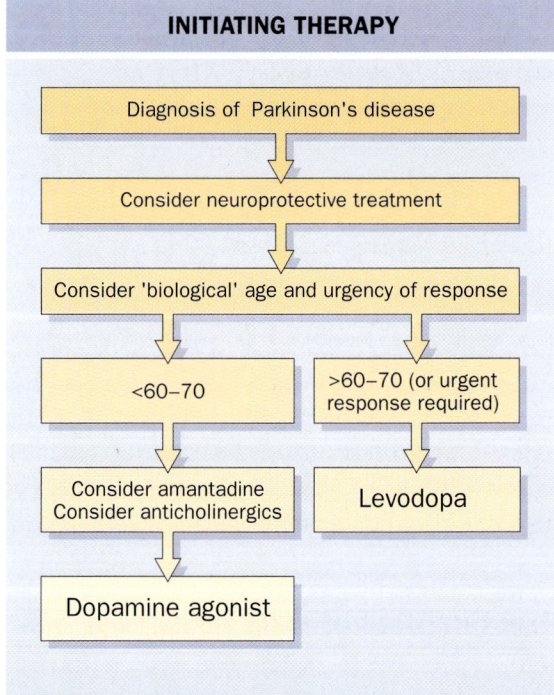

Figure 2.22. Simplified scheme for starting parkinsonian patients on therapy.

more of the agonist group develop early side-effects (nausea, vomiting, postural hypotension) than do the levodopa group. Furthermore, fewer of the agonist group derive sufficient symptomatic relief. The net effect is that whereas most of the levodopa treated group are still taking levodopa a few years later, more of the agonist group have changed to other treatment (typically levodopa). This colours the way that the 'better' long-term profile of agonists is viewed. A presently popular overall synthesis of the situation is that *if* a patient responds well to an agonist in the first place, then they are likely to do well in the long run. What we do not know is whether the same patient would have fared equally well if treated from the beginning with levodopa.

Many clinicians consider their patient's age when choosing between an agonist or levodopa. Younger patients are more likely to be given a trial of an agonist whereas many clinicians are more likely to go straight to levodopa when treating older patients.

Slow-release levodopa and longer-acting agonists

Most patients and doctors agree that it is easier for patients to take tablets once or twice a day, rather than at frequent intervals. So one attraction of these smoother-acting agents is obvious. An additional factor is the belief among some experts that the rapid ups and downs of dopamine stimulation which occur with regular levodopa and the shorter-acting agonists may be a contributory factor in the genesis of subsequent fluctuations and dyskinesias. Whether this theory will be borne out by ongoing trials is of course unknown. In the meantime, treating patients *de novo* with these potentially smoother-acting agents is a popular act of faith.

When given as monotherapy, sustained-release preparations of levodopa may not give rapid enough symptomatic benefit in the morning. Adding a single dose of standard levodopa in the morning may suffice to correct this problem.[112]

Taking a history of response fluctuations

One of the most difficult steps in managing complex response fluctuations is finding out quite how a patient changes during the day. It is helpful to begin by asking about how they are on waking, then when they take their first dose and what they take, how long it is before they

notice any change, what happens first, whether they get worse before they get better, when they first notice improvement, whether they develop peak-dose side-effects, how long the first dose lasts, what if any changes occur as the first dose loses its effect, and when they take the next dose and what they take. When armed with a detailed picture of the first dose of the day, move on to the second, bearing in mind that the picture is likely to become less clear as the day goes by. Bear in mind also that it can be quite hard for patients to distinguish between severe tremor and wild dyskinesias.

Occasionally one of several more extreme approaches may help. One option is to give patients an on–off chart marked out into hourly or half-hourly boxes and to ask them to fill in whether they are 'on' or 'off' or asleep for each half hour of the day (Table 2.5). This can be made more useful (but also more difficult for the patient) by asking for an additional indication of times during the day when they are dyskinetic. Another approach is to bring the patient up to the hospital for a few hours and to watch them through a whole day, or at least one or

Table 2.5. Patient on–off chart showing stable response to treatment

Time	Tablet	Day 1	Day 2	Day 3
05–06		Asleep	Asleep	Asleep
06–07		Asleep	Asleep	Asleep
07–08	*	On	Asleep	On
08–09		On	On	On
09–10		On	On	On
10–11		On	On	On
11–12		On	On	On
12–13	*	On	On	On
13–14		On	On	On
14–15		On	On	On
15–16		On	On	On
16–17		On	On	On
17–18	*	On	On	On
18–19		On	On	On
19–20		On	On	On
20–21		On	On	On
21–22		On	On	On
22–23		On	On	On
23–24		On	Asleep	Asleep
24–01		Asleep	Asleep	Asleep
01–02		Asleep	Asleep	Asleep
02–03		Asleep	Asleep	Asleep
03–04		Asleep	Asleep	Asleep
04–05		Asleep	Asleep	Asleep

two doses of medication, to ensure that you are 'speaking the same language'. Another option is for the doctor or a nurse specialist to visit the patient at home to observe part or all of a *more* typical day. Just occasionally we have asked patients if they or a friend has a video camera to make a short recording of their movements when at their worst; by this means we found that a university professor with Parkinson's disease was in profound 'off' at a time of the evening when we had gathered from our usual history-taking procedure that he was 'on' with extreme dyskinesias.

Dealing with 'wearing-off' (Table 2.6)

For patients who have been started on a non-controlled-release (CR) levodopa preparation, this is a sensible time to change to CR (bearing in mind that the CR preparations have only about a 70% bioavailability in comparison to the regular preparation). Selegiline may be added to reduce brain dopamine catabolism and it is likely that this will be an appropriate time to prescribe a central and/or peripheral COMT inhibitor. In some patients more frequent doses will be needed.

Another approach to wearing-off effects is to add a dopamine agonist to existing levodopa treatment. In patients with fairly mild fluctuations this is often a successful approach, yielding an increase in 'on' time.

Dealing with 'dose failures'

Levodopa competes with dietary amino acids for transport into the circulation. As their disease progresses, many patients find that levodopa medication is less effective if taken close to a high protein meal. In those patients who have their 'main meal' in the middle of the day, this can mean that their drugs are poorly absorbed and they are 'off' for much of the afternoon. Sometimes varying the timing of meals and eating the 'main meal' in the evening helps. Other patients find that reducing their total protein intake (to less than 1 g per kg per day) is helpful.

Gastric emptying is impaired in Parkinson's disease, especially in fluctuating patients who have 'delayed on' or dose failures.[113] A somewhat drastic solution to this problem is to deliver the drug directly into the duodenum via a nasogastric or gastrostomy tube, or to give the drug intravenously or subcutaneously. A less drastic approach is to give a drug to increase gut motility, such as cisapride[114] or domperidone, or to give a soluble formulation of levodopa.

● **Table 2.6.** Patient on–off chart showing wearing off

Time	Tablet	Day 1	Day 2	Day 3
05–06		Asleep	Asleep	Asleep
06–07		Asleep	Asleep	Asleep
07–08	*	Off	Off	Off
08–09		On	On	On
09–10		On	On	On
10–11		On	On	On
11–12		On	On	On
12–13	*	Off	Off	On
13–14		On	On	On
14–15		On	On	On
15–16		On	On	On
16–17		On	On	Off
17–18	*	Off	On	Off
18–19		On	On	On
19–20		On	On	On
20–21		On	On	On
21–22		On	On	On
22–23		Off	Off	On
23–24		Asleep	Off	Asleep
24–01		Asleep	Asleep	Asleep
01–02		Asleep	Asleep	Asleep
02–03		Asleep	Asleep	Asleep
03–04		Asleep	Asleep	Asleep
04–05		Asleep	Asleep	Asleep

Lastly a dose failure may be bypassed completely by taking a dose of (usually subcutaneous) apomorphine. This is likely to give 30–40 minutes of response to tide patients through to the beneficial effect of a further dose of oral medication.

Managing dyskinesias

The first step in managing dyskinesias is to determine whether they occur at peak dose, or else during the transition from 'off' to 'on' either at the beginning or end of a dose. Peak-dose dyskinesias may be lessened by steps taken to smooth out the delivery of drug throughout the day, such as by fractionation into smaller doses (such as 2 hourly, or even hourly doses of levodopa) or by using a controlled-release formulation.

Beginning and end of dose dyskinesias may be eased by steps taken to hasten the transformation from the 'off' to the 'on' state (soluble levodopa preparations, or at least avoiding controlled-release formulations taken alone as the first dose of the day), and by adequate dosing throughout the day in an effort to stop the transformation from 'on' to 'off'.

Neither of these approaches can be said to be wholly successful in the majority of patients and this in large part reflects the narrow dose threshold between being 'on' and dyskinetic. Patients may have to choose between being 'off', or being 'on' *and* dyskinetic. Of these two unattractive options, they generally prefer the latter.

Patients who suffer dystonic spasms on waking in the morning may benefit from a dose of slow-release levodopa or a long-acting agonist at bedtime.

Controlling on–off fluctuations

Once patients experience capricious swings in motor performance apparently unrelated to the timing of their drug treatment (Table 2.7), it can be extremely difficult to restore smooth treatment response. Nevertheless, it may be possible to iron out some of their motor swings.

Switching to a controlled-release levodopa formulation may help, as may long-acting agonists. The duration of benefit from single levodopa doses may be extended by blocking central MAOB activity (using selegiline), central COMT activity (tolcapone) or peripheral COMT activity (tolcapone or entacapone).

Where 'off' periods cannot be avoided, apomorphine (quickest) or soluble levodopa preparations (not so quick) may help deal with severe 'off' periods more quickly than slower-acting drugs; thus many patients at this stage are best served by a combination of slower- and faster-acting drugs.

● **Table 2.7.** Patient on–off chart showing on–off fluctuations

Time	Tablet	Day 1	Day 2	Day 3
05–06		Asleep	Asleep	Asleep
06–07		Asleep	Asleep	Asleep
07–08	*	Off	Off	Off
08–09		Off	On	On
09–10		On	On	Off
10–11		On	Off	On
11–12		On	Off	On
12–13	*	Off	Off	Off
13–14		On	Off	On
14–15		On	On	On
15–16		Off	On	Off
16–17		Off	On	On
17–18	*	Off	Off	On
18–19		Off	Off	Off
19–20		On	Off	Off
20–21		On	On	On
21–22		On	Off	Off
22–23		Off	Off	Off
23–24		Asleep	Asleep	Asleep
24–01		Asleep	Asleep	Asleep
01–02		Asleep	Asleep	Asleep
02–03		Asleep	Asleep	Asleep
03–04		Asleep	Off	Asleep
04–05		Asleep	Asleep	Off

References

1. Parkinson J. Essay on the shaking palsy. London: Whittingham and Rowland, for Sherwood, Neely and Jones, 1817

2. Hassler R. Zur pathologie de paralysis agitans und des postenzephalitischen parkinsonismus. J Psychol Neurol 1938; 48: 387–455

3. Gibb W R G, Lees A J. The relevance of the Lewy body to the pathogenesis of idiopathic Parkinson's disease. J Neurol Neurosurg Psychiatr 1988; 51: 745–752

4. Calne D B, Snow B J, Lee C. Criteria for diagnosing Parkinson's disease. Ann Neurol 1992; 32: S125–S127

5. Marek K L, Seibyl J P, Zoghbi S S et al. [^{123}I]β-CIT/SPECT imaging demonstrates bilateral loss of dopamine transporters in hemi-Parkinson's disease. Neurology 1996; 46: 231–237

6. McKeith I G, Galasko D, Kosaka K et al. Consensus guidelines for the clinical and pathologic diagnosis of dementia with Lewy bodies (DLB): Report of the consortium on DLB international workshop. Neurology 1996; 47: 1113–1124

7. Spillantini M G, Schmidt M L, Trojanowski J Q et al. Alpha-synuclein in Lewy bodies. Nature 1997; 388: 839–840

8. Polymeropoulos M H, Lavedan C, Leroy E et al. Mutation in the alpha-synuclein gene in families with Parkinson's disease. Science 1997; 276: 2045–2047

9. Kruger R, Kuhn W, Muller T et al. Ala30Pro mutation in the gene encoding alpha-synuclein in Parkinson's disease. Nature Genet 1998; 18: 106–108

10. Fearnley J M, Lees A J. Ageing and Parkinson's disease: Substantia nigra regional selectivity. Brain 1991; 114: 2283–2301

11. Gibb W R G, Lees A J. Anatomy, pigmentation, ventral and dorsal subpopulations of the substantia nigra, and differential cell death in Parkinson's disease. J Neurol Neurosurg Psychiatr 1991; 54: 388–396

12. Kish S J, Shannak K, Hornykiewicz O. Uneven pattern of dopamine loss in the striatum of patients with idiopathic Parkinson's disease. N Engl J Med 1988; 318: 876–880

13. Smith P E M, Irving D, Perry R H. Density, distribution and prevalence of Lewy bodies in the elderly: Influence of neuropsychiatric bias with epidemiological and diagnostic implications. Neurosci Res Comm 1991; 8: 127–135

14. Lowe J, Lennox G, Leigh P N. Disorders of movement and system degenerations. In: Graham D I, Lantos P L (eds). Greenfield's neuropathology (6th ed). London: Arnold, 1997: II: 281–366

15. Sage J I, Miller D C, Golbe L I et al. Clinically atypical expression of pathologically typical Lewy body parkinsonism. Clin Neuropharmacol 1990; 13: 36–47

16. Mark M H, Sage J I, Dickson D W et al. Levodopa-nonresponsive Lewy body-parkinsonism: Clinicopathological study of two cases. Neurology 1992; 42: 1323–1327

17. Takahashi K, Nakamura H, Okada E. Hereditary amyotrophic lateral sclerosis: Histochemical and electron microscopic study of hyaline inclusions in motor neurons. Arch Neurol 1972; 27: 292–299

18. Mjones H. Paralysis agitans: A clinical and genetic study. Acta Psychiat Neurol Scand 1949; 25(suppl. 54): 1–195

19. Gudmundsson K R. A clinical survey of parkinsonism in Iceland. Acta Neurol Scand 1967; 43 (Suppl. 33): 9–61

20. Ward C D, Duvoisin R C, Ince S E et al. Parkinson's disease in 65 pairs of twins and in a set of quadruplets. Neurology 1983; 33: 815–824

21. Koller W, O'Hara R, Nutt J et al. Monozygotic twins with Parkinson's disease. Ann Neurol 1986; 19: 402–405

22. Jankowic J, Reches A. Parkinson's disease in monozygotic twins. Ann Neurol 1986; 19: 405–408

23. Pahwa R, Busenbark K, Gray C, Koller W C. Identical twins with similar onset of Parkinson's disease: A case report. Neurology 1993; 43: 1159–1161

24. Johnson W G, Hodge S E, Duvoisin R. Twin studies and the genetics of Parkinson's disease — a reappraisal. Mov Dis 1990; 5: 187–194

25. Maraganore D M, Harding A E, Marsden C D. A clinical and genetic study of familial Parkinson's disease. Mov Dis 1991; 6: 205–211

26. Marder K, Tang M X, Mejia H et al. Risk of Parkinson's disease among first-degree relatives: A community-based study. Neurology 1996; 47: 155–160

27. Golbe L I, Di Iorio G, Bonavita V et al. A large kindred with autosomal dominant Parkinson's disease. Ann Neurol 1990; 27: 276–282

28. Hamouda M, Rad I. Grossesse, post-partum et infarctus cerebraux (pregnancy, post-partum and cerebral infarcts). Sang Thrombose Vaisseaux 1995; 7: 305–313

29. Gasser T, Wszolek Z K, Trofatter J et al. Genetic linkage studies in autosomal dominant parkinsonism: Evaluation of seven candidate genes. Ann Neurol 1994; 36: 387–396

30. Markopoulou K, Wszolek Z K, Pfeiffer R F. A Greek–American kindred with autosomal dominant, levodopa-responsive parkinsonism and anticipation. Ann Neurol 1995; 38: 373–378

31. Waters C H, Miller C A. Autosomal dominant Lewy body parkinsonism in a four-generation family. Ann Neurol 1994; 35: 59–64

32. Payami H, Bernard S, Larsen K et al. Genetic anticipation in Parkinson's disease. Neurology 1995; 45: 135–138

33. Golbe L I, Di Iorio G, Sanges G et al. Clinical genetic analysis of Parkinson's disease in the Contursi kindred. Ann Neurol 1996; 40: 767–775

34. Maraganore D M, Schaid D J, Rocca W A, Harding A E. Anticipation in familial Parkinson's disease: A reanalysis of 13 United Kingdom kindreds. Neurology 1996; 47: 1512–1517

35. Rubinsztein D C, Leggo J, Goodburn et al. Normal CAG and CCG repeats in the Huntington's disease genes of Parkinson's disease patients. Am J Med Gen — Neuropsychiat Gen 1995; 60: 109–110

36. CarreroValenzuela R, Lindblad K, Payami H et al. No evidence for association of familial Parkinson's disease with CAG repeat expansion. Neurology 1995; 45: 1760–1763

37. Sawle G V, Wroe S J, Lees A J et al. The identification of presymptomatic parkinsonism: Clinical and [^{18}F]Dopa PET studies in an Irish kindred. Ann Neurol 1992; 32: 609–617

38. Piccini P, Morrish P K, Turjanski N et al. Dopaminergic function in familial Parkinson's disease: A clinical and ^{18}F-dopa positron emission tomography study. Ann Neurol 1997; 41: 222–229

39. Polymeropoulos M H, Higgins J J, Golbe L I et al. Mapping of a gene for Parkinson's disease to chromosome 4q21–q23. Science 1996; 274: 1197–1199

40. Langston J W, Ballard P, Tetrud J K, Irwin I. Chronic parkinsonism in humans due to a product of meperidine-analog synthesis. Science 1983; 219: 979–980

41. Davis G C, Williams A C, Markey S P et al. Chronic parkinsonism secondary to intravenous injection of meperidine analogues. Psychiatr Rev 1979; 1: 249–254

42. Markey S P, Johannessen J N, Chiueh C C et al. Intraneuronal generation of a pyridinium metabolite may cause drug-induced parkinsonism. Nature 1984; 311: 464–467

43 Hekkila R E, Manzino L, Cabbat F S, Duvoisin R C. Protection against the dopaminergic neurotoxicity of 1-methyl-4-phenyl-1,2,3,6-tetrahydropyridine by monoamine oxidase inhibitors. Nature 1984; 311: 467–469

44. Schapira A H V. Evidence for mitochondrial dysfunction in Parkinson's disease — A critical appraisal. Mov Dis 1994; 9: 125–138

45. Di Monte D A. Mitochondrial DNA and Parkinson's disease. Neurology 1991; 41: 38–42

46. Parker W D, Boyson S J, Parks J D. Abnormalities of the electron transport chain in idiopathic Parkinson's disease. Ann Neurol 1989; 26: 719–723

47. Krige D, Carroll M T, Cooper J M et al. Platelet mitochondrial function in Parkinson's disease. Ann Neurol 1992; 32: 782–788

48. Mann V M, Cooper J M, Krige D et al. skeletal muscle and platelet homogenate mitochondrial function in Parkinson's disease. Brain 1992; 115: 333–342

49. Schapira A H V, Mann V M, Cooper J M et al. Anatomic and disease specificity of NADH CoQ reductase (complex I) deficiency in Parkinson's disease. J Neurochem 1990; 55: 2142–2145

50. Marttila R J, Lorentz H, Rinne U K. Oxygen toxicity protecting enzymes in Parkinson's disease: Increase of superoxide dismutase-like activity in the substantia nigra and basal nucleus. J Neurol Sci 1988; 86: 321–331

51. Saggu H, Cooksey J, Dexter A et al. A selective increase in particulate superoxide dismutase activity in parkinsonian substantia nigra. J Neurochem 1989; 53: 692–697

52. Dexter D T, Wells F R, Lees A J et al. Increased nigral oxygen content and alterations in other metal ions occurring in brain in Parkinson's disease. J Neurochem 1989; 52: 1830–1836

53. Jellinger K, Kienzl E, Rumpelmair G et al. Iron–melanin complex in substantia nigra of Parkinsonian brains: An X-ray microanalysis. J Neurochem 1992; 59: 1168–1171

54. Sian J, Dexter D T, Lees A J et al. Alterations in glutathione levels in Parkinson's disease and other neurodegenerative disorders affecting basal ganglia. Ann Neurol 1994; 36: 348–355

55. Zhang Z-x, Anderson D W, Lavine L, Mantel M. Patterns of acquiring parkinsonism-dementia complex on Guam 1944 through 1985. Arch Neurol 1990; 47: 1019–1024

56. Tanner C M. Epidemiological clues to the cause of Parkinson's disease. In: Marsden C D, Fahn S (ed). Movement disorders 3. Oxford: Butterworth Heinemann, 1994: 124–146

57. Rajput A H. Epidemiology of Parkinson's disease. Can J Neurol Sci 1984; 11: 156–159

58. Koller W, Vetere-Overfield B, Gray C et al. Environmental risk factors in Parkinson's disease. Neurology 1990; 40: 1218–1221

59. Hertzman C, Wiens M, Bowering D et al. Parkinson's disease: A case-control study of occupational and environmental risk factors. Am J Indust Med 1990; 17: 349–355

60. Semchuck K M, Love E J, Lee R G. Parkinson's disease and exposure to agricultural work and pesticide chemicals. Neurology 1992; 42: 1328–1335

61. Morens D M, Grandinetti A, Waslien C I et al. Case-control study of idiopathic Parkinson's disease and dietary vitamin E intake. Neurology 1996; 46: 1270–1274

62. Mouradian M M, Heuser I J E, Baronti F et al. Pathogenesis of dyskinesias in Parkinson's disease. Ann Neurol 1989; 25: 523–526

63. Riley D E, Lang A E. The spectrum of levodopa-related fluctuations in Parkinson's disease. Neurology 1993; 43: 1459–1464

64. Hillen M E, Sage J I. Nonmotor fluctuations in patients with Parkinson's disease. Neurology 1996; 47: 1180–1183

65. Shoulson I, The Parkinson Study Group. Effect of deprenyl on the progression of disability in early Parkinson's disease. N Engl J Med 1989; 321: 1364–1371

66. Lees A J, Abbott R, Banerji N et al. Comparison of therapeutic effects and mortality data of levodopa and levodopa combined with selegiline in patients with early, mild Parkinson's disease. Br Med J 1995; 311: 1602–1607

67. Lees A J, Stern G M. Sustained bromocriptine therapy in previously untreated patients with Parkinson's disease. J Neurol Neurosurg Psychiat 1981; 44: 1020–1023

68. Schachter M, Sheehy M P, Parkes J D, Marsden C D. Lisuride in the treatment of Parkinsonism. Acta Neurol Scand 1980; 62: 382–385

69. Lieberman A N, Goldstein M, Leibowitz M et al. Lisuride combined with levodopa in advanced Parkinson disease. Neurology 1981; 31: 1466–1469

70. Obeso J A, Luquin M R, Martinez Lage J M. Lisuride infusion pump: A device for the treatment of motor fluctuations in Parkinson's disease. Lancet 1986; 1: 467–470

71. Obeso J A, Luquin M R, Martinez Lage J M. Intravenous lisuride corrects oscillations of motor performance in Parkinson's disease. Ann Neurol 1986; 19: 31–35

72. Vaamonde J, Luquin M R, Obeso JA. Subcutaneous lisuride infusion in Parkinson's disease. Response to chronic administration in 34 patients. Brain 1991; 114: 601–614

73. Giovannini P, Scigliano G, Piccolo I et al. Lisuride in de novo Parkinsonian patients: A four-year follow-up. Acta Neurol Scand 1988; 77: 322–327

74. Rinne U K. Lisuride, a dopamine agonist in the treatment of early Parkinson's disease. Neurology 1989; 39: 336–339

75. Lieberman A, Goldstein M, Leibowitz M et al. Treatment of advanced Parkinson disease with pergolide. Neurology 1981; 31: 675–682

76. Lang A E, Quinn N, Brincat S et al. Pergolide in late-stage Parkinson disease. Ann Neurol 1982; 12: 243–247

77. Lieberman A N, Goldstein M, Gopinathan G et al. Further studies with pergolide in Parkinson disease. Neurology 1982; 32: 1181–1184

78. Mear J Y, Barroche G, De Smet Y et al. Pergolide in the treatment of Parkinson's disease. Neurology 1984; 34: 983–986

79. Rascol O, Lees A J, Senard J M et al. Ropinirole in the treatment of levodopa-induced motor fluctuations in patients with Parkinson's disease. Clin Neuropharmacol 1996; 19: 234–245

80. Rascol O. A double blind L-dopa controlled study of ropinirole in de novo patients with Parkinson's disease. Mov Dis 1996; 11 (Suppl. 1): 139

81. Brooks D J, Fuell D, Kreider M S. The efficacy and safety of ropinirole, a novel non-ergoline selective D2 agonist, for the treatment of early Parkinson's disease. Mov Dis 1997; 12 (Suppl. 1): 62

82. Lera G, Vaamonde J, Rodriguez M, Obeso J A. Cabergoline in Parkinson's disease: Long-term follow-up. Neurology 1993; 43: 2587–2590

83. Rabey J M, Nissipeanu P, Inzelberg R, Korczyn A D. Beneficial effect of cabergoline, new long-lasting D2 agonist in the treatment of Parkinson's disease. Clin Neuropharmacol 1994; 17: 286–293

84. Ahlskog J E, Muenter M D, Maraganore D M et al. Fluctuating Parkinson's disease: Treatment with the long-acting dopamine agonist cabergoline. Arch Neurol 1994; 51: 1236–1241

85. Steiger M J, El-Debas T et al. Double-blind study of the activity and tolerability of cabergoline versus placebo in parkinsonians with motor fluctuations. J Neurol 1996; 243: 68–72

86. Hutton J T, Koller W C, Ahlskog J E et al. Multicenter, placebo-controlled trial of cabergoline taken once daily in the treatment of Parkinson's disease. Neurology 1996; 46: 1062–1065

87. Rinne U K, Bracco F, Chouza C et al. Cabergoline in the treatment of early Parkinson's disease: Results of the first year of treatment in a double-blind comparison of cabergoline and levodopa. Neurology 1997; 48: 363–368

88. Inzelberg R, Nisipeanu P, Rabey J M et al. Double-blind comparison of cabergoline and bromocriptine in Parkinson's disease patients with motor fluctuations. Neurology 1996; 47: 785–788

89. Molho E S, Factor S A, Weiner W J et al. The use of pramipexole, a novel dopamine (DA) agonist, in advanced Parkinson's disease. J Neural Transm (Suppl.) 1995; 45: 225–230

90. Hubble J P, Koller W C, Cutler N R et al. Pramipexole in patients with early Parkinson's disease. Clin Neuropharmacol 1995; 18: 338–347

91. Van Laar T, Jansen E N H, Essink A W G, Neef C. Intranasal apomorphine in Parkinsonian on–off fluctuations. Arch Neurol 1992; 49: 482–484

92. Dewey Jr R B, Maraganore D M, Ahlskog J E, Matsumoto J Y. Intranasal apomorphine rescue therapy for parkinsonian 'off' periods. Clin Neuropharmacol 1996; 19: 193–201

93. Van Laar T, Jansen E N H, Neef C et al. Pharmacokinetics and clinical efficacy of rectal apomorphine in patients with Parkinson's disease: A study of five different suppositories. Mov Dis 1995; 10: 433–439

94. Van Laar T, Neef C, Danhof M et al. A new sublingual formulation of apomorphine in the treatment of patients with Parkinson's disease. Mov Dis 1996; 11: 633–638

95. Schwab R S, Amador L V, Lettvin J Y. Apomorphine in Parkinson's disease. Trans Am Neurol Assoc 1951; 76: 251–253

96. Cotzias G C, Papavasiliou P S, Fehling C et al. Similarities between neurologic effects of L-dopa and apomorphine. N Engl J Med 1970; 282: 31–33

97. Pramipexole hydrochloride. Drugs of the Future 1996; 21: 449

98. Kempster P A, Frankel J P, Stern G M, Lees A J. Comparison of motor response to apomorphine and levodopa in Parkinson's disease. J Neurol Neurosurg Psychiat 1990; 53: 1004–1007

99. Davis T L, Roznoski M, Burns R S. Effects of tolcapone in Parkinson's patients taking L-dihydroxyphenylalanine/carbidopa and selegiline. Mov Dis 1995; 10: 349–351

100. Hughes A J, Bishop S, Kleedorfer B et al. Subcutaneous apomorphine in Parkinson's disease: Response to chronic administration for up to five years. Mov Dis 1993; 8: 165–170

101. Obeso J A, Grandas F, Vaamonde J et al. Apomorphine infusion for motor fluctuations in Parkinson's disease. Lancet 1987; 1: 1376–1377

102. Gancher S T, Nutt J G, Woodward W R. Apomorphine infusional therapy in Parkinson's disease: Clinical utility and lack of tolerance. Mov Dis 1995; 10: 37–43

103. Poewe W, Kleedorfer B, Wagner M et al. Side effects of subcutaneous apomorphine in Parkinson's disease. Lancet 1989; 1: 1084–1085

104. Hughes A J, Lees A J, Stern G M. Apomorphine test to predict dopaminergic responsiveness in parkinsonian syndromes. Lancet 1990; 336: 32–34

105. Guttman M, Leger G, Reches A et al. Administration of the new COMT inhibitor OR-611 increases striatal uptake of fluorodopa. Mov Dis 1993; 8: 298–304

106. Sawle G V, Burn D J, Morrish P K et al. The effect of entacapone (OR-611) on brain [^{18}F]-6-L-fluorodopa metabolism: Implications for levodopa therapy of Parkinson's disease. Neurology 1994; 44: 1292–1297

107. Ruottinen H M, Rinne U K. A double-blind pharmacokinetic and clinical dose-response study of entacapone as an adjuvant to levodopa therapy in advanced Parkinson's disease. Clin Neuropharmacol 1996; 19: 283–296

108. Nutt J G, Woodward W R, Beckner R M et al. Effect of peripheral catechol-O-methyltransferase inhibition on the pharmacokinetics and pharmacodynamics of levodopa in parkinsonian patients. Neurology 1994; 44: 913–919

109. Kurth M C, Adler C H, St Hilaire M et al. Tolcapone improves motor function and reduces levodopa requirement in patients with Parkinson's disease experiencing motor fluctuations: A multicenter, double-blind, randomized, placebo-controlled trial. Neurology 1997; 48: 81–87

110. Tetrud J W, Langston J W. The effect of deprenyl (selegiline) on the natural history of Parkinson's disease. Science 1989; 245: 519–522

111. Ward C D. Does selegiline delay progression of Parkinson's disease? A critical re-evaluation of the DATATOP study. J Neurol Neurosurg Psychiat 1994; 57: 217–220

112. Pahwa R, Lyons K, McGuire D et al. Early morning akinesia in Parkinson's disease: Effect of standard carbidopa/levodopa and sustained-release carbidopa/levodopa. Neurology 1996; 46: 1059–1062

113. Djaldetti R, Baron J, Ziv I, Melamed E. Gastric emptying in Parkinson's disease: Patients with and without response fluctuations. Neurology 1996; 46: 1051–1054

114. Djaldetti R, Koren M, Ziv I et al. Effect of cisapride on response fluctuations in Parkinson's disease. Mov Dis 1995; 10: 81–84

chapter 3

Parkinsonism: *Parkinson's plus*

Guy Sawle

The accurate diagnosis of parkinsonism *not due to Parkinson's disease* can be of critical therapeutic importance, or an issue of seemingly academic trivia. In one case misdiagnosis may deprive the patient of specific life- and disability-saving treatment, whereas in another case accurate diagnosis may seem for the moment to bring little more than the realization of poor prognosis and certain therapeutic failure. Precision in diagnosis is warranted, however, in separating the former group with certainty and in the hope and expectation that current and future research endeavours will enable therapeutic success across the range of these serious and disabling conditions.

Wilson's disease

The single cause of parkinsonism 'never to be missed' is Wilson's disease, an autosomal recessive disorder of copper metabolism.

Whilst the clinical features are varied and there may even be a characteristic pattern in younger parkinsonian patients with prominent hand and bulbar impairments, the only sensible diagnostic approach to this condition is to screen all patients who present with parkinsonism below a certain age (I choose the age of 50) by checking their blood copper and caeruloplasmin levels. This *must* be the minimum level of investigation of a young parkinsonian patient; the outcome without treatment is invariably fatal.

Genetics and clinical chemistry

Wilson's disease is an autosomal recessive disorder caused by a variety of (insertion or deletion) mutations in the gene on chromosome 13 which encodes copper transporting P-type ATPase.[1,2] Disruption of this gene leads to accumulation of excess body copper, with low serum caeruloplasmin, high serum copper, and increased urine copper excretion. Copper accumulation in the liver can lead to cirrhosis, and in the brain there may be destruction of basal ganglia structures.

Psychiatric symptoms are common. Renal and joint changes also occur. Accumulation in the cornea leads to Kayser–Fleischer rings which are a (very nearly but not quite[3]) invariable accompaniment of neurological Wilson's disease (Fig. 3.1). It is likely that the variable presentation of this disorder reflects the range of mutations responsible for the gene defect.

Neurological symptoms and signs

Around a third of patients with Wilson's disease present with psychiatric symptoms including depression and personality change. A similar number present with an extrapyramidal syndrome which may appear as parkinsonism though many patients show dystonia (CD 3.1) leading sometimes to extreme postures and contractures. Almost all patients with a

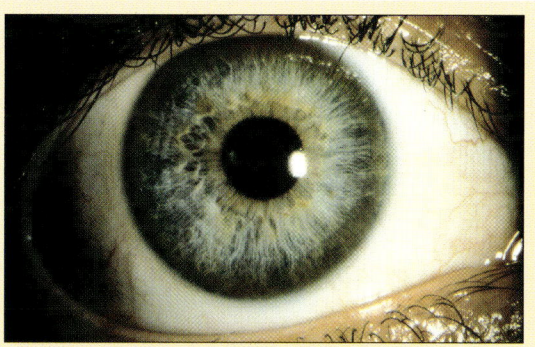

Figure 3.1. Kayser–Fleischer ring in Wilson's disease. (Courtesy of S. Vernon.)

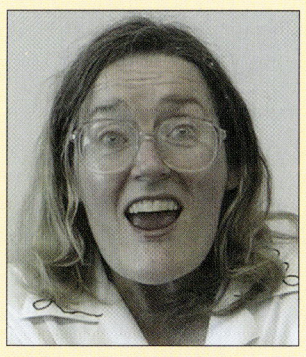

CD 3.1. Wilson's disease.

neurological presentation have dysarthria. Speech is often slurred and monotonous; a facile grin and lip retraction may be seen. Others present with liver disease (usually in childhood) or through the genetic screening of asymptomatic family members.

Diagnostic testing

All patients in whom Wilson's disease is a possibility should have serum copper and caeruloplasmin concentrations assessed. Patients with a neurological condition which *suggests* Wilson's disease should have an ophthalmological slit-lamp examination to look for Kayser–Fleischer rings (deposits of copper in Descemet's membrane; at the outer border of the cornea). When these tests give ambiguous results, measures of urinary copper excretion or a liver biopsy (using a copper-free needle) to measure dry copper weight may be necessary.

T2-weighted MRI scans may show either an area of decreased signal intensity with an increased signal surround, or increased signal intensity alone[4] (Fig. 3.2).

Treatment

The key to drug treatment in Wilson's disease is to tip the patient into negative copper balance.[5] Chelating agents are used to achieve this goal. British anti-Lewisite (BAL) was the first agent to be used; but it must be given by intramuscular injections which are painful and it is rarely used today. Once a patient has been successfully decoppered, lifelong treatment is necessary to prevent deterioration.

D-penicillamine

Taken together with pyridoxine (because it has an incidental antipyridoxine effect) on an empty stomach, penicillamine binds copper and leads to increased urinary copper excretion. After starting penicillamine, around a third of patients initially deteriorate;[5,6] most recover the lost ground, but a minority are left with residual deficits which are worse than their condition when they started treatment.[6] Even patients who are neurologically asymptomatic at the time of starting treatment can develop severe and permanent symptoms on starting penicillamine.[7]

Side-effects are common, including hypersensitivity, skin reactions, systemic lupus erythematosus (SLE), Goodpasture's syndrome and myasthenia gravis. When acute hypersensitivity reactions occur

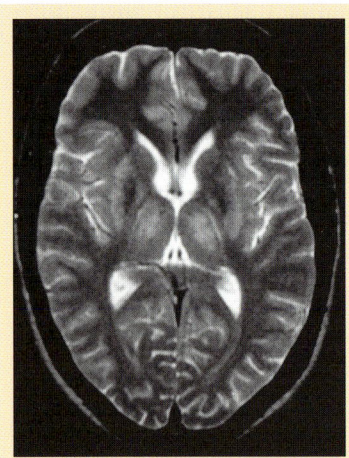

Figure 3.2. MRI scan in Wilson's disease. Note signal change in striatum. (Courtesy of R. Lenthall.)

(fever, rash, eosinophilia etc.) the drug should be stopped to allow resolution of the symptoms, and it may be possible to successfully reintroduce the drug at a lower dose under steroid cover.[8] Sudden discontinuation of penicillamine can lead to a rapid deterioration.

Trientene

Trientene is another effective but less powerful chelating agent.[9] Side-effects are less common but do include lupus nephritis and sideroblastic anaemia. It is more expensive than penicillamine.

Zinc

Although not a chelating agent, dietary zinc supplements reduce body copper by reducing dietary copper absorption. The commonest side-effect of zinc therapy is gastrointestinal irritation. Zinc acetate or sulphate are most commonly used to keep tissue copper levels low after decoppering with a chelating agent. If used as primary treatment, the copper levels fall more slowly than with either penicillamine or trientene. Zinc is favoured as first-line treatment for asymptomatic patients.

Tetrathiomolybdate

This agent chelates copper in the gut, preventing its absorption. It also chelates plasma copper, increasing copper excretion. It is a powerful, but experimental agent.[10]

Family screening

The gene frequency is around 1%. Asymptomatic homozygous individuals should be sought because decoppering treatment at this stage may prevent disease presentation. All first-degree relatives should be seen and examined and should have liver function tests, serum copper and caeruloplasmin assessment, 24-hour urine copper excretion and a slit lamp examination.

Multiple system atrophy

After a rocky history over the nosology of multiple-system atrophy (MSA) there is now general agreement on what is meant by this term.[11] Having been originally coined to describe a single patient with autonomic failure, cerebellar ataxia and probably pyramidal signs but no parkinsonism,[12] the term is now used to describe a conglomerate of clinical syndromes which were previously described as the Shy–Drager syndrome,[13] striatonigral degeneration[14] and olivopontocerebellar atrophy.[15] The reason for this conglomeration at a time in neurological history when we are mostly struggling to *separate* different disorders rather than lump them together has been the realization that they share a similar pathology, together with symptoms and signs indicating a combination of pyramidal, extrapyramidal, autonomic and cerebellar degeneration. It is the variable severity of these component degenerations that previously led to the description of apparently separate disorders.

The pathological unity of this condition was first suggested by the occurrence of overlapping patterns of neuronal loss with gliosis in some or all of the inferior olives, pons, cerebellum, striatum (mainly putamen) and the intermediolateral columns and Onuf's nucleus of the spinal cord. More recently, the identification and characterization of glial cytoplasmic inclusions has added further weight to this definition[16] (Fig. 3.3). Initially, these inclusions were reported to be specific to multiple system atrophy, but subsequent reports have described similar inclusions in a minority of patients with other conditions including corticobasal degeneration, progressive supranuclear palsy,[17] and spinocerebellar ataxia type 1 (SCA 1).[18] The glial cytoplasmic inclusions of MSA stain with anti-α-synuclein (Fig. 3.4). Perhaps glial cytoplasmic inclusions will be as specific as the Lewy body in Parkinson's disease; essential for the clinicopathological diagnosis, but not quite restricted to patients who have the characteristic clinical picture in life.

Clinical diagnosis of MSA

In the context of parkinsonism it is now conventional to *consider* MSA as a possible diagnosis in patients who do not quite match the clinical criteria we use for diagnosing Parkinson's disease. It is important to remember, however, that patients with MSA may have symptoms and signs indistinguishable from those of Parkinson's disease early on in their clinical course; if we are to correctly diagnose these patients in life, we must maintain a watchful eye throughout their illness.

The median age of onset is in the early 50s. Patients with MSA nearly all show parkinsonism.[19] More than half have pyramidal signs, and half have cerebellar

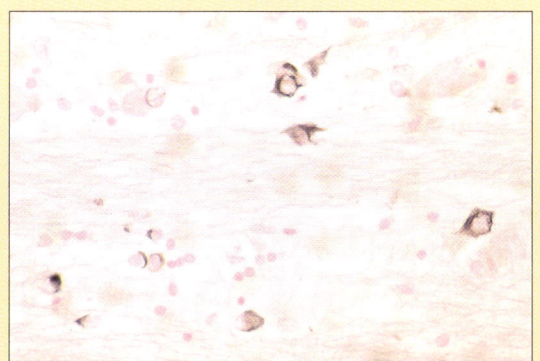

Figure 3.3. Glial cytoplasmic inclusion from basis pontis in MSA (Gallyas silver impregnation). (Courtesy of J. Lowe.)

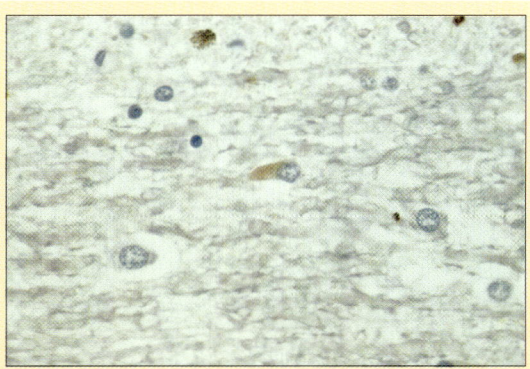

Figure 3.4. Glial cytoplasmic inclusion from basis pontis in MSA (anti-α-synuclein stain). (Courtesy of J. Lowe.)

signs. Most have symptoms of autonomic dysfunction (Fig. 3.5). Of those with parkinsonism, a quarter have *no* clinical features of either pyramidal or cerebellar dysfunction and these are the hardest group to diagnose in life. Of those with parkinsonism, many have either no response to levodopa, or else they respond poorly (CD 3.2).

The pyramidal signs reported in MSA comprise hyperreflexia and extensor plantar responses (not the *spontaneous* toe extension seen in parkinsonism). Clinically significant weakness and spasticity are not usually seen.

Autonomic features may antedate the movement disorder by up to several years. Impotence, urinary symptoms and postural hypotension are common; snoring and stridor sufficient to demand tracheostomy may occur; the latter can even be the presenting symptom.[20] Patients who in reality are developing postural hypotension may have a recent history of (presumably compensatory) supine hypertension. Dementia is not a feature.

Some patients develop a disproportionate antecollis. Prominent orofacial dyskinesias and dystonia develop in around a quarter of treated patients. Pain unrelieved by levodopa, contractures and pseudobulbar crying spells have all been described.

There is no absolute diagnostic test, though basal ganglia changes (such as putaminal hypointensity) on high field MRI have been reported[21] and a variety of changes have been reported using positron emission tomography (PET) and single photon emission computed tomography (SPECT). Published findings from PET include reduced fluorodopa uptake (which may differ in pattern from the changes seen in Parkinson's disease),[22,23] reduced striatal raclopride binding (Fig. 3.6)[24] and impaired diprenorphine (opiate receptor) binding.[25] SPECT findings include reduced IBZM (dopamine receptor) binding.[26,27] The pattern of presynaptic and postsynaptic external urethral or anal sphincter EMG may be pathological, and if so, this is highly suggestive of the condition[28] (Fig. 3.7).[29]

Treatment and prognosis

The response of parkinsonian features to levodopa may be transiently good, but it is usually modest or absent and it is often short lived. The response to dopamine agonists is no better. The mild antiparkinsonian effect of amantadine seems to work as well in MSA as in Parkinson's disease, and whilst such subtle improvement may lead us towards more efficacious therapy in Parkinson's disease, it must not be ignored in patients with MSA. Anticholinergic drugs may help the parkinsonism a little, and benefit the urinary symptoms somewhat more. Sometimes a penile sheath or a urethral catheter is necessary for the latter. Intermittent (self) catheterization is preferable if dexterity permits. Nocturnal diuresis may be helped by desmopressin (DDAVP). If urinary retention intervenes on anticholinergics they may need to be stopped — but if catheterization becomes necessary, then the anticholinergics can usually be started again.

If dopaminergic drugs do help the motor aspects of the disease, they may still precipitate or worsen postural hypotension, sometimes to a dramatic extent. Elastic stockings or a head-up tilt of the bed with an

THE COMPONENTS OF MSA

Parkinsonism

Cerebellar degeneration

MSA

Autonomic failure

Pyramidal signs

Figure 3.5. Relationship between the components of MSA.

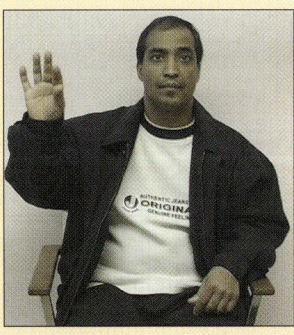

CD 3.2. Parkinsonism in multiple system atrophy.

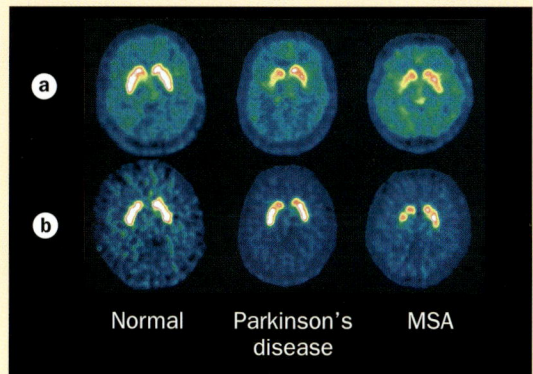

Figure 3.6. (a) Fluorodopa uptake and (b) raclopride (dopamine D2) binding in right hemi-parkinsonism and MSA. The Parkinson's disease patient has increased raclopride binding at the site of reduced fluorodopa uptake, indicating upregulation of receptors. The patient with MSA has reduced raclopride binding at the site of reduced fluorodopa uptake, indicating loss of striatal neurons.

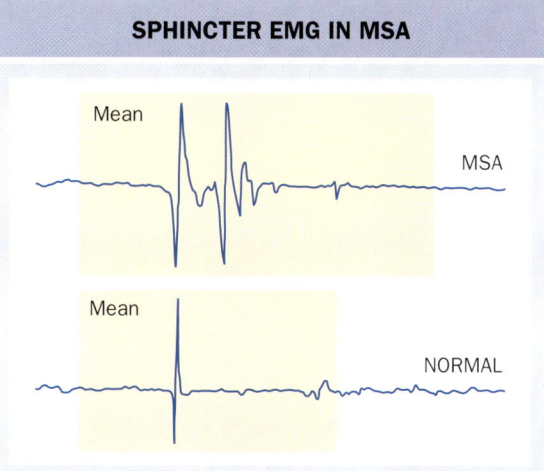

Figure 3.7. Sphincter EMG in MSA. Motor unit of MSA patient is prolonged and polyphasic in comparison with control subject.

increased salt intake and possibly a small dose of fludrocortisone are often sufficient to prevent catastrophic postural faintness.

Some patients with erectile impotence are helped through intracavernosal papaveretum injections or penile implants. The role of sildenafil in this condition is not yet known.

Patients with MSA present earlier, and die sooner, than their parkinsonian counterparts. The median survival from symptom onset is around 8 years.

The relationship with familial olivopontocerebellar atrophy

MSA as defined above is not thought to be an hereditary disorder.

The classification of adult onset cerebellar syndromes is presently in a state of flux and falls outside the scope of this chapter. The safest label for patients who present with a pure cerebellar syndrome in adult life (i.e. without features of autonomic failure or other signs of MSA) is idiopathic late (adult) onset cerebellar ataxia. One form of this condition, comprising atrophy limited to the cerebellum and olive *without* atrophy of other brainstem structures is confusingly called cerebellar cortical atrophy (CCA) when sporadic or dominant, and olivopontocerebellar atrophy (OPCA) when recessive. The use of both of these terms is controversial.

Progressive supranuclear palsy

In 1964, Steele, Richardson and Olszewski described a group of patients with a late onset progressive neurodegenerative disorder comprising supranuclear gaze palsy, pseudobulbar palsy, dystonic rigidity of the neck and trunk, dysarthria and dementia.[30] Their patients had neurofibrillary degeneration with neuronal loss and gliosis in a number of central grey matter structures. Although much less common than Parkinson's disease, progressive supranuclear palsy has been reported from many countries and it is one of the more common conditions misdiagnosed as Parkinson's disease.

Clinical features

The early signs and symptoms of progressive supranuclear palsy are usually distinctive, with unsteadiness and falls being very common. Speech is often affected with quiet and spastic vocal output (CD 3.3a). Visual symptoms are common. Some patients complain that they cannot move their eyes but the symptoms reported may not be such an obvious hint at the diagnosis. Others complain of dry eyes, photophobia or diplopia. Clinically significant early memory impairment and personality change are more common in progressive supranuclear palsy than in Parkinson's disease.

Limb and axial signs

Examination findings include axial rigidity and sometimes dystonia, with early loss of postural reflexes. The axial tone changes are much more severe than any limb changes, although limb bradykinesia is usual (CD 3.3b). A minority of patients present with an akinetic-rigid syndrome indistinguishable from Parkinson's disease (and progressive supranuclear palsy is represented pathologically in series of patients who have carried a clinically confident diagnosis of Parkinson's disease in life). Some degree of pseudobulbar palsy is common with slow tongue movements, brisk facial and jaw reflexes and even forced laughter or crying.

Eye signs

The eye signs may be the most suggestive, although they are not quite diagnostic. The commonest signs are impairment of upgaze and convergence, but since both of these movements are impaired to some extent in many otherwise healthy elderly people, if mild then these eye signs alone do not provide robust diagnostic information until downgaze is affected. The downgaze palsy is supranuclear (hence progressive *supranuclear* palsy) and movements to command are more affected than pursuit movements. Oculocephalic movements are affected least of all (CD 3.4). Ultimately all eye movements may be lost, including those in the horizontal plane. Examination to show the preservation of the oculocephalic vertical eye movements is sometimes difficult because of nuchal rigidity.

Many patients with progressive supranuclear palsy have a rather staring appearance due to lid retraction (Fig. 3.8). Other lid abnormalities are also seen,

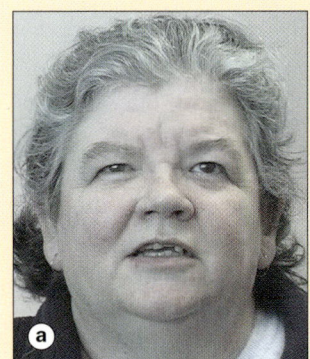
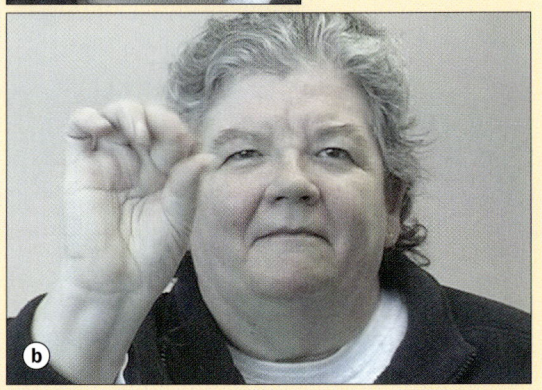

CD 3.3. Speech (a) and limb signs (b) in progressive supranuclear palsy.

including blepharospasm and apraxia of either lid opening or closing. Not all patients have a supranuclear palsy,[31] and some patients with the ophthalmological signs usually associated with progressive supranuclear palsy have been shown at postmortem to have other conditions. Furthermore, patients with MSA may have a mild reduction of downgaze,[32] typically with concurrent horizontal gaze paresis.[33] Some patients with corticobasal degeneration also develop a severe supranuclear gaze palsy.[34]

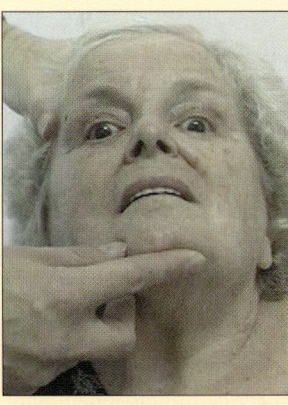

CD 3.4. Eye movement in progressive supranuclear palsy.

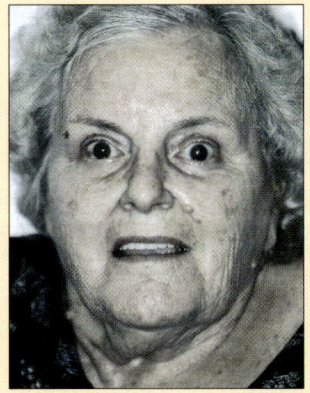

Figure 3.8. Lid reaction in progressive supranuclear palsy.

Cognitive and personality changes

The cognitive changes seen in progressive supranuclear palsy have been referred to as an example of so-called subcortical dementia. This comprises cognitive change believed to depend on abnormal subcortical neuronal activity. The implication of this term is that in patients with subcortical dementia, cortical function is normal or at least preferentially spared. Yet in many of those conditions formerly referred to as subcortical dementias, histopathological studies have shown that significant cortical involvement is more common and widespread than previously thought. Even so, there is still support for the notion that in progressive supranuclear palsy, much of the cognitive change is due to impairment of frontal-basal ganglia loops rather than direct damage to the cortex.

Part of the apparent difficulty that patients with progressive supranuclear palsy have in cognitive tests may be explained by either a difficulty in visual scanning (due to their ophthalmoparesis) or to a defect in the orientation of visual attention.

Neuropathology

Macroscopically, brains from patients with progressive supranuclear palsy show depigmentation of the substantia nigra and locus coeruleus. Third and lateral ventricular dilatation and pallor with atrophy of the globus pallidus may also be visible to the naked eye (Fig. 3.9).

The definitive histopathological diagnosis of progressive supranuclear palsy still depends upon comparison with the features noted in Steele,

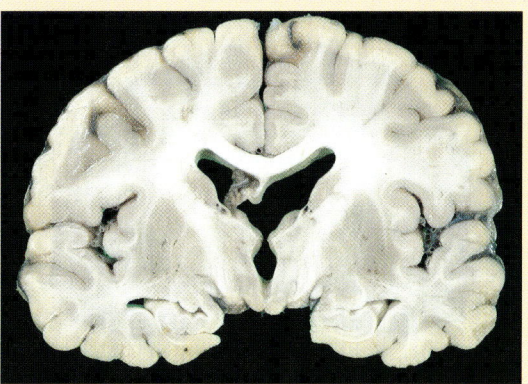

Figure 3.9. Coronal section of brain in progressive supranuclear palsy. Slight shrinkage and discoloration of basal ganglia, most marked in putamen. (Courtesy of J. Lowe.)

Richardson and Olszewski's original manuscript. Briefly stated, the predilection of pathology for globus pallidus, subthalamus and substantia nigra, in the setting of cortical, subcortical and brainstem tangles is a useful pathological pointer to this pathological diagnosis.

Nerve cell loss with gliosis and neurofibrillary tangles are seen chiefly in the globus pallidus, subthalamic nucleus, substantia nigra, and other brainstem regions including the superior colliculi, pretectal area, periaqueductal grey matter and pontine nuclei. Many patients also show cell loss and tangles in the caudate, putamen, red nucleus, locus coeruleus, dentate, thalamus, and selected regions of cortex (frontal, insular, hippocampal and parahippocampal) (Figs. 3.10, 3.11).

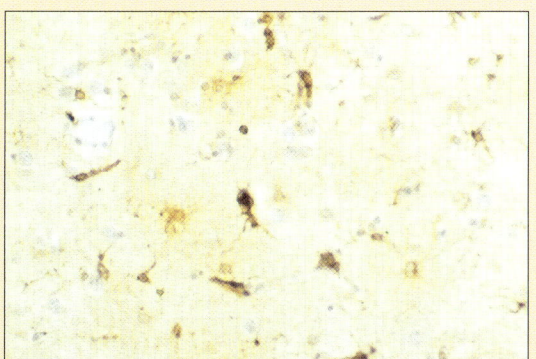

Figure 3.10. Astrocytic tau immunoreactivity within dentate nucleus in progressive supranuclear palsy. (Courtesy of J. Lowe.)

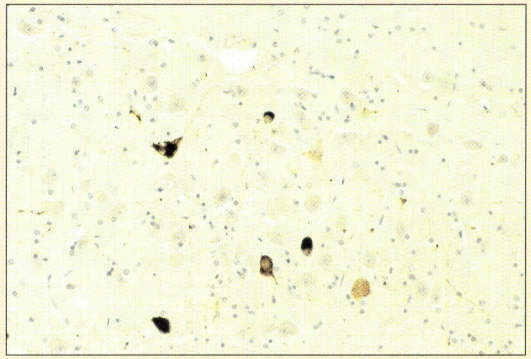

Figure 3.11. Tau staining of tangles within pontine nuclei in progressive supranuclear palsy. (Courtesy of J. Lowe.)

Widespread abnormal tau storage is seen in the nerve cell soma, neuronal processes, and fibre tracts of the internal capsule, subcortical nuclei and brachium conjunctivum. Tau also accumulates in astrocytes, oligodendrocytes and microglia.

Treatment and prognosis

A small minority of patients with progressive supranuclear palsy derive some functional benefit from levodopa or other dopamine agonists. The benefit, if seen at all, is usually slight and evident only in the early phase of the illness. Such benefit as occurs is manifest as an improvement in rigidity and gait; the eye signs are almost without exception unaffected. Small improvements on amantadine have been reported. Occasional patients in whom dystonia is a problem (such as causing blepharospasm) may benefit from botulinum toxin injections. Amitriptyline is of benefit in some patients, with reported improvement in the emotional distress of pseudobulbar failure.

Physiotherapy, occupational therapy and speech therapy can all help ease the suffering to some extent. Some patients need help with feeding via a nasogastric or gastrostomy tube. Occasional patients benefit from cricopharyngeal myotomy (for dystonic dysphagia) or tracheostomy (for sleep apnoea).

Disease progression is relentless. Patients become helpless with both axial and limb rigidity, complete failure of voluntary eye movements, almost unintelligible speech, and sometimes profound emotional lability. The mean survival from clinical onset to death is around 6 years.

Corticobasal degeneration

Of the differential diagnoses most commonly considered alongside Parkinson's disease, corticobasal degeneration is perhaps the most recent arrival. That is not to say that it is a new disease; but its widespread recognition has increased substantially in the last decade, almost certainly due to changes in diagnostic process, rather than disease incidence.

History

The first classical description of this disorder is credited to Rebeiz and associates in 1968 who reported three Irish patients who presented in late middle age with variable combinations of an asymmetric akinetic-rigid syndrome, involuntary movements, apraxia, dysarthria and dysphagia, supranuclear palsy and frontal lobe signs. Mental impairment occurred late and the patients came to postmortem in 6–8 years.

Clinical features

The illness is manifest as a combination of cortical and basal ganglia associated symptoms. Most commonly, patients present with a highly asymmetrical akinetic rigid ('basal') syndrome together with one or more of a variety of 'cortical' signs such as apraxia, alien limb, myoclonus, or cortical sensory change. Some patients show dystonia, dysphasia, or an irregular jerky tremor (though the jerkiness of the tremor may be evidence of coincident myoclonus, and sometimes patients with marked myoclonus are incorrectly described as tremulous) (CD 3.5). A supranuclear gaze palsy may occur, in which case patients may at first sight be misdiagnosed as having progressive supranuclear palsy. Some patients have prominent frontal lobe release signs including grasp responses and facial reflexes. Occasionally cerebellar signs are evident. Intellectual failure is neither a prominent, nor an early, feature.

Symptom onset is most frequently after the age of 60. Men and women are equally affected.

Extrapyramidal syndrome

The akinetic-rigid syndrome of corticobasal degeneration is at least as asymmetrical as in Parkinson's disease, if not more so. Some patients progress to complete functional redundancy of one side of the body with only subtle contralateral signs. With further progression, however, the initially spared limbs become

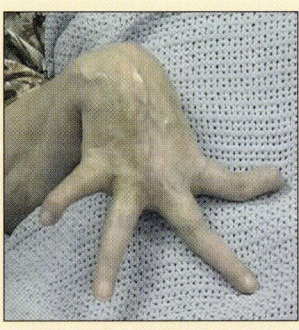

CD 3.5. Clinical signs in corticobasal degeneration.

affected similarly. It is common for the affected limb to eventually assume a position of flexed contracture. Tremor may be seen but is not always present. Postural instability and dysarthria both occur.

Cortical dysfunction

The range of so-called cortical signs in corticobasal degeneration is considerable. I have used the term 'so-called', because some of these signs may in reality arise from abnormal function in one of several anatomical sites.

Alien limb

This refers to a limb (most usually one arm) which seems in a colloquial sense to have developed a will of its own. The limb may interfere with its opposite partner and may even make quasi-purposeful movements directed towards nearby people or objects.

Myoclonus

The myoclonus seen in corticobasal degeneration is usually initially focal. It may appear at 'rest', though this is usually on a background of almost continual muscular contraction (the basis of the underlying rigidity and dystonia). Myoclonus becomes more obvious during voluntary movement and it can also be stimulus sensitive. Electrophysiological measurements of stimulus sensitive myoclonus in corticobasal degeneration suggest enhancement of a direct sensory input to the motor cortex.[35]

Apraxia

The most striking and consistent cortical sign in corticobasal degeneration is apraxia. It is the combination of apraxia, bradykinesia and rigidity in one (usually upper) limb that so often gives the first suggestion of the correct diagnosis. Ideomotor apraxia (difficulty in the performance of pantomime actions) is common and can usually be detected in the clinically least affected hand.[36] Some patients also have apraxia for performing sequential acts (often referred to as ideational apraxia). Buccofacial apraxia is uncommon, but has been described.[37]

Other 'cortical' signs

Some patients have dysgraphaesthesia; others have simultagnosia. With disease progression, mild or moderate pyramidal signs such as hyperreflexia, spasticity and extensor plantar responses are common.

Investigations

Standard laboratory investigations (blood, urine, cerebrospinal fluid [CSF]) are normal. The changes seen on CT and MRI are variable; both are classically normal in early disease, but asymmetrical focal atrophy is seen with progression.

When a tremor is present, electrophysiological studies show a frequency of 6–8 Hz.

Functional imaging studies including both PET and SPECT have shown a mixture of cortical and subcortical defects. Fluorodopa PET studies have shown reduced uptake into the striatum and medial frontal cortex[38] (Fig. 3.12). Blood flow and oxygen/glucose metabolic studies have shown a characteristic pattern of asymmetrical abnormalities including parts of the frontal cortex (medial and posterior), inferior parietal cortex and thalamus[38–41] (Fig. 3.13).[38]

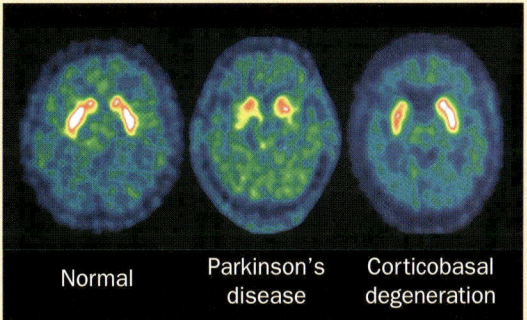

Figure 3.12. Fluorodopa uptake in corticobasal degeneration. Note asymmetrical loss of uptake into caudate and putamen (in Parkinson's disease, loss of caudate signal is less striking).

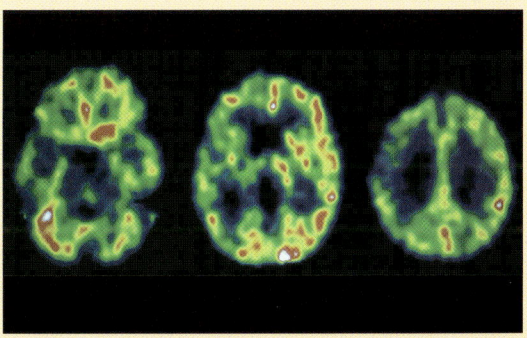

Figure 3.13. Asymmetrical cortical oxygen hypometabolism in corticobasal degeneration.

Pathology and relationship with Pick's disease

The neuropathological features of corticobasal degeneration are a mixture of asymmetric cortical atrophy (Fig. 3.14) with neuronal swelling and achromasia of pyramidal neurons, together with loss of melanin-containing neurons of the substantia nigra pars compacta and neuronal loss with gliosis in a variety of other sites (subcortical, brainstem and cerebellar grey). Lewy bodies are not usually seen. Glial cytoplasmic inclusions (believed initially to be specific for MSA) are occasionally seen in patients who have the otherwise typical pathological features of corticobasal degeneration.

The particular cellular feature of corticobasal degeneration is the swollen pale (achromatic) cells (Fig. 3.15) which have been likened to so-called Pick cells as described in Pick's disease. Many of the ballooned cells in corticobasal degeneration stain with anti-α,β-crystallin. Small inclusion bodies may also be seen in the nigra (Fig. 3.16).

Current clinicopathological understanding of Pick's disease is blurred at the edges, in part because some patients present, not with the usual frontal dementia, but with an anatomically highly restricted 'focal atrophy'. The pathology of Pick's disease accounts, therefore, for a subset of those patients with primary progressive aphasia and similar localized cortical disorders. A so-called 'generalized' variant of Pick's disease has also been described with both cortical and subcortical atrophy. The exact relationship, if any, between these two conditions has yet to be clarified.

Treatment and prognosis

Most patients with corticobasal degeneration show no useful response to levodopa or dopamine agonist treatment. Patients with troublesome myoclonus may benefit from clonazepam and rarely baclofen can provide relief from symptomatic spasticity.

The progression of corticobasal degeneration leads often to contractures, particularly of the hands. Physiotherapy and occupational therapy may be helpful in maintaining posture and movement so far as is possible.

Disease progression is relentless. After slowly losing the battle against apraxia, myoclonus and rigidity in one limb, the patient generally succumbs to the same sequence of functional failure on the other side. Most patients die 5–10 years from symptom onset.

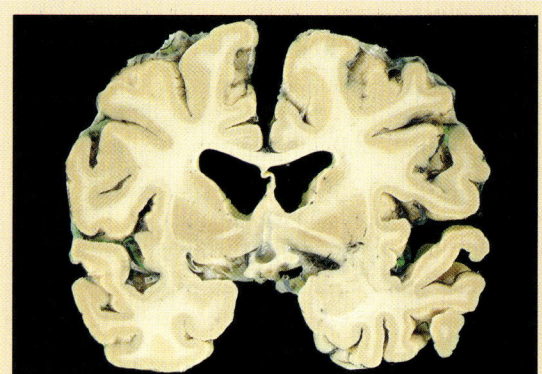

Figure 3.14. Focal cortical atrophy in corticobasal degeneration. (Courtesy of J. Lowe.)

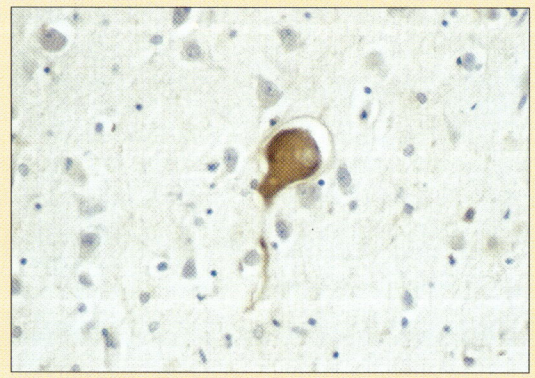

Figure 3.15. Ballooned cells from temporal neocortex in corticobasal degeneration stained with anti-α,β-crystallin. (Courtesy of J. Lowe.)

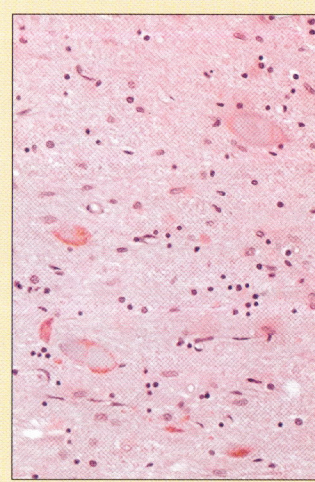

Figure 3.16. Nigral neuronal inclusions in corticobasal degeneration (H&E stain). (Courtesy of J. Lowe.)

Postencephalitic parkinsonism

Previously a common cause of a parkinsonian syndrome, this entity has now all but vanished from diagnostic working memory. Most cases arose after the 'flu' pandemics earlier this century and the patients affected at that time have now almost all died.

History

Between 1916 and 1927 around three-quarters of a million patients worldwide developed encephalitis lethargica (sleeping sickness). Around one-third died acutely. Of the survivors, half were left with chronic neurological problems. Constantin Von Economo is credited with the classical description of the neurological aspects of this disorder.[42] Some patients developed external ophthalmoplegia, oculogyric crises and nystagmus. Others showed bradykinesia, catalepsy and mutism; still others were impulsive, restless, dyskinetic and suffered visual hallucinations. Amongst those who recovered to some extent, parkinsonism was the most disabling symptom complex. Of those who seemingly recovered fully, a proportion went on to develop parkinsonism up to 20 years later (but mostly in the first 5–10 years). Other patients were left with sleep disorders, depression, obsessional ideation and repetitive motor behaviour.

A variety of other kinds of encephalitis with known aetiology have exceptionally been reported as causing parkinsonism. But none of these conditions (such as Western equine encephalitis, coxsackie B, measles, chicken pox, mycoplasma) have led to the clinical pattern seen after sleeping sickness.

More recent data

Unlike patients with Parkinson's disease, those with postencephalitic parkinsonism have been observed to have comparatively fixed deficits. Decades after symptom onset, postmortem examination of the nigra shows almost total pigment loss. Many of the surviving nigral cells contain neurofibrillary tangles. Fluorodopa PET scans in elderly subjects have shown almost no residual fluorodopa uptake.

Occasional patients are still encountered in whom a diagnosis of encephalitis lethargica seems appropriate.[43,44] The diagnosis is suggested in patients with an acute or subacute encephalitic illness, typically including signs of basal ganglia involvement, oculogyric crises, ophthalmoplegia and/or pupillary changes, obsessive-compulsive behaviour, akinetic mutism, central respiratory irregularities and either somnolence or sleep inversion.

No aetiological viral agent has ever been identified, but some patients who fit the above description have oligoclonal bands in their CSF.

Treatment

Many of the older patients with encephalitis lethargica were unable to tolerate very large doses of levodopa because of psychiatric side-effects. Many were said to respond better to anticholinergic agents. Unlike Parkinson's disease, some patients derived undiminished benefit from the same modest dose of levodopa taken without increase over a period of decades.

Arteriosclerotic parkinsonism

Writing in 1895, Brissaud included arteriosclerosis in his list of causes of Parkinson's disease.[45] Some while later in 1929 'arteriosclerotic parkinsonism' was described by Critchley[46] and it was gradually accepted that classical parkinsonism may be caused by cerebrovascular disease.

Over the years, neurologists have become more sceptical about whether a patient who fulfils the clinical diagnostic criteria for Parkinson's disease can have cerebrovascular disease as the underlying cause. And over the same period it has become very clear that patients with a variety of brain diseases including cerebrovascular disease, hydrocephalus, or frontal parasagittal meningiomas may present with 'lower body parkinsonism' which appears different to clinically defined Parkinson's disease.

'Lower body parkinsonism'

Patients with 'lower body parkinsonism'[47,48] classically have an erect posture with short, wide-based stance and straight legs. Most have a shuffling gait, with reduced arm-swing and start hesitation, freezing and difficulty turning corners. The classical festinant gait of Parkinson's disease is not seen. Only one-third have arm akinesia, though some do show slight loss of finger and upper limb dexterity. Some have facial masking. Tremor is not seen.

Many such patients have a history of hypertension and brain scans most commonly show diffuse symmetrical low attenuation white matter changes, with or without visible lacunar infarcts. Such patients do not usually respond to levodopa. Other features which suggest a vascular cause for symptoms include accompanying upper motor neuron signs, an abrupt onset, a history of transient ischaemic attacks or strokes, and radiological evidence of ventricular dilatation, ischaemic white matter change (Figs. 3.17, 3.18) and/or lacunar infarction.

'True' arteriosclerotic parkinsonism

Yet there are also occasional patients in whom the clinical features do not allow differentiation from Parkinson's disease during life, but who turn out at postmortem to have vascular disease rather than Lewy bodies.[49] Histopathologically, the brains of such patients show fibrohyalinosis of small arteries and arterioles

(Fig. 3.19) with relative sparing of large arteries. They typically have microvascular ischaemic damage affecting the basal ganglia and hemispheric white matter, with a few cases having additional damage to the substantia nigra.

Patients who have the typical clinical features of Parkinson's disease in life and in whom the postmortem pathological findings are of vascular disease alone, are unusual. More commonly, patients have dual pathology. When basal ganglia lacunar damage occurs in patients with Parkinson's disease, it may impair their response to treatment, and hence cloud the clinical picture.

Juvenile parkinsonism

The divide between juvenile parkinsonism, young-onset parkinsonism, and otherwise unspecified Parkinson's disease is arbitrary. By convention the term 'juvenile

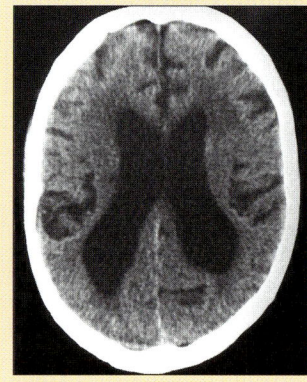

Figure 3.17. CT scan of deep white matter vascular changes in arteriosclerotic parkinsonism. (Courtesy of A. Nisbet.)

Figure 3.18. CT scan of brain to show infarction adjacent to ventricle in arteriosclerotic parkinsonism. (Courtesy of A. Nisbet.)

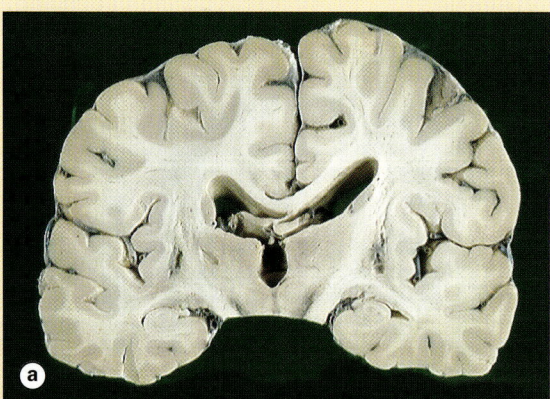

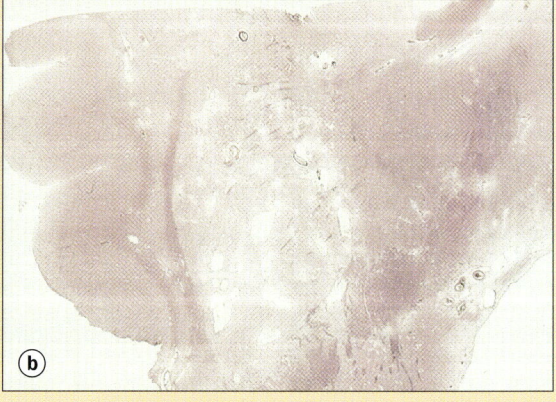

Figure 3.19. Arteriosclerotic parkinsonism. Coronal brain section (a) and stained section through sub-insular region (b) showing extensive lacunar infarction of putamen. (Courtesy of J. Lowe.)

parkinsonism' is used when the symptom onset is up to the age of 20 and many patients in this group have something *other than* idiopathic Parkinson's disease. 'Young onset' parkinsonism relates to symptom onset between 21 and 40, and most of the patients in this group have Parkinson's disease which is indistinguishable from that seen in older patients.

Head trauma

There can be few neurological conditions in which patients do not ask their physicians whether a blow to the head several years earlier might have been a causative factor. Repetitive head trauma may be relevant in parkinsonism, at least in so far as parkinsonism may be a component of the pugilist's encephalopathy. The pathological features of this condition are diffuse cortical atrophy with severe neuronal loss from the locus coeruleus and substantia nigra with numerous neurofibrillary tangles, but no senile plaques, spread throughout the central nervous system.

A temporary (few weeks) worsening of parkinsonian symptomatology has been reported following head trauma from motor vehicle accidents,[50] although it is difficult to disentangle the effects of the associated stress from the head trauma. The most widely held view at the present time is that prior head trauma is not relevant to the pathogenesis of idiopathic Parkinson's disease.

There have been occasional reports of direct trauma to the substantia nigra (e.g. bullet injury) causing parkinsonism. In such cases, the aetiology must surely be quite obvious.

Structural lesions

A broad range of histological tumour types (meningioma, epidermoid, astrocytoma, oligodendroglioma, glioma and others) have been reported to cause parkinsonism when arising in critical sites. Classical examples include sphenoid wing meningiomas and frontal paramedian tumours involving the supplementary motor area. Most of these cases have been reported in the neurosurgical literature; detailed clinical descriptions have not always been provided and

it is difficult to be sure whether these patients would fulfill current clinical diagnostic criteria. In those cases where the supplementary motor area is involved in the pathology, patients are most probably refractory to levodopa therapy; and in patients with idiopathic Parkinson's disease who develop incidental frontal tumours levodopa response may be lost.[51]

Infections

Aside from the vexed issue of whether a viral or other infective agent is responsible for idiopathic Parkinson's disease, parkinsonism has been reported as one of the symptoms in the course of otherwise typical infections due to a variety of organisms. Neurosyphilis can cause parkinsonism, which may be reversible after appropriate antibiotic treatment. Rarely, parkinsonism has been reported in patients with enteric fever (*Salmonella typhi*), with presumed *Mycoplasma pneumoniae*,[52] or brucellosis.

Parkinsonism has also been reported after amphotericin and/or cytosine arabinoside treatment of cryptococcal meningitis or fungal non-CNS infection following bone marrow transplantation.

A wide variety of movement disorders have been described in patients with AIDS complicated by an assortment of coincident infections (including viral encephalitis, tuberculosis and toxoplasmosis), vacuolar myelopathy and Whipples disease.[53] Slowed rapid voluntary alternating hand movements have been described in patients with HIV infection with no other neurological symptoms, and with normal MRI appearances.[54]

Toxins

Several toxic agents are known to cause parkinsonism, including 1-methyl-4-phenyl-1,2,3,6-tetrahydropyridine (MPTP), manganese, cyanide, methanol, and carbon monoxide.

MPTP

The MPTP story is well known. In brief, a chemist in California in the early 1980s was trying to synthesize an illicit opioid analgesic. But something went wrong in the manufacturing process, and in the summer of 1982, several young heroin addicts developed a severe parkinsonian syndrome. More cases were identified, and a chemical analysis of the drugs they were injecting showed that it contained MPTP. Giving the same drug to monkeys turned out to cause a similar motor disturbance. Ultimately around 400 subjects were identified who had probably been exposed to MPTP in the early 1980s. Most did not develop acute parkinsonism, presumably because of difference in total dosage and dosage schedule as well as other factors.

In those patients who developed parkinsonism, the initial clinical picture was indistinguishable from that seen in patients with advanced idiopathic Parkinson's disease. The pathology of MPTP parkinsonism is distinct, however, since the pathology is limited to the substantia nigra and definite Lewy bodies have not been reported. One interesting point which these patients therefore demonstrate is that the nigral lesion *alone* may well be sufficient to cause all of the cardinal motor features of Parkinson's disease. Dementia has not occurred to any major extent in MPTP-exposed subjects, though depression has.

Manganese

Manganese poisoning causes degeneration in the globus pallidus and striatum, and to a lesser extent in the substantia nigra. In patients with mild parkinsonism due to manganese intoxication, fluorodopa PET scans show normal uptake in the striatum, implying a normal nigrostriatal projection.[55] Patients in the early stages of intoxication show mood change with emotional lability, compulsive laughter, hallucinations and neuropsychological impairment. Speech disorder, gait disturbance, slowness and clumsy movement with postural imbalance follow, and then dystonia, chorea and tremor. Exposure to manganese has been reported in miners and ore-crushers, those involved in smelting, alloy manufacturing and steel workers.[56] Welders may be affected and there have been occasional reports of exposure through water contamination.

Other toxins

Survivors of cyanide poisoning (of whom there are few) may develop a severe parkinsonian syndrome[57] but usually also suffer major intellectual decline. Bilateral pallidal lesions may be seen on imaging[57] (Fig. 3.20) and at postmortem.[58]

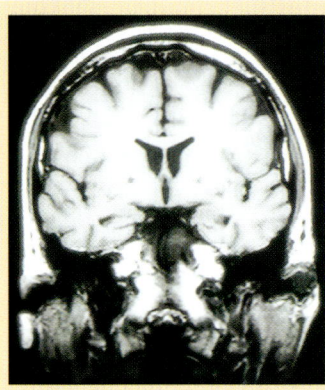

Figure 3.20. MRI scan. Bilateral pallidal lesions following carbon monoxide poisoning.

Methanol poisoning causes multisystem derangements related to metabolic acidosis. Visual loss is common; as are headache, dizziness, confusion and seizures. Bilateral putaminal lesions are typical. Survivors may be blind, parkinsonian,[59] dystonic and demented. Peripheral neuropathy, pseudobulbar palsy and a pyramidal syndrome have all been described.

Inhalation of less than 1% carbon monoxide can cause headache, dizziness, tachycardia, tachypnoea and coma. Death follows within minutes unless exposure is terminated. Survivors subsequently show disorientation, lethargy, hypertonia, and sometimes bradykinesia. Some patients are left with permanent symptoms including dementia, psychosis, chorea, Tourette syndrome, obsessive behaviour, generalized dystonia, mutism, inertia, hemiplegia, cortical blindness, apraxia and agnosia, peripheral neuropathy, incontinence and parkinsonian symptoms. A pure parkinsonian syndrome can occur.[60] Some patients recover quite well from their initial problems, only to deteriorate abruptly 1–4 weeks later with a similar range of neuropsychiatric symptoms.[61]

Parkinsonian dementia on Guam

Guam is the largest of the Mariana islands, which lie in the western Pacific ocean south-east of Japan and north-east of the Philippines (Fig. 3.21). Guam is about 15 km long and up to 14 km wide. The island is volcanic and vegetation is tropical with dense cycad forests growing in limestone areas. The indigenous Chamorro people are of special neurological interest because many have developed either amyotrophic lateral sclerosis (ALS) or a parkinsonism–dementia complex, or both together. These disorders formerly accounted for up to 7% of deaths on the island, though the incidence of both has been reducing over the last several decades. For those affected, it is believed that the critical age of exposure to an unknown environmental factor was during childhood.[62] The parkinsonism–dementia complex comprises a movement disorder very similar to Parkinson's disease but usually with little, if any, tremor. All have dementia and many also have signs of ALS. The same condition has also been reported in the nearby Kii peninsula (of Japan) and western New Guinea.

The pathological features are of cerebral atrophy with neuronal loss in the cortex, basal ganglia, brainstem (including substantia nigra and locus coeruleus) and cerebellum. Neurofibrillary tangles and rare Lewy bodies are seen but not senile plaques. Hirano bodies (bright eosinophilic intracytoplasmic inclusions with a characteristic crystalloid fine structure) may be seen although they are not specific for this condition, occurring also in patients with Alzheimer's disease, Pick's disease and 'normal' elderly individuals.

Candidate explanations for the malady are the ingestion of toxic material derived from cycads, and chronic nutritional manganese and calcium deficiency.

Calcification of the basal ganglia

Favourite questions for the neurological trainee include lists of causes of either basal ganglia calcification, or basal ganglia holes. The latter term is becoming more complex with the variable meaning of the word holes in the context of MRI. When it comes to calcification, the basic list is well established (Table 3.1). In some cases basal ganglia calcification is an incidental finding on a CT or MRI scan performed for some quite separate reason (as much as 1% of otherwise normal scans; possibly a higher percentage of scans in patients with otherwise typical Parkinson's disease). But there are other occasions where calcification has diagnostic significance. Of those patients in whom CT shows calcification, in very few cases can

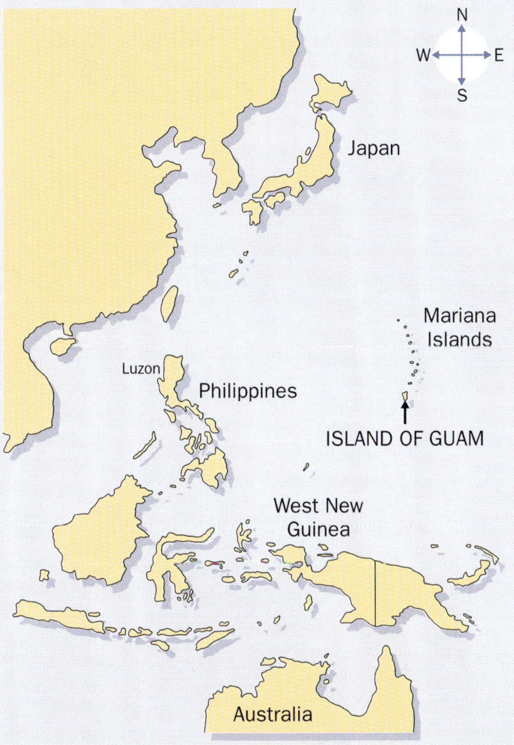

Figure 3.21. The island of Guam.

● **Table 3.1.** Recognized causes of basal ganglia calcification	
Physiological	(Idiopathic)
Familial disorders	Bilateral striopallidodentate calcinosis (Fahr's disease)
	Tuberous sclerosis
	Cockayne's syndrome
	Familial encephalopathies
Metabolic	Hypoparathyroidism
	Anoxia
Mitochondrial disease	
Infection	AIDS
	Cysticercosis
	Toxoplasma
Postinfection	
Toxins/drugs	Lead
	Carbon monoxide
	Methotrexate
	Radiation
Others	Down's syndrome

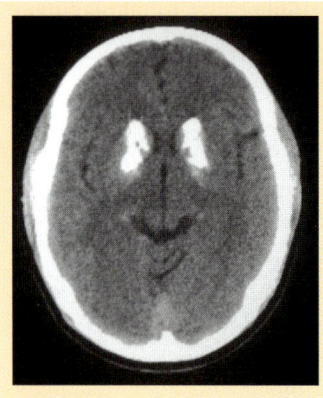

Figure 3.22. CT scan. Basal ganglia calcification.

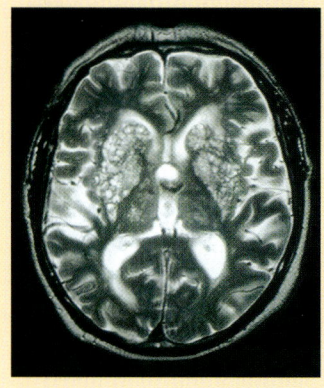

Figure 3.23. MRI scan. Basal ganglia calcification.

the changes been seen on plain X-rays. Cerebral infections, carbon monoxide poisoning and cerebral trauma are all causes of basal ganglia calcification which are dealt with elsewhere (Figs. 3.22, 3.23).

Fahr's syndrome (bilateral striopallidodentate calcinosis)

This is a familial disorder characterized by symmetrical striopallidodentate calcinosis. Histologically, the calcium is deposited in small cerebral vessels and in addition to the sites included in the title, there may be excess deposition in the thalamus, cerebral cortex, cerebral and cerebellar white matter (Fig. 3.24).[63] Symptom onset is typically in the fourth to sixth decade and patients may develop a movement disorder with parkinsonism or sometimes dystonia, chorea, or ataxia. Some develop epilepsy and both pyramidal signs and mental deterioration can occur. Biochemical indices including serum calcium, phosphorus and parathyroid hormone levels are normal. PET fluorodopa studies have shown no change in striatal tracer uptake, indicating that the nigrostriatal projection is intact. Increased CSF homocarnosine (a CNS specific peptide) has been reported in some patients.

Metabolic disorders

Patients with primary hyperparathyroid disease may have symmetric calcification of the basal ganglia. Likewise such calcification may be present in patients with pseudohypoparathyroidism in whom parkinsonism may remit with correction of the serum calcium level. Basal ganglia calcification and reversible parkinsonism has also been reported in a patient with iatrogenic post-thyroidectomy hypoparathyroidism as long

as 26 years after surgery. Rarely, to complicate matters still further, patients may have pseudohypoparathyroidism and parkinsonism in early adult life *without* basal ganglia calcification. Rarely, patients with hypoparathyroidism and parkinsonism may respond to levodopa, although the possibility that such patients have coincident hypoparathyroidism and idiopathic Parkinson's disease cannot be discounted.[64]

In one family with autosomal dominant striopallidodentate calcification and late onset (age 20–57) parkinsonism with or without choreoathetoid movement, affected members were shown to have an inborn error of vitamin D metabolism.[65]

Pure akinesia

It is not clear whether pure akinesia is really a separate pathological entity. The term refers to patients in whom

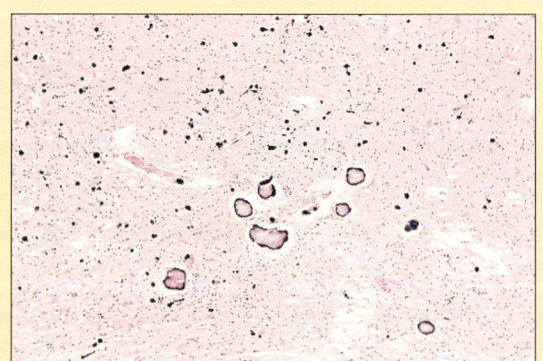

Figure 3.24. Brain calcification. Note the purple staining mineralization in basal ganglia, both in vessels and within the parenchyma. (Courtesy of J. Lowe.)

akinesia is manifest by freezing of gait, micrographia and festinating speech, but without any evidence of rigidity or tremor and without response to levodopa. The condition has been described more frequently in Japan than elsewhere. Some patients who have 'pure akinesia' in life turn out to have the pathological changes of progressive supranuclear palsy at postmortem.[66] Likewise, MRI appearances (atrophy of the pretectum and dorsal pons), PET fluorodopa and deoxyglucose scans show similar appearances in patients carrying these two diagnostic labels in life.[67]

Hemiparkinsonism–hemiatrophy syndrome

Mild physiological asymmetry of both brain and body is the norm, whereas gross asymmetry is usually taken as a sign of abnormal development. Occasionally, patients without any obvious prior history of brain insult present with body hemiatrophy. Attention was first drawn to the fact that some such patients also develop hemiparkinsonism in 1981.[68] This is a heterogeneous condition and some patients also have hemidystonia.[69]

Marked brain asymmetry may be seen on MRI and may include the substantia nigra.[69] Although few such patients have been PET scanned, most (but not all) fluorodeoxyglucose scans have shown marked asymmetry of glucose metabolism. Striatal fluorodopa uptake has been reduced,[69] confirming the presence of a nigral lesion, but there has been no asymmetry of striatal dopamine D2 receptors.[70]

With the passage of time, the parkinsonism may become bilateral, although the disease usually runs a fairly benign course. Most, but not all, patients respond to levodopa.[71] Many show signs of dystonia prior to levodopa therapy. They do not generally develop complications from long-term levodopa.

Despite the absence of obvious brain injury, it is assumed that this heterogeneous group of patients have indeed suffered some kind of brain insult in early life.

Pallidal degenerations

This refers to a collection of conditions in which atrophy of the globus pallidus is a striking feature.

Hunt, writing in 1917, described four patients with juvenile parkinsonism, one of whom developed rigidity and tremor at the age of 15 and who died at age 38 after an accrual of disability including generalized bradykinesia, tremor, rigidity, and flexion dystonia of the limbs.[72] He was noted to have facial masking, but preserved intellect. The pathology in this single autopsied case showed neuronal loss and gliosis in the globus pallidus, caudate, putamen, and nucleus basalis of Meynert. One of Hunt's other cases later died and her autopsy findings were described by Davison in 1954.[73] She showed similar changes, but also some neuronal loss in the substantia nigra and the pyramidal tracts; so the condition was referred to as 'pallido-pyramidal degeneration'.

With the passage of time, a number of further disorders have been described. Some are clearly inherited disorders, whilst others are sporadic. Multiple anatomical structures are commonly affected, whilst broadly speaking the most affected regions are the globus pallidus and/or subthalamic nucleus and their efferent fibre systems. Various efforts to coax these conditions into a diagnostic classification have been made, including a division into 'pure pallidal degeneration', 'pure pallidoluysian atrophy', 'extended pallidal degeneration', 'pallidonigral degeneration', 'pallidoluysionigral degeneration', and various combinations of the above.[74] Recently described cases have been classified variously as 'rapidly progressive autosomal dominant parkinsonism and dementia with pallidopontonigral degeneration',[75] and 'pallidonigroluysian degeneration with iron deposition'.[76] Linkage to chromosome 17 has been shown in a number of families with frontotemporal dementia associated with parkinsonism. Some have tau-rich inclusions in neurons and glia (Fig. 3.25).

Is there a 'typical presentation' for such a wide range of individually very rare disorders? In truth, these conditions are so rare that except in families with a known histological diagnosis, classification in life must remain imperfect. One suggested omnibus description is 'the combination of progressive rigidity and postural anomalies associated with choreoathetosis and torsion dystonia or rhythmical tremor with or without pyramidal signs and mental deterioration with onset at the end of the first or beginning of the second decade, or later, and gradually

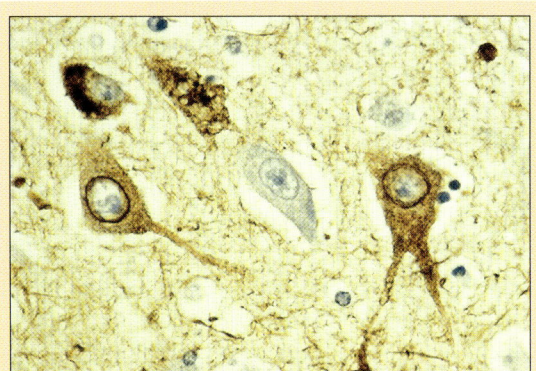

Figure 3.25. Chromosome 17 neurodegeneration. Tau staining in hippocampus. (Courtesy of J. Lowe.)

resulting in semiflexed contractures of the limbs'.[74] In a recent case of adult onset pure pallidal degeneration the symptoms were of 'extreme slowness in motion without rigidity, which was distinct from the akinesia of parkinsonism; later the patient developed dystonia in the neck and fingers with mild "rigidospasticity"'.[77]

In several patients where nigral involvement has been suspected *in vivo*, levodopa has been of some therapeutic benefit.

In a small number of cases where nigral involvement has been suspected in life, and/or later confirmed at autopsy, fluorodopa PET has confirmed a nigral defect.[75,78]

Miscellanea

Golby and colleagues reported a single patient with paraneoplastic degeneration of the substantia nigra leading to refractory parkinsonism.[79]

References

1. Bull P C, Thomas G R, Rommens J M et al. The Wilson disease gene is a putative copper transporting P-type ATPase similar to the Menkes gene. Nature Genet 1993; 5: 327–337

2. Yamaguchi Y, Heiny M E, Gitlin J D. Isolation and characterization of a human liver cDNA as a candidate gene for Wilson disease. Biochem Biophys Res Comm 1993; 197: 271–277

3. Demirkiran M, Jankovic J, Lewis R A, Cox D W. Neurologic presentation of Wilson disease without Kayser–Fleischer rings. Neurology 1996; 46: 1040–1043

4. Magalhaes A C A, Caramelli P, Menezes J R et al. Wilson's disease: MRI with clinical correlation. Neuroradiology 1994; 36: 97–100

5. Walshe J M, Yealland M. Chelation treatment of neurological Wilson's disease. Q J Med 1993; 86: 197–204

6. Brewer G J, Terry C A, Aisen A M, Hill G M. Worsening of neurologic syndrome in patients with Wilson's disease with initial penicillamine therapy. Arch Neurol 1987; 44: 490–493

7. Brewer G J, Turkay A, YuzbasiyanGurkan V. Development of neurologic symptoms in a patient with asymptomatic Wilson's disease treated with penicillamine. Arch Neurol 1994; 51: 304–305

8. Chan C-Y, Baker A L. Penicillamine hypersensitivity: Successful desensitization of a patient with severe hepatic Wilson's disease. Am J Gastroenterol 1994; 89: 442–443

9. Walshe J M. Treatment of Wilson's disease with trientine (triethylene tetramine) dihydrochloride. Lancet 1982; 1: 643–647

10. Brewer G J, Johnson V, Dick R D et al. Treatment of Wilson disease with ammonium tetrathiomolybdate: II. Initial therapy in 33 neurologically affected patients and follow-up with zinc therapy. Arch Neurol 1996; 53: 1017–1025

11. Quinn N. Multiple system atrophy — the nature of the beast. J Neurol Neurosurg Psychiat 1989; 52: 78–89

12. Graham J C, Oppenheimer D R. Orthostatic hypotension in a case of multiple system atrophy. J Neurol Neurosurg Psychiat 1969; 32: 28–34

13. Shy G M, Drager G A. A neurological syndrome associated with orthostatic hypotension. Arch Neurol 1960; 2: 511–527

14. Adams R, Van Bogaert L, Van Der Ecken H. Striatonigral degeneration. J Neuropathol Exp Neurol 1964; 23: 219–259

15. Dejerine J, Thomas A A. L'atrophie olivo-ponto-cérébelleusse. Nouv Iconogr Salpêtrière 1990; 13: 330–370

16. Papp M I, Lantos P L. The distribution of oligodendroglial inclusions in multiple system atrophy and its relevance to clinical symptomatology. Brain 1994; 117: 235–243

17. Daniel S E, Geddes J F, Revesz T. Glial cytoplasmic inclusions are not exclusive to multiple system atrophy. J Neurol Neurosurg Psychiat 1995; 58: 262

18. Gilman S, Sima A A F, Junck L et al. Spinocerebellar ataxia type 1 with multiple system degeneration and glial cytoplasmic inclusions. Ann Neurol 1996; 39: 241–255

19. Quinn N P, Marsden C D. The motor disorder of multiple system atrophy. J Neurol Neurosurg Psychiat 1993; 56: 1239–1242

20. Kew J, Gross M, Chapman P. Shy–Drager syndrome presenting as isolated paralysis of vocal cord abductors. Br Med J 1990; 300: 1441

21. Drayer B P, Olanow W, Burger P et al. Parkinson plus syndrome: Diagnosis using high field MR imaging of brain iron. Radiology 1986; 159: 493–498

22. Brooks D J, Ibañez V, Sawle G V et al. Differing patterns of striatal ^{18}F-dopa uptake in Parkinson's disease, multiple system atrophy and progressive supranuclear palsy. Ann Neurol 1990; 28: 547–555

23. Burn D J, Sawle G V, Brooks D J. Differential diagnosis of Parkinson's disease, multiple system atrophy, and Steele–Richardson–Olszewski syndrome: Discriminant function analysis of striatal ^{18}F-dopa PET data. J Neurol Neurosurg Psychiat 1994; 57: 278–284

24. Sawle G V, Playford E D, Brooks D J et al. Asymmetrical presynaptic and postsynaptic changes in the striatal dopamine projection in dopa-naïve parkinsonism: Diagnostic implications of the D2 receptor status. Brain 1993; 116: 853–867

25. Burn D J, Rinne J O, Quinn N P et al. Striatal opioid receptor binding in Parkinson's disease, striatonigral degeneration and Steele–Richardson–Olszewski syndrome — A [^{11}C]diprenorphine PET study. Brain 1995; 118: 951–958

26. Schulz J B, Klockgether T, Petersen D et al. Multiple system atrophy: Natural history, MRI morphology, and dopamine receptor imaging with ^{123}I-IBZM-SPECT. J Neurol Neurosurg Psychiat 1994; 57: 1047–1056

27. van Royen E, Verhoeff N F L G, Speelman J D et al. Multiple system atrophy and progressive supranuclear palsy. Diminished striatal D_2 receptor activity demonstrated by ^{123}I-IBZM single photon emission computed tomography. Arch Neurol 1993; 50: 513–516

28. Eardley I, Quinn N P, Fowler C J et al. The role of urethral sphincter electromyography in the differential diagnosis of parkinsonism. J Neurol Neurosurg Psychiat 1990; 53: 177

29. Beck R, Fowler C J, Mathias C J. Genitourinary dysfunction in disorders of the autonomic nervous system. In: Rushton D N (ed) Handbook of neuro-urology. New York: Marcel Dekker, Inc., 1994: 281–301

30. Steele J C, Richardson J C, Olszewski J. Progressive supranuclear palsy. Arch Neurol 1964; 10: 333–359

31. Dubas F, Gray F Escourolle R. Maladie de Steele–Richardson–Olszewski sans ophthalmoplegie. Rev Neurol 1983; 139: 407–416

32. Wenning G K, Ben-Shlomo Y, Magalhães M et al. Clinicopathological study of 35 cases of multiple system atrophy. J Neurol Neurosurg Psychiat 1995; 58: 160–166

33. Litvan I, Campbell G, Mangone C A et al. Which clinical features differentiate progressive supranuclear palsy (Steele–Richardson–Olszewski syndrome) from related disorders? A clinicopathological study. Brain 1997; 120: 65–74

34. Rinne J O, Lee M S, Thompson P D, Marsden C D. Corticobasal degeneration. A clinical study of 36 cases. Brain 1994; 117: 1183–1196

35. Thompson P D, Day B L, Rothwell J C et al. The myoclonus in corticobasal degeneration: Evidence for two forms of cortical reflex myoclonus. Brain 1994; 117: 1197–1207

36. Leiguarda R, Lees A J, Merello M et al. The nature of apraxia in corticobasal degeneration. J Neurol Neurosurg Psychiat 1994; 57: 455–459

37. Lang A E. Cortical basal ganglionic degeneration presenting with 'progressive loss of speech output and orofacial dyspraxia'. J Neurol Neurosurg Psychiat 1992; 55: 1101

38. Sawle G V, Brooks D J, Marsden C D, Frackowiak R S J. Corticobasal degeneration: A unique pattern of regional cortical oxygen metabolism and striatal fluorodopa uptake demonstrated by positron emission tomography. Brain 1991; 114: 541–556

39. Eidelberg D, Dhawan V, Moeller J R et al. The metabolic landscape of cortico-basal ganglionic degeneration: Regional asymmetries studied with positron emission tomography. J Neurol Neurosurg Psychiat 1991; 54: 856–862

40. Blin J, Vidailhet M-J, Pillon B et al. Corticobasal degeneration: Decreased and asymmetrical glucose consumption as studied with PET. Mov Dis 1992; 7: 348–354

41. Markus H S, Lees A J, Lennox G et al. Patterns of regional cerebral blood flow in corticobasal degeneration studied using HMPAO SPECT; comparison with Parkinson's disease and normal controls. Mov Dis 1995; 10: 179–187

42. von Economo C. Encephalitis lethargica. Its sequelae and treatment (Translated by K D Newman). London: Oxford University Press, 1931.

43. Rail D, Scholtz C, Swash M. Post-encephalitic Parkinsonism: Current experience. J Neurol Neurosurg Psychiat 1981; 44: 670–676

44. Howard R S, Lees A J. Encephalitis lethargica. Brain 1987; 110: 19–33

45. Brissaud E. Vingt-deuxieme le Aon: Pathogenie et symptomes de la maladie de Parkinson. In: Meige H (ed) Le Aons sur les maladies nerveuses (Salpetriere 1893–1894). Paris: G Masson, 1895: 469–487

46. Critchley M. Arteriosclerotic parkinsonism. Brain 1929; 52: 23–83

47. Thompson P D, Marsden C D. Gait disorder of subcortical arteriosclerotic encephalopathy. Binswanger's disease. Mov Dis 1987; 2: 1–8

48. Fitzgerald P M, Jankovic J. Lower body parkinsonism: Evidence for a vascular etiology. Mov Dis 1989; 4: 249–260

49. Hughes A J, Daniel S E, Kilford L, Lees A J. Accuracy of clinical diagnosis of idiopathic Parkinson's disease: A clinico-pathological study of 100 cases. J Neurol Neurosurg Psychiat 1992; 55: 181–184

50. Goetz C G, Stebbings G T. Effects of head trauma from motor vehicle accidents on Parkinson's disease. Ann Neurol 1991; 29: 191–193

51. Fabbrini G, Baronti F, Ruggieri S, Lenzi G L. Meningioma-induced loss of antiparkinsonian response to levodopa. Mov Dis 1995; 10: 231–232

52. Kim J S, Choi I L S, Lee M C. Reversible parkinsonism and dystonia following probable Mycoplasma pneumoniae infection. Mov Dis 1995; 10: 510–512

53. Nath A, Jankovic J, Pettigrew L C. Movement disorders and AIDS. Neurology 1987; 37: 37–41

54. Arendt G, Hefter H, Elsing C et al. Motor dysfunction in HIV-infected patients without clinically detectable central-nervous deficit. J Neurol 1990; 237: 362–368

55. Wolters E Ch, Huang C, Clark C et al. Positron emission tomography in manganese intoxication. Ann Neurol 1989; 26: 647–651

56. Huang C C, Chu N S, Lu C S et al. Chronic manganese intoxication. Arch Neurol 1989; 46: 1104–1106

57. Rosenberg N L, Myers J A, Martin W R. Cyanide-induced parkinsonism: Clinical, MRI, and 6-fluorodopa PET studies. Neurology 1989; 39: 142–144

58. Uitti R J, Rajput A H, Ashenhurst E M, Rozdilsky B. Cyanide-induced parkinsonism: A clinicopathologic report. Neurology 1985; 35: 921–925

59. Oliveras Ley C, Gali F G. Parkinsonian syndrome after methanol intoxication. Eur Neurol 1983; 22: 405–409

60. Klawans H L, Stein R W, Tanner C M, Goetz C G. A pure Parkinsonian syndrome following acute carbon monoxide intoxication. Arch Neurol 1982; 39: 302–304

61. Lee M S, Marsden C D. Neurological sequelae following carbon monoxide poisoning: clinical course and outcome according to the clinical types and brain computed tomography scan findings. Mov Dis 1994; 9: 550–558

62. Zhang Z-X, Anderson D W, Lavine L, Mantel M. Patterns of acquiring parkinsonism–dementia complex on Guam 1944 through 1985. Arch Neurol 1990; 47: 1019–1024

63. Manyam B V, Bhatt M H, Moore W D et al. Bilateral striopallidodentate calcinosis: Cerebrospinal fluid, imaging and electrophysiological studies. Ann Neurol 1992; 31: 379–384

64. Vaamonde J, Legarda I, Jimenez-Jimenez J et al. Levodopa-responsive parkinsonism associated with basal ganglia calcification and primary hypoparathyroidism. Mov Dis 1993; 8: 398–400

65. Martinelli P, Giuliani S, Ippoliti M et al. Familial idiopathic strio-pallido-dentate calcifications with late onset extrapyramidal syndrome. Mov Dis 1993; 8: 220–222

66. Honma Y, Takahashi H, Takeda S, Ikuta F. An autopsy case of progressive supranuclear palsy showing 'pure akinesia without rigidity and tremor and with no effect by L-Dopa therapy'. Brain Nerve 1987; 39: 183–187

67. Taniwaki T, Hosokawa S, Goto I et al. Positron emission tomography (PET) in 'pure akinesia'. J Neurol Sci 1992; 107: 34–39

68. Klawans H L. Hemiparkinsonism as a late complication of hemiatrophy: A new syndrome. Neurology 1981; 31: 625–628

69. Lang A E. Hemiatrophy, juvenile-onset exertional alternating leg paresis, hypotonia, and hemidystonia and adult-onset hemiparkinsonism: The spectrum of hemiparkinsonism–hemiatrophy syndrome. Mov Dis 1995; 10: 489–495

70. Przedborski S, Goldman S, Levivier M et al. Brain glucose metabolism and dopamine D2 receptor analysis in a patient with hemiparkinsonism–hemiatrophy syndrome. Mov Dis 1993; 8: 391–395

71. Giladi N, Burke R E, Kostic V, et al. Hemiparkinsonism–hemiatrophy syndrome: Clinical and neuroradiologic features. Neurology 1990; 40: 1731–1734

72. Hunt J R. Progressive atrophy of the globus pallidus (primary atrophy of the pallidal system). A system disease of the paralysis agitans type, characterised by atrophy of the motor cells of the corpus striatum. Brain 1917; 40: 58–148

73. Davison C H. Pallido-pyramidal disease. J Neuropathol Exp Neurol 1954; 13: 50–59

74. Jellinger K. Pallidal, pallidonigral and pallidoluysionigral degenerations including association with thalamic and dentate degenerations. In: Vinken P J, Bruyn G W, Klawans I I L (eds) Handbook of clinical neurology, Vol 5 (49): Extrapyramidal disorders. Amsterdam: Elsevier Science, 1986: 445–463

75. Wszolek Z K, Pfeiffer R F, Bhatt M H et al. Rapidly progressive autosomal dominant parkinsonism and dementia with pallido-ponto-nigral degeneration. Ann Neurol 1992; 32: 312–320

76. Kawai J, Sasahara M, Hazama F et al. Pallidonigroluysian degeneration with iron deposition: A study of three autopsy cases. Acta Neuropathol 1993; 86: 609–616

77. Aizawa H, Kwak S, Shimuzu T et al. A case of adult onset pure pallidal degeneration. I Clinical manifestations and neuropathological observations. J Neurol Sci 1991; 102: 76–82

78. Remy P, Hosseini H, Degos J-D et al. Striatal dopaminergic denervation in pallidopyramidal disease demonsrated by positron emission tomography. Ann Neurol 1995; 38: 954–956

79. Golbe L I, Miller D C, Duvoisin R C. Paraneoplastic degeneration of the substantia nigra with dystonia and parkinsonism. Mov Dis 1989; 4: 147–152

chapter 4

Surgery for Parkinson's disease

Robert Hauser and Thomas Freeman

Introduction

Surgical therapies for Parkinson's disease fall into three broad categories: destructive lesioning, chronic stimulation and reconstruction. Destructive therapies improve symptoms by disrupting abnormal pathways, chronic stimulation therapies mimic lesioning but are potentially reversible, and reconstructive therapies seek to replace missing neurons. Modern destructive therapies include thalamotomy and pallidotomy. Sites subject to chronic stimulation include the nucleus ventralis intermedius (VIM), the pallidum, and the subthalamic nucleus (STN). Reconstructive strategies include implantation of biologically active cells such as fetal tissue, cell lines, encapsulated cells, progenitor cells, trophic factors or trophic factor producing cells, and somatically or surgically delivered gene therapy.

History

Many of the early surgical procedures for Parkinson's disease targeted the corticospinal tract. Bucy[1] undertook extirpation of Brodmann's cortical area 4, Putnam performed cervical pyramidotomy[2] and Walker sectioned the lateral two-thirds of the cerebral peduncle using a subtemporal approach.[3] These procedures provided tremor relief only at the expense of weakness, and tremor usually recurred as weakness resolved over time. Other features of Parkinson's disease were not improved.[4] Attention was then directed toward lesioning the extrapyramidal motor system in an effort to avoid motor weakness.

Meyers introduced surgery of the basal ganglia for Parkinson's disease in 1942.[5] A transventricular approach was used to lesion the caudate nucleus, anterior limb of the internal capsule, and pallidothalamic fibres. This procedure reduced tremor in more than 60% of patients but was associated with a 12% mortality and therefore not recommended for general use. Fenelon,[6] Fenelon and Theibant,[7] and Guiot and

Brion[8] undertook freehand coagulation of the ansa lenticularis utilizing a variety of surgical approaches. Improvement in tremor and rigidity was reported in up to 72% of patients but mortality rates were still unacceptably high.

In 1952, Cooper[9] attempted a pedunculotomy on a young patient with postencephalitic parkinsonism. He accidentally ruptured and then ligated the anterior choroidal artery (AChA) and abandoned the procedure. Surprisingly, the patient experienced relief of contralateral tremor and rigidity without motor or sensory deficits. This unexpected improvement was attributed to an ischaemic lesion of the medial globus pallidus, the ansa and fasciculus lenticularus, and the ventrolateral nucleus of the thalamus.[10] Cooper went on to perform more than 50 AChA ligations to treat parkinsonism between 1952 and 1955. Tremor and rigidity were improved but mortality remained high at 10%.

The development of a stereotactic apparatus by Spiegel and Wycis[11] allowed more precise targeting of brain regions while reducing intracerebral trauma. A metal ring was fixed to the patient's shaved head using a cap made of plaster of Paris. The plaster cast was later replaced by fixation pins screwed to the head.[12] Pneumoencephalography was used to provide an outline of the ventricular system which served as an internal landmark for target localization. Spiegel and Wycis[13] used this apparatus to perform stereotactic electrolytic lesioning of the ansa and noted reduced tremor and rigidity without paralysis in four of six Parkinson's disease patients. These early stereotactic procedures carried a mortality of approximately 2%.

Over the next several years, surgeons performed pallidotomies and ansotomies.[14–16] The pallidal target was the anterodorsal and medial part of the nucleus. Medial pallidotomy was reported to improve rigidity but benefit for tremor was inconsistent.

Hassler and Richert[17] introduced stereotactic thalamotomy as a treatment for Parkinson's disease in 1954. Cooper performed chemopallidectomy between 1954 and 1958, chemothalamectomy beginning in 1956, and most successfully cryothalamotomy beginning in 1957. Using cryothalamotomy, surgical mortality dropped to 1.3%.[18] After its introduction, thalamotomy became the surgical procedure of choice. Thalamotomy provided tremor relief in approximately 90% of patients whereas pallidotomy relieved tremor in only 60–75% of patients. In addition, Cooper[19] noted recurrence of tremor and rigidity in 25% of patients after pallidotomy compared with only 11% after thalamotomy.

With the introduction of levodopa and other medical therapies for Parkinson's disease, interest in surgical procedures declined dramatically. However, attention has recently refocused on surgical procedures for a number of reasons. The shortcomings of chronic medical therapy have become clear over time. Tremor is variably responsive to medication, signs and symptoms of Parkinson's disease continue to progress despite medical therapy, many patients develop drug associated motor fluctuations and dyskinesia, and features such as postural instability and freezing that are not amenable to medical therapy become more prominent. Technological advances including computed tomography (CT) and magnetic resonance imaging (MRI) localization, intraoperative electrophysiological monitoring and stimulation, and improved instrumentation have combined to improve target localization and reduce morbidity and mortality. Increased understanding of the functional anatomy of the basal ganglia has provided a rationale for the investigation of lesioning anatomic targets. Advances in transplant biology have permitted the evaluation of implantation of dopamine-producing cells to replace degenerating neurons.

Thalamotomy

The target for modern thalamotomy is the VIM, which lies posterior to the ventrolateral nucleus and anterior to the ventroposterior sensory nucleus. Surgery is performed under local anaesthesia with the patient awake to allow physiological and clinical monitoring during the procedure. A stereotactic frame is fixed to the patient's head and a CT or MRI is performed to localize the target area in relationship to a grid coordinate system. In the operating room, a burr hole is drilled and an electrode is advanced into the target region. The final

site for lesioning is determined by either macrostimulation or a combination of microelectrode recording and stimulation. Using macrostimulation, the target is identified as the site at which stimulation at high frequency relieves tremor (and may evoke paraesthesias in the hand, especially the thumb and index finger). Stimulation at the target using low frequency signals drives the tremor. Proper placement of the electrode based on physiological testing is often slightly different from that predicted using imaging alone.[20] Some centres employ microelectrode recording. This may provide more precise target localization but requires a trained neurophysiologist and sophisticated equipment, and lengthens the surgical procedure. Within the thalamus, the VIM nucleus exhibits high background activity,[21] and kinaesthetic, voluntary motor and tremor cells can be identified.[21–31] Whether 'tremor' cells drive the tremor in a pacemaker fashion or are part of a pathological feedback loop that includes abnormal firing of kinaesthetic cells is unclear.[26,27] Microelectrode recording can also be used to establish the medial and lateral boundaries of the ventroposterior sensory nucleus to serve as landmarks for lesioning of the VIM nucleus located immediately anterior. The final site for lesioning is confirmed by stimulation. The site at which the lowest intensity of stimulation suppresses tremor and does not cause a side-effect is lesioned using radiofrequency to heat the electrode tip. During this time the patient is monitored clinically, particularly for the development of weakness or dysarthria. If there is residual tremor without side-effects, the lesion can be modified or expanded.[20,32]

Reported results from thalamotomy vary considerably, presumably due to differences in the surgical procedure, and pre- and postoperative evaluations. Nonetheless, it is clear that thalamotomy can improve contralateral tremor and to a lesser extent rigidity. Other features of Parkinson's disease, including bradykinesia, postural stability and ipsilateral tremor are not improved.[20,33,34] Tremor abolition has been reported in 45.8–92% of patients with improvement in rigidity in 41% to 92%.[33–44] Bilateral thalamotomies are reported to improve tremor in 33–73.6% of patients and rigidity in 22.7–74%.[22,33,37,38,45,46]

Perioperative mortality associated with thalamotomy has varied from 0.4–6% and is usually due to haemorrhage at the lesion site.[33,34,36,37,45,47,48] Mortality currently is expected to be less than 1%.[20–22] The common complications of thalamotomy are related to the fact that the effective site for lesioning is just medial to the motor fibres for the leg in the internal capsule and just rostral to the sensory thalamus. The incidence of contralateral hemiparesis has ranged from 0.5–22.34%.[20,22,35,37,39–41,47] Paraesthesias, usually of the fingers or lips, are a common immediate complication but resolve within 1 year in all but 1–3% of patients.[22,33] Seizures occur in less than 2%.[22,40,45,47] Other uncommon complications include ataxia, apraxia, hypotonia, abulia and gait disturbances.[22]

Bilateral thalamotomies are associated with a higher incidence of speech and swallowing complications, particularly in patients with preoperative dysfunction.[19] Tasker[22] noted worsening of dysarthria in 29% of patients following bilateral thalamotomy. In addition, neuropsychological deficits are common.[46] An interval of 6–12 months between operations is now usually employed to allow resolution of transient symptoms and permit evaluation of residual dysfunction from the initial procedure.[22,45] The use of modern stereotactic techniques and performing the surgeries in staged procedures have reduced but not eliminated these complications.

Jankovic et al.[20] recently reported the results of stereotactic thalamotomy in 42 Parkinson's disease patients (of whom two underwent bilateral surgery) performed between 1982 and 1994. Complete abolition of tremor was reported in 72% and significant improvement in tremor and ability to function in an additional 14%. There was a trend for decreased rigidity, but this change was not statistically significant. Weakness immediately following surgery was noted in 34% and persisted in 15% of patients. Dysarthria occurred in 29% and persisted in 10%.

Fox et al.[32] used modern stereotactic techniques, including microelectrode recording to perform thalamotomy in 36 patients. Persistent abolition of tremor was achieved in 86% and substantial improvement in 5%. Persistent complications occurred in 14% of patients and included arm dyspraxia, dysarthria, dysphasia and abulia. Disability persisted in only two patients (5%).

The long-term effect of thalamotomy was investigated by Diederich et al.[49] who performed blinded evaluations of patients who had undergone thalamotomy a mean of 10.9 years earlier. Resting tremor in the upper extremity contralateral to the surgery was significantly less than on the ipsilateral side. As surgery had been undertaken contralateral to the side with greatest tremor, this reversal of asymmetry was felt to be indicative of long-term tremor suppression.

Thalamotomy may also reduce dyskinesia although the reliability and duration of this effect is unclear. Page[50] evaluated the effect of thalamotomy in 1-methyl-4-phenyl-1,2,3,6-tetrahydropyridine (MPTP)-monkeys made dyskinetic with levodopa. Thalamotomy was carried out in the pallidal innervation territory of the thalamus as determined by anatomic studies. Levodopa-induced chorea was usually abolished and always reduced. Lesions placed elsewhere in the thalamus had no effect on chorea, and dystonia was not relieved. Several investigators have noted partial or complete resolution of medication-induced dyskinesia following surgery in Parkinson's disease patients.[20,32,34,36,39,51–53] In addition, others have noted that patients with a history of prior thalamotomy have not gone on to develop dyskinesia.[34,38,46,51,54] In contrast, Diederich et al. did not detect a side to side difference in dyskinesia ten years after thalamotomy.[49]

Thus, thalamotomy is very effective to relieve contralateral tremor in Parkinson's disease and the effect is often long-lasting. Rigidity may also be reduced. However, disease progression continues as reflected by a gradual worsening of other parkinsonian features.[22] Thalamotomy may reduce contralateral dyskinesia but this has not been systematically evaluated.

Thalamic stimulation

Chronic high-frequency thalamic stimulation has emerged as an alternative to thalamotomy for the treatment of tremor. Chronic thalamic stimulation was first used to treat intractable pain related to somatosensory deafferentation[55–57] and later, various movement disorders.[58,59] Transient high-frequency (>100 Hz) VIM stimulation was used to localize the most effective target for thalamotomy[29,60]. Benabid and co-workers initially developed chronic VIM stimulation for use contralateral to prior thalamotomy to treat bilateral tremor and possibly avoid the complications associated with bilateral thalamotomy.[61] Initial results were encouraging and chronic thalamic stimulation was then assessed as primary therapy.

The first part of the procedure is similar to thalamotomy. The VIM nucleus is targeted using CT or MRI. An electrode is advanced into the target area and the site at which the least electrical stimulation most effectively suppresses tremor is sought. Placing the electrode more on the anterior than posterior border of the VIM may diminish or avoid induction of paraesthesias by spreading current to the primary somatosensory relay, the ventroposterior nucleus.[62] Some centres also employ microelectrode recording to help guide electrode placement. If satisfactory tremor suppression is achieved, a permanent electrode is fixed in position and connected to an external lead. This lead is connected to a stimulator placed in the chest wall. Several days after surgery, parameters for electrical stimulation are optimized using a programmer with an electromagnetic head. Stimulation frequencies of 100–250 Hz are generally employed.[63,64] The lowest intensity of stimulation that will effectively control tremor is used to spare battery power. In some patients, surgical trauma from electrode implantation itself may reduce or eliminate tremor independent of electrical stimulation (microthalamotomy effect). If this occurs, optimization of stimulation parameters is delayed until tremor recurs, often within 1–2 weeks.[63] The intensity of stimulation required to effectively control tremor often increases during the first few months after surgery but then stabilizes.[63,64] When effective, tremor reduction occurs within a few seconds following activation of stimulation and the effect is lost within seconds after the stimulator has been turned off.[64] Patients are able to turn the stimulator on and off using a hand-held magnet (CD 4.1) and many elect to turn the stimulator off at night in order to prolong battery life. Current batteries are expected to last between 3 and 6 years depending on the intensity of stimulation and the number of hours each day the stimulator is switched on.

The mechanism by which chronic electrical stimulation of the VIM nucleus reduces tremor is not known. Stimulation may create a functional ablation of a 'firing centre' or 'tremor loop'. Alternatively, stimulation may desynchronize neuronal firing which has become overactive and autonomous.[64] Suppression of

tremor by thalamic stimulation is associated with decreased regional cerebral blood flow (rCBF) medially and paramedially in the rostral cerebellum, suggesting that thalamic stimulation may disrupt a cerebellothalamocortical oscillatory mechanism.[65]

Benabid et al.[63] initially evaluated chronic thalamic stimulation as primary therapy in 26 patients with Parkinson's disease. Total tremor suppression was reported in 68% and major improvement in an additional 26%. Side-effects included paraesthesias in three, dystonia in two, cerebellar ataxia in two, disequilibrium in two and dysarthria in five. These effects were mild and resolved when stimulation was stopped or reduced. Blond and Siegfried[66] similarly reported total suppression of tremor in 12 of 19 Parkinson's disease patients and partial improvement in the remainder.

More recently, Benabid and co-workers reported results of chronic thalamic stimulation in 80 Parkinson's disease patients followed for up to 8 years.[62] Complete or almost complete control of upper extremity tremor was achieved in 92% at 3 months and 88% at last follow-up. Lower extremity tremor was completely or almost completely controlled in 86% at 3 months and 85% at last follow-up. Resting and postural tremor were better controlled than action tremor. In addition, distal tremor was better controlled than proximal tremor. Side-effects included paraesthesias (9%), dysarthria (19.6%), disequilibrium (9%), and dystonia (5%). Dysarthria was observed in 27.5% of bilaterally stimulated patients compared with 40% of those who underwent thalamotomy on one side and stimulation on the other. Of note, bilateral stimulation

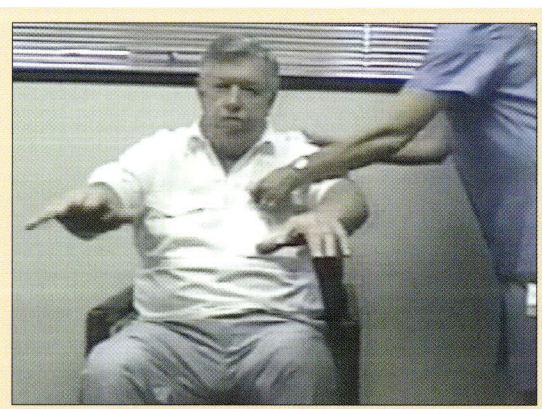

CD 4.1. Parkinsonian patient with a thalamic stimulator.

did not induce neuropsychological deficits usually associated with bilateral thalamotomy. These observations suggest that stimulation may be particularly advantageous when bilateral procedures are contemplated.

Koller *et al.* performed a blinded assessment of tremor reduction following unilateral thalamic stimulation.[67] Twenty-four Parkinson's disease patients were randomized to stimulation 'on' or stimulation 'off' 3 months after surgery. Patients randomized to stimulation 'on' experienced a significant decrease in contralateral tremor ($p<0.5$). Moreover, 71% of patients exhibited moderate or marked tremor reduction and 58% exhibited total resolution of tremor. Benefit was sustained through the 12-month observation period.

Chronic thalamic stimulation has also been reported to improve rigidity,[63] unilateral pain, and dyskinesia,[64] although these benefits have not been studied systematically. Akinesia is unchanged.[63]

Thus, chronic thalamic stimulation is effective in controlling tremor in Parkinson's disease. The principal advantage of stimulation is that it is adjustable. Side-effects due to stimulation can be reduced or eliminated by decreasing the intensity of stimulation. In addition, if tremor begins to re-emerge over time, stimulation can be increased. Long-term benefit can be achieved in most patients. Chronic stimulation may afford fewer persistent side-effects than thalamotomy, particularly when bilateral procedures are indicated.

Functional anatomy

An increased understanding of the functional anatomy of the extrapyramidal system has provided a rationale for lesioning certain anatomic targets in Parkinson's disease. Cortical outflow is modulated by a striatopallidothalamocortical circuit in which the striatum receives input from descending cortical efferents (Fig. 4.1). Striatal output is directed to the medial globus pallidus (GPi) through a direct and an indirect pathway. In Parkinson's disease, loss of striatal dopamine secondary to degeneration of substantia nigra pars compacta (SNc) neurons diminishes inhibition of the GPi by the direct pathway and increases stimulation of the GPi via the indirect pathway. This leads to an increase in GPi inhibition of thalamocortical neurons. This model is consistent with the finding of increased tonic discharges and

metabolic activity in the GPi and subthalamic nucleus (STN) in MPTP-treated monkeys.[68–70] The model suggests that the GPi and the STN (which provides the main excitatory drive to the GPi) are rational targets for lesioning in Parkinson's disease. Overactivity of the GPi and resultant excessive inhibition of the thalamocortical pathway may be returned toward normal by pallidotomy or STN lesioning.

Pallidotomy

Lars Leksell began to perform anterodorsal pallidotomies in 1952.[71] He deliberately varied the target location within the pallidum and a preliminary analysis of 32 patients indicated that the best results came from lesions in the posteromedial part of the pallidum.[16] Analysis of 81 cases performed between 1953 and 1957 including both anterodorsal and posterior lesions of the pallidum revealed lasting remission of tremor in 82%, lasting relief of rigidity in 79% and lasting relief of both tremor and rigidity in 77%. Benefit was largely confined to the contralateral limbs although improvement in gait and mobility were also noted. Twenty-five percent of unemployed patients were able to resume work and of the last 20 patients to undergo posterior pallidotomy, 95% experienced complete relief of rigidity and tremor.

Based on discussions with Leksell, Laitinen performed stereotactic posteroventral pallidotomies from 1985 to 1990 in 38 patients whose main complaint was hypokinesia.[71] The target was identified using macrostimulation. At a mean observation period of 28 months, complete or almost complete relief of rigidity and hypokinesia was reported in 92% of the patients. Eighty-one percent experienced complete or almost complete relief of tremor. Gait, speech, and levodopa-induced dyskinesia were also improved. Six patients experienced permanent partial homonymous hemianopsia, one patient experienced transient dysphagia and facial weakness, and one developed transient hemiparesis.

More recently, microelectrode recording and stimulation have been used to identify the sensorimotor territory of the GPi, the optic tract, and internal capsule in an effort to reduce side-effects and maximize benefit. Lozano *et al.*[72] evaluated 14 patients followed for 6 months. In the 'off' state total motor score improved by

BASAL GANGLIA CIRCUITRY

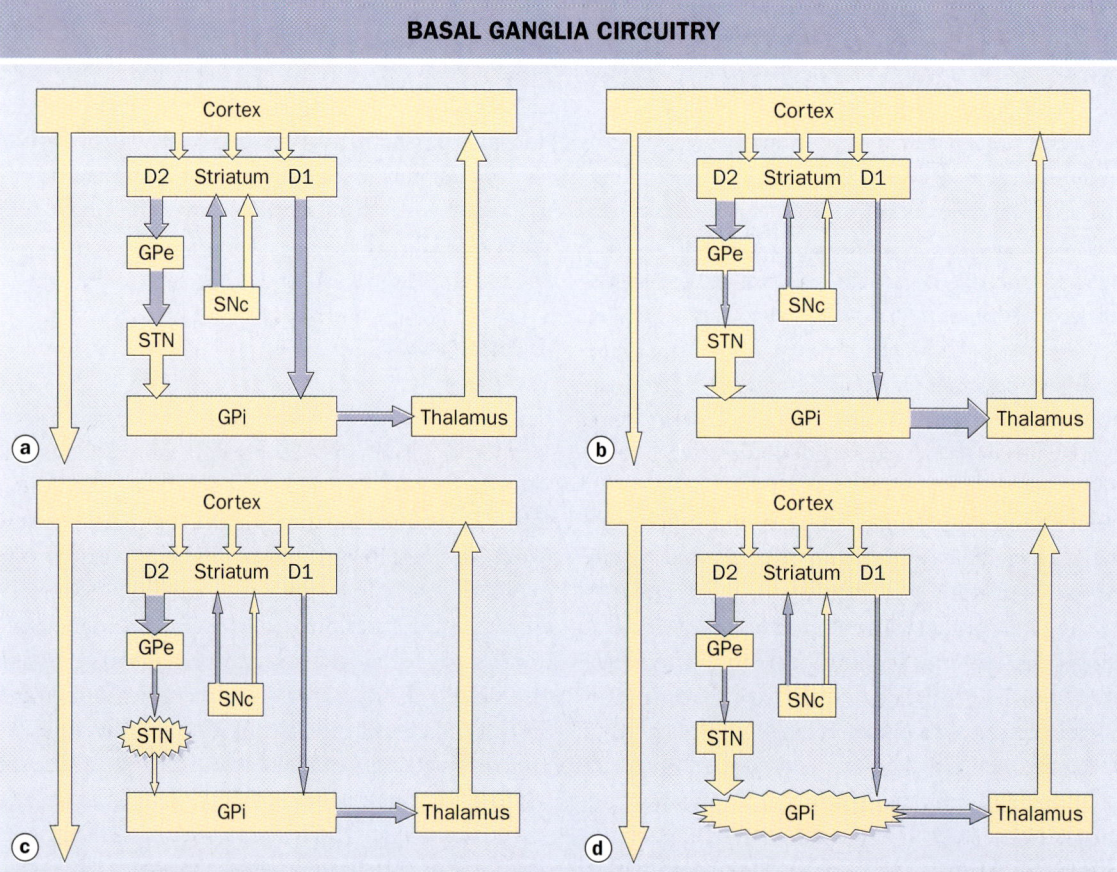

SNc – substantia nigra pars compacta; GPe – globus pallidus externa; STN – subthalamic nucleus; GPi = globus pallidus interna

Figure 4.1. Simplified diagram of basal ganglia circuitry. Orange arrows represent excitatory pathways and purple arrows represent inhibitory pathways. The relative 'strength' of a pathway is denoted by arrow thickness. (a) Cortical outflow is modulated by a striatopallidolthalamocortical circuit in which the striatum receives input from descending cortical efferents. Striatal output is directed to the medial globus pallidus (GPi) through a direct and an indirect pathway. Output from the GPi exerts a chronic inhibitory effect on thalamocortical neurons. Dopamine, derived from substantia nigra pars compacta (SNc) neu-rons, stimulates the direct pathway and inhibits the indirect pathway. (b) In Parkinson's disease loss of striatal dopamine diminishes inhibition of the GPi by the direct pathway and increases stimulation of the GPi via the indirect pathway. Increased GPi output causes excessive inhibition of thalamocortical neurons and diminishes cortical outflow. (c) A lesion of the subthalamic nucleus (STN) reduces excessive stimulation of the GPi and decreases inhibition of thalamocortical neurons. (d) A lesion of the GPi reduces excessive inhibition of thalamocortical neurons, thereby restoring cortical outflow toward normal.

30% ($p<0.005$) and total akinesia score by 22% ($p<0.01$). 'Off' state contralateral tremor and rigidity were significantly reduced. Dyskinesia was reduced by 92% on the contralateral side and 32% on the ipsilateral side. Dogali et al.[73] identified benefit in 18 patients followed for 1 year. Unified Parkinson's Disease Rating Scale (UPDRS) motor scores while 'off' improved by 65% ($p<0.0001$) and timed tests of motor function improved 38.2% in the contralateral limb and 24.2% in the ipsilateral limb (both $p<0.0001$). Contralateral dyskinesia was reported to be resolved.

Baron et al.[74] reported results of posterior GPi pallidotomy in 15 patients with advanced Parkinson's disease. Significant improvement was observed in Activities of Daily Living (ADL) and motor scores during the 'off' state 1 year following surgery. ADL 'off' scores were improved at 3 months (34.1%, $p=0.008$) and 1 year (14.9%, $p=0.035$). Motor 'off' scores were also improved at 3 months (24.9%, $p=0.001$) and 1 year (21.3%, $p=0.002$). All cardinal features were improved and contralateral drug-induced dyskinesias were dramatically ameliorated. Patient age was inversely related to improvement in total UPDRS scores at 3 months. Scores decreased by an average of 52.2% in younger patients (38–52 years) and by 13.8% in older patients (58–69 years). ADL and motor scores during the 'on' state were only transiently improved. Adverse events related to surgery were generally mild. Several patients experienced transient postoperative confusion or contralateral facial weakness. One patient experienced persistent worsening of dysarthria and another exhibited persistent superior quadrantanopia.

Quantitative ^{18}F-fluorodeoxyglucose (FDG) positron emission tomography (PET) following unilateral pallidotomy indicates that improvement in contralateral limb motor performance correlates significantly with reductions in thalamic metabolism and increases in lateral frontal metabolism.[75] These findings are consistent with the functional anatomic model as one would expect a decline in thalamic metabolism as a result of decreased afferent activity. Following surgical disinhibition of the thalamus, motor and premotor frontal metabolism increases.

Thus, several series indicate that consistent benefit can be obtained with pallidotomy. The most striking benefit is the marked reduction of contralateral peak-dose dyskinesia. In addition, there is improvement in both activities of daily living and motor function with improvement in all of the cardinal features of Parkinson's disease (tremor, rigidity, bradykinesia) on the contralateral side during the 'off' state. Improvement on the ipsilateral side is modest. Benefits in the 'on' state (other than a reduction in dyskinesia) are limited. Patients who are experiencing marked dyskinesia or contralateral bradykinesia and tremor are most likely to benefit. Younger patients may improve the most. Despite these observations, questions concerning the magnitude and longevity of benefit remain.[76] In their open-label study, Baron et al. noted that total UPDRS 'off' score was improved by 30.1% at 3 months but only 19.7% at 1 year. Long-term follow-up and controlled studies are necessary to better define the benefits of this procedure. Preliminary results of pallidal stimulation also appear promising.[77]

Pallidal stimulation

The clinical response to pallidal stimulation varies depending on the region stimulated.[78,79] High-frequency stimulation in the dorsal GPi improves akinesia, rigidity and gait when patients are in the 'off' state and can induce dyskinesia. Stimulation in the posteroventral GPi reduces rigidity but worsens akinesia and gait for patients in the 'off' state and dramatically reduces dyskinesia but worsens akinesia and gait for patients in the 'on' state, thereby negating some of the positive effects of levodopa. Optimal benefit for dyskinesia and rigidity are achieved with stimulation of the ventral GPi whereas the best effect for akinesia usually occurs with stimulation of the dorsal GPi. Thus, the cardinal symptoms of Parkinson's disease appear to have functional somatotopy within the GPi.

Chronic pallidal stimulation provides clinical benefit similar to pallidotomy.[67,78–80] Stimulation parameters are adjusted to provide the best combination of benefit. Patients commonly require slightly more levodopa and it may be necessary to accept the presence of mild dyskinesia to maintain an optimal levodopa effect. Krack et al. evaluated three patients with unilateral and five patients with bilateral pallidal stimulation at 6 months.[79] Patients were taking 25% more levodopa and experienced a 72% reduction in dyskinesia during on-drug periods. Motor scores off drug improved 32% and significant benefit was observed in gait (46%), contralateral tremor (46%), contralateral rigidity (52%) and akinesia (25%). That stimulation in different areas of the GPi provides different benefits suggests that the ability to adjust stimulation parameters including which contacts to activate may allow for a better clinical outcome than pallidotomy. However, this remains to be evaluated in a randomized clinical trial.

Subthalamic nucleus stimulation

Monkeys rendered parkinsonian by injection of MPTP exhibit hyperactivity of the STN[68–70] and lesions or high-frequency stimulation of the STN reverse akinesia and rigidity.[81] As there is concern that lesioning the STN in Parkinson's disease patients might cause permanent hemiballism, STN stimulation has been undertaken as the primary investigation of STN surgery. Limousin *et al.* reported results of bilateral STN stimulation in three patients.[82] Electrodes were implanted in two separate sessions for the first two patients and at the same time for the third patient. Targeting was performed using MRI, electrophysiological recording and stimulation. 'Off' motor scores were improved 42% to 84% 3–4 months after surgery and benefit persisted for up to 15 months.[82,83] Levodopa was reduced by 40–50% in two patients and withdrawn completely in the third. Unilateral stimulation provided some improvement in contralateral akinesia and rigidity but bilateral stimulation provided major improvement in akinesia, rigidity, gait and posture.[83] Dyskinesias could be elicited with greater electrical stimulation than was necessary for motor improvement.

Krack *et al.* compared subthalamic and internal pallidal stimulation in 13 young onset patients with motor fluctuations and dyskinesia 6 months after surgery.[84] In the off-drug state, UPDRS motor scores improved 71% with STN stimulation compared to 39% with GPi stimulation ($p<0.05$). STN stimulation provided significantly greater improvement for akinesia, gait and hand-tapping scores (CD 4.2). Improvement in motor symptoms from STN stimulation was close or equal to the best levodopa response. In contrast, GPi stimulation only improved akinesia approximately 50% compared to levodopa. Dyskinesia elicited by an acute levodopa test was significantly decreased with GPi stimulation (–82%) compared to STN stimulation (–41%). However, maintenance levodopa doses were reduced in the STN group by 56% compared to an increase of 29% in the GPi group, leading to a similar reduction of everyday dyskinesia in both groups. Thus, preliminary comparison greatly favours STN stimulation in this population as the improvement for tremor, rigidity and dyskinesia was approximately the same in both groups but STN stimulation provided about twice the benefit for akinesia.

Fetal tissue transplantation

Fetal nigral transplantation was first utilized in the treatment of Parkinson's disease because: (1) the disease is primarily related to selective degeneration of

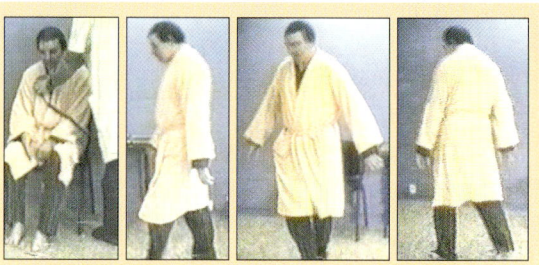

CD 4.2. A parkinsonian patient with bilateral subthalamic stimulators. (Courtesy of Professors P. Pollak and A. Benabid.)

dopamine-containing nigrostriatal neurons; (2) replacement therapy with levodopa provides significant clinical benefit; (3) dopaminergic neurons provide tonic neuromodulatory input to the striatum, and do not carry primary neural information; (4) the target area for neural transplantation is limited in size; and (5) similar dopaminergic neural grafts induce behavioural recovery in rodent and non-human primate models of parkinsonism.[85]

Lindvall *et al.*[86] reported the short-term follow-up of two patients with Parkinson's disease receiving unilateral suspension nigral grafts. Four embryonic donors aged 7–9 weeks postconception (PC) were transplanted into the caudate and anterior putamen. Storage of tissue before transplantation was prolonged and the needle catheter diameter was suboptimal. A small amount of blood was seen in the needle tracts of one of the patients on MR image. Clinical improvement at 6 months was significant, but minimal. Furthermore, striatal fluorodopa uptake as determined by positron emission tomography (FD-PET) was not significantly increased in the graft site. Two additional patients subsequently underwent a modification of this protocol.[87,88] In these patients, tissue storage time and the diameter of the stereotactic transplant needle were decreased, and three needle tracts separated by about 9 mm were utilized in the putamen. These two patients experienced a more pronounced clinical improvement starting approximately 2 months after surgery. Improvement was noted over a 4–6 year observation period,[89–91] including the ability to withdraw levodopa from one of the two patients. Improvements in bradykinesia, rigidity and percent 'off' time were noted. Mild clinical deterioration, primarily on the side ipsilateral to the transplant, was noted starting 4–6 years after transplantation. Contralateral benefits were stable long-term.[91] FD-PET revealed a significant improvement on the side of the graft, for up to 6 years, with progressive decline on the contralateral, ungrafted side (Figs. 4.2, 4.3).[89–92] In four subsequent subjects, the use of more needle tracts, more donors or inclusion of the caudate as a transplant site in addition to the putamen did not result in marked additional improvement compared with these earlier results.[90,91] Peschanski *et al.*[93–95] have replicated many of Lindvall's results, demonstrating that this technique is reproducible between centres.

Freed *et al.*[96,97] transplanted dopamine neurons from a single early gestational embryo unilaterally in two patients and bilaterally in five patients. A linear array of graft deposits separated by 5 mm was utilized. Twelve-month follow-up revealed statistically significant improvement in activities of daily living, scores of facial expression, postural control, gait and bradykinesia. Levodopa doses were reduced on average by 39%.

Spencer *et al.*[98] utilized cryopreserved fetal nigral tissue transplanted unilaterally into the caudate nucleus in four patients with severe Parkinson's disease. Donor age ranged from 5–9 weeks PC. Clinical improvement was marginal, and not significantly different than the comparison medically-controlled group. A patient from this series who died 4 months after surgery had pathological features of striatonigral degeneration, and there was no significant survival of tyrosine hydroxylase positive (dopaminergic) neurons.[99]

Widner *et al.*[91,100] performed fetal nigral transplantation in two patients with parkinsonism secondary to the neurotoxin MPTP. These patients received bilateral transplants derived from three to four donors per side, transplanted into both the caudate and putamen. Donor age was 6–8 weeks PC. These patients experienced progressive improvement in motor function starting 3 months after transplantation, and striatal FD uptake was markedly improved 1 year after transplantation. The investigators reported that the magnitude of improvement was greater than observed in their Parkinson's disease patients. This could have been secondary to the use of bilateral rather than unilateral transplants, the age of the recipients (who were comparatively younger in the case of the MPTP patients) or differences in the underlying diseases.

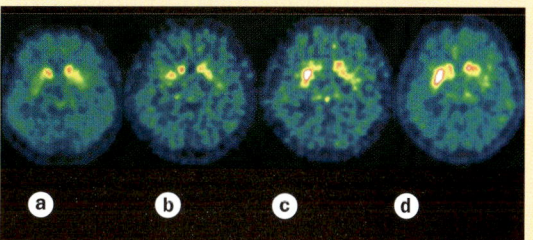

Figure 4.2. Sequential fluorodopa PET images from patient scanned before (a) and then at 5 (b), 8 (c) and 13 (d) months after implantation of fetal cells into left putamen.

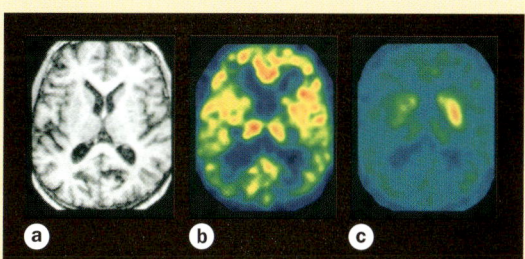

Figure 4.3. MRI (a), PET oxygen metabolism (b) and PET fluorodopa (c) images 3 years after transplantation of fetal cells into right putamen (shown on right).

Widner *et al.*[101] have also preliminarily reported clinical improvement following transplantation in a single unmedicated patient with MPTP-induced parkinsonism who did not tolerate levodopa. This suggests that graft-induced recovery is due, at least in part, to graft-induced reinnervation of the recipient's brain, and is not necessarily dependent on levodopa therapy.

The authors performed an open-label clinical trial of fetal tissue transplantation in six patients with Parkinson's disease.[102,103] Three to four donors per side were transplanted bilaterally into the postcommissural putamen. Solid grafts were utilized from donor ages 6.5–9 weeks PC. Grafts were separated by 5 mm in a three-dimensional array. Patients were immunosuppressed for a 6-month period. All patients experienced clinically meaningful improvement that generally began at 1 month, increased over a 3-month period and persisted for the length of the study (mean of 20 months). Mean total UPDRS 'off' scores improved 32%, and each patient experienced at least a 19% improvement. The percent time 'on' without dyskinesia improved from 22% to 60%. FD-PET revealed progressive improvement in putaminal uptake in 11 of the 12 implanted putamina. Each patient exhibited at least a 42% increase in putaminal FD uptake (Ki). Increased FD-uptake correlated with improvement in UPDRS 'off' scores and percent 'on' time without dyskinesia.[104] Patient number 6, in whom cyclosporine was discontinued before his second transplant procedure because of reversible cyclosporine-induced renal dysfunction, demonstrated a 118% increase in putaminal Ki at 1 year in the side where transplantation was performed without cyclosporine.

Two of the patients in our series died 18 months following transplantation from causes unrelated to the procedure. The first patient died from a pulmonary embolism following ankle surgery for post-traumatic degenerative arthritis.[103,105,106] The second patient died presumably secondary to aspiration.[103,107–109] These cases demonstrated, for the first time, robust graft survival following fetal tissue transplantation in patients with Parkinson's disease. Between 82 000 and 135 000 transplanted dopaminergic neurons were seen in each transplanted putamen. Up to three-quarters of the transplanted target area within the postcommissural putamen was reinnervated by the grafts in a 'patch-matrix' fashion, similar to what is observed in the normal brain. Synapses between graft and host were demonstrated using tyrosine hydroxylase (TH)-immunoelectron microscopy. Grafted regions elaborated dopamine transporter, tyrosine hydroxylase messenger RNA and increased cytochrome oxidase activity. These findings suggest that grafts are metabolically active and capable of synthesizing and taking up dopamine. For the three putamina evaluated pathologically, increased uptake on FD-PET correlated with the number of TH-immunoreactive cells.[103,106]

Wenning et al.[90] reported clinical and PET scan results very similar to the authors' following unilateral fetal nigral transplantation into the putamen or putamen plus caudate in six patients through 1 year and four patients through 2 years. Both groups attempted to maintain antiparkinsonian medications unchanged and the mean levodopa reduction was 10% (1 year) and 20% (2 years) in their series compared with 16% (20.5 months) in ours. UPDRS 'off' scores were decreased by 18% and 26% in their series compared with 32% in ours. 'Off' time was reduced by 34% and 43% in their series compared

with 43% in ours. After 8–12 months, FD uptake in the transplanted putamen was increased by 68% in their patients compared with 61% after 12 months in ours. These investigators postulated that the long-term decline (4–6 years after transplantation) they observed in some patients might be due to continued degeneration on the non-grafted side. Whether bilateral grafting will provide a better long-term outcome remains to be determined.

Kopyov et al.[110] reported dramatic clinical improvement following bilateral transplantation in patients with Parkinson's disease. These authors utilized one to two donors per side, transplanted utilizing four needle tracts. UPDRS scores improved by approximately 75% in the 'on' state and 55% in the 'off' state at 2 years following surgery. No other groups have noted significant improvement in the 'on' state, making the degree of improvement reported by these authors quite remarkable. One patient on a low dose of levodopa (400 mg per day) prior to transplantation was able to discontinue medical therapy. The investigators also noted improvement in Hoehn–Yahr stage as well as measures of activities of daily living and dyskinesia. PET scans were not performed in this study.

Direct comparison between programmes is difficult due to different variables utilized between programmes. These variables include donor age, methods of tissue storage, the use of solid versus suspension grafts, the number of donors, the distribution of grafted tissue, the site of implantation, unilateral vs bilateral transplantation, the use of immunosuppression, the source of donor tissue, patient selection and the method of clinical assessment of patients with Parkinson's disease.[85] The single most important variable for graft survival, however, has been demonstrated to be donor age.[102,103,106,111–113] Improvement on FD-PET or autopsy evidence of graft survival has only been demonstrated in programmes that utilize donors within a narrowly defined donor age window. Much research is necessary both in the laboratory as well as the clinic to further define the importance of other variables to the ultimate outcome of the transplantation procedure.[85]

Fetal nigral transplantation has never been demonstrated to be efficacious in a prospective randomized trial. It is also important to note that improvement in FD-PET or autopsy-proven graft survival are surrogate endpoints rather than primary clinical endpoints. Further, although our group has demonstrated preliminary clinical efficacy in an open-label trial, improved FD-PET, and graft survival at autopsy, two of our first six patients died 18 months after surgery. This underscores the need for controlled clinical trials to evaluate transplantation's clinical utility. Two such trials, funded by the National Institutes of Health, are currently under way. Both utilize a surgical placebo control arm, consisting of burr holes without transplantation.

One group is based out of the University of Colorado and Columbia Presbyterian Medical Center in New York, and the second group utilizes a collaboration between Mt Sinai Medical Center in New York, Rush Presbyterian Medical Center in Chicago and the University of South Florida in Tampa.

Of concern, both patients in our group that came to autopsy had multiple immune markers within the grafts.[108] Markers for T-cells, B-cells, macrophages and activated microglia were present in all grafts. Nonetheless, these patients exhibited robust graft survival by TH-immunohistochemistry, improved FD uptake on PET, and experienced significant clinical improvement. Therefore, it is difficult to evaluate the meaning of these immunological markers, and it is unclear if a chronic rejection process is ongoing in these patients in the absence of immunosuppression.

However, there is significant indirect evidence that grafts are likely to be viable long-term. Progressive improvements in FD-PET has been observed in 12 patients in three centres for at least 6 months after cessation of all immunosuppression.[90,95,102,103,113] Clinical improvement has been stable for up to 6 years.[90] In our two patients that have come to autopsy, robust graft survival has been seen from all 13 unrelated donors transplanted into two separate patients in staged procedures. This indicates that the likelihood of unrelated allografts in the brain undergoing rejection is low, and that unrelated allografts are unlikely to induce second-set rejection.[114] Finally, similar immunological markers have been noted in animal allograft models in the absence of graft rejection.[115,116]

In conclusion, fetal tissue transplantation has preliminarily been demonstrated to be efficacious and definitive trials to prove this point are ongoing. Grafts transplanted into patients with Parkinson's disease can survive and reinnervate the brain. Graft survival been demonstrated to correlate with clinical improvement as well as improvement on FD-PET scan. Transplantation can be performed reliably both within and between centres. Clinical improvement appears to be long-term.

Among all the currently utilized surgical therapies for the treatment of Parkinson's disease, fetal tissue transplantation perhaps has the most potential for improvement in results in the future based on further laboratory and clinical research.

References

1. Bucy P C. Cortical extirpation in the treatment of involuntary movements. Am J Surg 1948; 75: 257–263

2. Putnam T J. Treatment of unilateral paralysis agitans by section of the lateral pyramidal tract. Arch Neurol Psych 1940; 44: 950–976

3. Walker A E. Cerebral pedunculotomy for the relief of involuntary movements. J Nerv Ment Dis 1952; 116: 766–775

4. Cooper I S. Parkinsonism: Its medical and surgical therapy. Springfield, Ill: Charles C. Thomas, 1961

5. Meyers R. The modification of alternating tremors, rigidity and festination by surgery of the basal ganglia. Res Publ Assoc Res Nerv Ment Dis 1942; 20: 602–665

6. Fenelon F. Essais de traitement neurochirurgical du syndrome parkinsonien par intervention direct sur les voies extrapyramidales immediatement sous-striopallidales (anse lenticulaire). Rev Neurol 1950; 83: 437–440

7. Fenelon F, Theibant F. Resultats du traitement neurochirurgical d'une rididite parkinsonienne par intervention striopallidale unilaterale. Rev Neurol 1950; 83: 280

8. Guiot G, Brion S. Traitement des mouvements anormaux par la coagulation pallidale. Rev Neurol 1953; 83: 578–580

9. Cooper I S. The neurosurgical alleviation of parkinsonism. Springfield, Ill: Charles C. Thomas, 1956

10. Abbie A A. Morphology of forebrain arteries, with especial reference to evolution of basal ganglia. J Anat 1934; 68: 433–470

11. Spiegel E A, Wycis H T, Marks M, Lee A S T. Stereotaxic apparatus for operations on the human brain. Science 1947; 106: 349–350

12. Spiegel E A, Wycis H T, Thur C. The stereoencephalotome. J Neurosurg 1951; 8: 452–453

13. Spiegel E A, Wycis H T. Ansotomy in paralysis agitans. Arch Neurol Psych 1954; 71: 598–614

14. Cooper I S, Bravo G. Chemopallidectomy and chemothalamectomy. J Neurosurg 1958; 15: 244–250

15. Narabayashi H, Okum T. Procaine-oil blocking of the globus pallidus for the treatment of rigidity and tremor of parkinsonism. Proc Jpn Acad 1953; 29: 134–137

16. Svennilson E, Torvik A, Lowe R et al. Treatment of parkinsonism by stereotactic thermolesions in the pallidal region. Acta Psychiat Neurol Scand 1960; 35: 358–377

17. Hassler R, Reichert T. Indikationen und lokalisations methode der gezielten Hirnoperationen. Nevenarzt 1954; 25: 411–447

18. Cooper I S. Involuntary movement disorders. New York: Harper & Row, 1969

19. Cooper I S. Surgical treatment of parkinsonism. Ann Rev Med 1965; 16: 309–330

20. Jankovic J, Cardoso F, Grossman R G, Hamilton W J. Outcome after stereotactic thalamotomy for parkinsonian, essential, and other types of tremor. Neurosurg 1995; 37: 680–687

21. Ohye C, Shibazaki T, Hirato M et al. Strategy of selective VIM thalamotomy guided by microrecording. Stereotact Funct Neurosurg 1990; 54&55: 186–191

22. Tasker R R. Thalamotomy. Neurosurg Clin North Am 1990; 1: 841–864

23. Alberts W W, Libet B, Wright E W et al. Physiological mechanisms of tremor and rigidity in parkinsonism. Confina Neurologica 1965; 26: 318–327

24. Guiot G, Hardy J, Albe-Fessard D. Delimitation precise des structures sous-corticales et identification de noyaux thalaminques chez l'homme par l'electrophysiologie stereotaxique. Neurochirurgia 1962; 5: 1–18

25. Lenz F A, Tasker R R, Kwan H C et al. Cross-correlation analyses of thalamic neurons and EMG activity in parkinsonian tremor. Appl Neurophysiol 1985; 48: 305–308

26. Lenz F A, Tasker R R, Kwan H C et al. Selection of the optimal site for the relief of parkinsonian tremor on the basis of spectral analysis of neuronal firing patterns. Appl Neurophysiol 1987; 50: 338–343

27. Lenz F A, Tasker R R, Kwan H C et al. Single unit analysis of the human ventral thalamic nuclear group: Correlation of thalamic 'tremor cells' with the 3–6 Hz component of parkinsonian tremor. J Neurosci 1988; 8: 754–764

28. Narabayashi H. Tremor mechanisms. In: Schaltenbrand G, Walker A E (eds) Stereotaxy of the human brain. Stuttgart: Georg Thieme Verlag, 1982: 510–514

29. Ohye C, Narabayashi H. Physiological study of presumed ventralis intermedius neurons in the human thalamus. J Neurosurg 1979; 50: 290–297

30. Ohye C, Shibazaki T, Hirai T et al. Further physiological observations on the ventralis intermedius neurons in the human thalamus. J Neurophysiol 1989; 16: 488–500

31. Tasker R R, Lenz F, Yamashiro K et al. Microelectrode techniques in localization of stereotactic targets. Neurol Res 1987; 9: 105–112

32. Fox M W, Ahlskog J E, Kelly P J. Stereotactic ventrolateralis thalamotomy for medically refractory tremor in post-levodopa era Parkinson's disease patients. J Neurosurg 1991; 75: 723–730

33. Tasker R R. Surgical aspects symposium on extrapyramidal diseases. Applied Therapeutics 1967; 9: 454–462

34. Tasker R R, Siqueira J, Hawrylyshyn P, Organ L W. What happened to VIM thalamotomy for Parkinson's disease? Appl Neurophysiol 1983; 46: 68–83

35. Kelly P J, Ahlskog J E, Goerss S J et al. Computer-assisted stereotactic ventralis lateralis thalamotomy with microelectrode recording control in patients with Parkinson's disease. Mayo Clin Proc 1987; 62: 655–664

36. Kelly P J, Gillingham F J. The long-term results of stereotactic surgery and L-dopa therapy in patients with Parkinson's disease. J Neurosurg 1980; 53: 332–337

37. Matsumoto K, Schichijo F, Fukami T. Long-term follow-up review of cases of Parkinson's disease after unilateral or bilateral thalamotomy. J Neurosurg 1984; 60: 1033–1044

38. Miyamoto T, Bekku H, Moriyama E et al. Present role of sterotactic thalamotomy for parkinsonism. Retrospective analysis of operative results and thalamic lesions in computed tomograms. Appl Neurophysiol 1985; 48: 294–304

39. Mundinger F. Postoperative and long-term results of 1,561 sterotactic operations in parkinsonism. Appl Ncurophysiol 1985; 48: 293

40. Narabayashi H, Maeda T, Yokochi F. Long-term follow-up study of nucleus ventralis intermedius and ventrolateralis thalamotomy using a microelectrode technique in parkinsonism. Appl Neurophysiol 1987; 50: 330–337

41. Nagaseki Y, Shibazaki T, Hirai T et al. Long-term follow-up results of selective VIM-thalamotomy. J Neurosurg 1986; 65: 296–302

42. Scott R M, Brody J A, Cooper I S. The effect of thalamotomy on the progress of unilateral Parkinson's disease. J Neurosurg 1970; 32: 286–288

43. Selby G. Stereotactic surgery for the relief of Parkinson's disease. Part I: A critical review. J Neurol Sci 1967; 5: 315–342

44. Riechert T. Stereotactic brain operations: Methods, clinical aspects, indications. Bern, Hans Huber 1980: 213–304

45. Krayenbuhl H, Wyss O A M, Yasargil M G. Bilateral thalamotomy and pallidotomy as treatment for bilateral parkinsonism. J Neurosurg 1961; 18: 429–444

46. Matsumoto K, Asano T, Baba T et al. Long-term follow-up results of bilateral thalamotomy for parkinsonism. Appl Neurophysiol 1976; 39: 257–260

47. Laitinen L V. Thalamic targets in stereotaxic treatment of Parkinson's disease. J Neurosurg 1966; 24: 82–85

48. Stellar S, Cooper I S. Mortality and morbidity in cryothalamectomy for Parkinson's disease: A statistical study of 2868 consecutive operations. J Neurosurg 1968; 28: 459–467

49. Diederich N, Goert C G, Stebbins G T et al. Blinded evaluation confirms long-term aysmmetric effect of unilateral thalamotomy or subthalamotomy on tremor in Parkinson's disease. Neurology 1992; 42: 1311–1314

50. Page R D. The use of thalamotomy in the treatment of levodopa-induced dyskinesia. Acta Neurochir 1992; 114: 77–117

51. Narabayashi H, Yokochi F, Nakajima Y. Levodopa-induced dyskinesia and thalamotomy. J Neurol Neurosurg Psychiatry 1984; 47: 831–839

52. Nittner K. Auswirkungen stereotaktischer hirnoperationen auf tremor, rigor und hypokinese in abhaengigkeit vom ort der laesion. In: Gainshirt H, Berlit P, Haack G (eds) Pathophysiologie, klinik und therapie des parkinsonismus. Berlin: Editiones Roche 1983: 359–364

53. Riechert T. Stereotactic surgery for treatment of Parkinson's syndrome. Prog Neurol Surg 1973; 5: 1–78

54. Hughes R C, Polgar J G, Weightman D, Walton J N. L-dopa in parkinsonism and the influence of previous thalamotomy. Br Med J 1971; 1: 7–13

55. Bechtereva N P, Bondartchuk A N, Smirnov V M et al. Method of electrostimulation of the deep brain structures in treatment of some chronic diseases. Confin Neurol 1975; 37: 136–140

56. Mazars G, Merienne L, Cioloca C. Control of dyskinesias due to sensory deafferentation by means of thalamic stimulation. Acta Neurochir 1980; (Suppl. 30): 239–243

57. Siegfried J. Stimulation of thalamic nuclei in human: Sensory and therapeutical aspects. In: Besson J M, Guilbault G, Peschanski M (eds) Thalamus and pain. Amsterdam: Elsevier, 1987: 271–278

58. Andy O J. Thalamic stimulation for control of movement disorders. Appl Neurophysiol 1983; 46: 107–111

59. Brice J, McLellan L. Suppression of intention tremor by contingent deep-brain stimulation. Lancet 1980; 1: 1221–1222

60. Narabayashi H. Stereotaxic VIM thalamotomy for treatment of tremor. Eur Neurol 1989; 29: 29–32

61. Benabid A L, Pollak P, Louveau A et al. Combined (thalamotomy and stimulation) stereotactic surgery of the VIM thalamic nucleus for bilateral Parkinson's disease. Appl Neurophysiol 1987; 50: 344–346

62. Benabid A L, Pollak P, Gao D et al. Chronic electrical stimulation of the ventralis intermedius nucleus of the thalamus as a treatment of movement disorders. J Neurosurg 1996; 84: 203–214

63. Benabid A L, Pollak P, Gervason C et al. Long-term suppression of tremor by chronic stimulation of the ventral intermediate thalamic nucleus. Lancet 1991; 337: 403–406

64. Blond S, Caparros-Lefebvre D, Parker F et al. Control of tremor and involuntary movement disorders by chronic stereotactic stimulation of the ventral intermediate thalamic nucleus. J Neurosurg 1992; 77: 62–68

65. Deiber M P, Pollak P, Passingham R et al. Thalamic stimulation and suppression of parkinsonian tremor. Evidence of a cerebellar deactivation using positron emission tomography. Brain 1993; 116: 267–279

66. Blond S, Siegfried J. Thalamic stimulation for the treatment of tremor and other movement disorders. Acta Neurochir 1991; 52: 109–111

67. Koller W, Pahwa R, Busenbark K et al. High-frequency unilateral thalamic stimulation in the treatment of essential and parkinsonian tremor. Ann Neurol 1997; 42: 292–299

68. Miller W C, DeLong M R. Altered tonic activity of neurons in the globus pallidus and subthalamic nucleus in the primate MPTP model of parkinsonism. In: Carpenter M B, Jayaraman A (eds) The basal ganglia II. New York: Plenum Press, 1987: 415–427

69. Filion M, Boucher R, Bedard P. Globus pallidus unit activity in the monkey during the induction of parkinsonism by 1-methyl-4-phenyl-1,2,3,6-tetrahydropyridine (MPTP). Soc Neurosci 1985; 11: 1160

70. Alexander G E, Crutcher M D, DeLong M R. Basal ganglia-thalamocortical circuits: parallel substrates for motor, oculomotor, 'prefrontal' and 'limbic' functions. Prog Brain Res 1990; 85: 119–146

71. Laitinen L V, Bergenheim A T, Hariz M I. Leksell's posteroventral pallidotomy in the treatment of Parkinson's disease. J Neurosurg 1992; 76: 53–61

72. Lozano A M, Lang A E, Galvez-Jimenez N et al. Effect of GPi pallidotomy on motor function in Parkinson's disease. Lancet 1995; 346: 1383–1387

73. Dogali M, Fazzini E, Kolodny E et al. Stereotactic ventral pallidotomy for Parkinson's disease. Neurology 1995; 45: 753–761

74. Baron M S, Vitek J L, Bakay R A E et al. Treatment of advanced Parkinson's disease by posterior GPi pallidotomy: 1-year results of a pilot study. Ann Neurol 1996; 40: 355–366

75. Eidelberg D, Moeller J R, Ishikawa T et al. Regional metabolic correlates of surgical outcome following unilateral pallidotomy for Parkinson's disease. Ann Neurol 1996; 39: 450–459

76. Olanow C W. GPi pallidotomy – have we made a dent in Parkinson's disease? Ann Neurol 1996; 40: 341–342

77. Siegfried J, Lippitz B. Bilateral chronic electrostimulation of ventroposterolateral pallidum: a new therapeutic approach for alleviating all parkinsonian symptoms. Neurosurgery 1994; 35: 1126–1130

78. Bejjani B, Damier P, Arnulf L et al. Pallidal stimulation for Parkinson's disease: two targets? Neurology 1997; 49: 1564–1569

79. Krack P, Pollack P, Limousin P et al. Opposite motor effects of pallidal stimulation in Parkinson's disease. Ann Neurol 1998; 43: 180–192

80. Pahwa R, Wilkinson S, Smith D et al. High-frequency stimulation of the globus pallidus for the treatment of Parkinson's disease. Neurology 1997; 49: 249–253

81. Bergman H, Wichmann T, DeLong M R. Reversal of experimental parkinsonism by lesions of the subthalamic nucleus. Science 1990; 249: 1436–1438

82. Limousin P, Pollak P, Benazzouz A et al. Effect on parkinsonian signs and symptoms of bilateral subthalamic nucleus stimulation. Lancet 1995; 345: 91–95

83. Limousin P, Pollak P, Benazzouz A et al. Bilateral subthalamic nucleus stimulation for severe Parkinson's disease. Mov Dis 1995; 10: 672–674

84. Krack P, Pollak P, Limousin P, Hoffman D, Xie J, Benazzouz A L, Benabid AL. Subthalamic nucleus or internal pallidal stimulation in young onset Parkinson's disease. Brain 1998; 121: 451–457

85. Olanow C W, Kordower J H, Freeman T B. Fetal nigral transplantation as a therapy for Parkinson's disease. Trends Neurosci 1996; 19: 102–109

86. Lindvall O, Rehncrona S, Brundin P et al. Human fetal dopamine neurons grafted into the striatum in two patients with severe Parkinson's disease: A detailed account of methodology and a 6-month follow-up. Arch Neurol 1989; 46: 615–631

87. Lindvall O, Brundin P, Widner H et al. Grafts of fetal dopamine neurons survive and improve motor function in Parkinson's disease. Science 1990; 247: 574–577

88. Lindvall O, Widner H, Rehncrona S et al. Transplantation of fetal dopamine neurons in Parkinson's disease: One-year clinical and neurophysiological observations in two patients with putaminal implants. Ann Neurol 1992; 31: 155–165

89. Lindvall O, Sawle G, Widner H et al. Evidence for long-term survival and function of dopaminergic grafts in progressive Parkinson's disease. Ann Neurol 1994; 35: 172–180

90. Wenning G K, Odin P, Morrish P et al. Short- and long-term survival and function of unilateral intrastriatal dopaminergic grafts in Parkinson's disease. Ann Neurol 1997; 42: 95–107

91. Widner H. The Lund transplant program for Parkinson's disease and patients with MPTP-induced parkinsonism. In: Freeman T B, Wider H (eds) Cell transplantation for neurological disorders: toward reconstruction of the human central nervous system. New Jersey: Humana Press, 1998: 1–18

92. Sawle G V, Bloomfield P M, Bjorklund A et al. Transplantation of fetal dopamine neurons in Parkinson's disease: Positron emission tomography [18F]-6-L-fluorodopa studies in two patients with putaminal implants. Ann Neurol 1992; 31: 166–173

93. Peschanski M, Defer G, N'Guyen J P et al. Bilateral motor improvement and alteration of L-dopa effect in two patients with Parkinson's disease following intrastriatal transplantation of foetal ventral mesencephalon. Brain 1994; 177: 487–499

94. Defer G L, Geny C, Ricolfi F et al. Long-term outcome of unilaterally transplanted parkinsonian patients. I. Clinical approach. Brain 1996; 119: 41–50

95. Remy P, Samson Y, Hantray P et al. Clinical correlates of [18F] fluorodopa uptake in five grafted parkinsonian patients. Ann Neurol 1995; 38: 580–588

96. Freed C R, Breeze R E, Rosenberg N L et al. Transplantation of human fetal dopamine cells for Parkinson's disease: results at one year. Arch Neurol 1990; 47: 505–512

97. Freed C R, Breeze R E, Rosenberg N L et al. Survival of implanted fetal dopamine cells and neurologic improvement 12 to 46 months after transplantation for Parkinson's disease. N Engl J Med 1992; 327: 1549–1555

98. Spencer D D, Robbins R J, Naftolin F et al. Unilateral transplantation of human fetal mesencephalic tissue into the caudate nucleus of patients with Parkinson's disease. N Engl J Med 1992; 327: 1541–1548

99. Redmond D E Jr, Leranth C, Spencer D D et al. Fetal neural graft survival. Lancet 1990; 336: 820–822

100. Widner H, Tetrud J, Rehncrona S et al. Bilateral fetal mesencephalic grafting in two patients with parkinsonism induced by 1-methyl-4-phenyl-1,2,3,6-tetrahydropyridine (MPTP). N Engl J Med 1992; 327: 1556–1563

101. Widner H, Rehncrona S, Snow B et al. Neural grafting into a L-dopa untreated, severely MPTP-lesioned patient. Mov Dis 1996; 11(Suppl. 1): 249

102. Freeman T B, Olanow C W, Hauser R A et al. Bilateral fetal nigral transplantation into the postcommissural putamen in Parkinson's disease. Ann Neurol 1995; 38: 379–388

103. Hauser R A, Freeman T B, Snow B J et al. Long-term evaluation of fetal nigral transplantation in Parkinson's disease. Arch Neurol 1999; 56: 179–187

104. Snow B J, Vingerhoets F J G, Hauser R A et al. PET studies of bilateral fetal nigral transplantation for Parkinson's disease. Mov Dis 1996; 11(Suppl. 1): 250

105. Kordower J H, Freeman T B, Snow B J et al. Neuropathologic evidence of graft survival and striatal reinnervation after the transplantation of fetal mesencephalic tissue in a patient with Parkinson's disease. N Engl J Med 1995; 332: 1118–1124

106. Kordower J H, Rosenstein J M, Collier T J et al. Functional fetal nigral grafts in a patient with Parkinson's disease: Chemoanatomic, ultrastructural, and metabolic studies. J Comp Neurol 1996; 370: 203–230

107. Freeman T B, Olanow W C, Hauser R A et al. Human fetal tissue transplantation. In: Germano I M (ed) Neurosurgical treatment of movement disorders. Park Ridge: Amercian Association of Neurological Surgeons, 1998: 177–192

108. Kordower J H, Styren S, Dekosky S T et al. Fetal grafting for Parkinson's disease expression of immune markers of two patients with functional fetal nigral implants. Cell Transplant, 1997; 6: 213–219

109. Kordower J H, Freeman T B, Chen E-Y et al. Fetal nigral grafts survive and mediate clinical benefit in a patient with Parkinson's disease. Mov Dis 1998; 13: 383–393

110. Kopyov O V, Jacques D, Lieberman A et al. Clinical study of fetal mesencephalic intracerebral transplants for the treatment of Parkinson's disease. Cell Transplant 1996; 5: 327–337

111. Freeman T B, Spence M S, Boss B D et al. Development of dopaminergic neurons in the human substantia nigra. Exp Neurol 1991; 113: 344–353

112. Freeman T B, Sanberg P R, Nauert G M et al. The influence of donor age on the survival of human embryonic nigral grafts. Cell Transplant 1995; 4: 141–154

113. Langston J W, Widner H, Brooks D et al. Core assessment program for intracerebral transplantations (CAPIT). Mov Dis 1992; 7: 2–13

114. Duan W-M, Widner H, Bjorklund A, Brundin P. Sequential intrastriatal grafting of allogeneic dopamine-rich neuronal tissue in adult rats: Will the second graft be rejected? Neuroscience 1993; 57: 261–274

115. Duan W-M, Widner H, Frodl E M, Brundin P. Immune reactions following systemic immunization prior or subsequent to intrastriatal transplantation of allogeneic mesencephalic tissue in adult rats. Neuroscience 1995; 64: 629–641

116. Shinoda M, Hudson J L, Stromberg I et al. Allogeneic grafts of fetal dopamine neurons: Immunological reactions following active and adoptive immunizations. Brain Res 1995; 680: 180–195

chapter 5

Tremor

Guy Sawle

Tremor is generally regarded as an involuntary movement which is approximately rhythmic and roughly sinusoidal.[1] It has long been recognized that some types of tremor are more obvious when the patient is at rest, whilst others are most noticeable during activity. This division into 'rest' versus 'other' tremors has enabled generations of doctors to recognize Parkinson's disease when it is accompanied by its characteristic resting tremor. It does not, however, provide a sufficient framework to enable us to deal with the wide variety of non-parkinsonian tremors. For this we must divide our non-resting state in a more detailed way, at least into efforts to maintain a steady posture, and during intentional movement. The following classification is that agreed upon by the International Tremor Foundation, Tremor Investigation Group (TRIG).[2]

Rest tremor (CD 5.1)

Tremor which is present when a limb is fully supported against gravity and the relevant muscles are not voluntarily activated.

An important point about the resting state is that it cannot always be achieved in the doctor's office. In the consulting room some patients can relax with their arms on their legs and their feet on the floor. Others are able to achieve a state of physical relaxation lying on an examination couch. But just as our workplace can add several millimetres of mercury to an anxious patient's blood pressure, so it can make the resting state simply unattainable for a proportion of patients. Because of this, I ask patients whether they notice their tremor when they are at home, sitting relaxed and watching their favourite television programme.

Action tremor

Tremor occurring during any voluntary muscle contraction which includes postural, kinetic, intention, isometric and task specific tremors.

Postural tremor (CD 5.2)

Tremor apparent during the voluntary maintenance of a particular posture which is opposed by the force of gravity.

Some everyday tasks demand that we hold our arm out, maintaining an approximately static position. Such is the action necessary to carry a cup and saucer from room to room. The approximately equivalent task in the neurological examination is to ask patients to hold their arms out in front of themselves. It is worthwhile

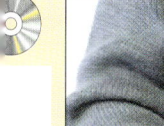
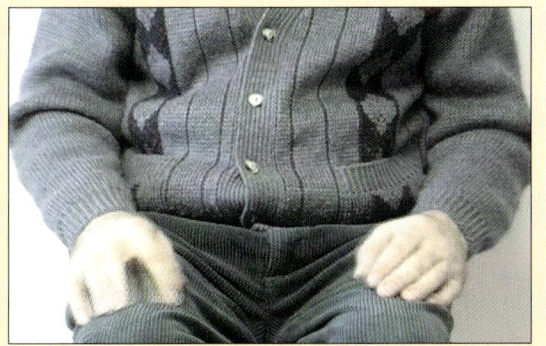

CD 5.1. Rest tremor.

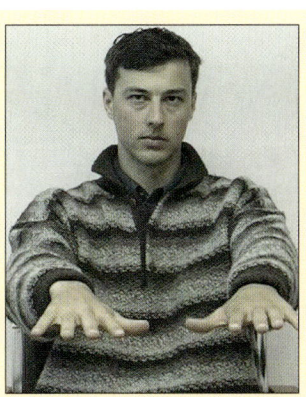

CD 5.2. Postural tremor.

watching whilst patients hold several different positions, such as palms up, palms down, and palms facing one another. Tremor in any of these positions may be accentuated by asking patients to close their eyes and perform a distracting cognitive task, such as counting backwards out loud. One of the most dramatic ways to accentuate postural tremor, which illustrates just how frustrating the condition can be, is to pass the patient an almost full beaker of water.

Kinetic tremor

Tremor evident during any kind of movement.

Intention (terminal) tremor (CD 5.3)

The pronounced exacerbation of kinetic tremor towards the end of a goal-directed movement.

The finger–nose and heel–shin tests of coordination illustrate what is meant by intention tremor when the tremor occurs as the limb approaches a target. This must be distinguished, however, from the postural tremor which can occur during the same test once the target has been reached. Intention tremor is usually easy to identify.

Task-specific tremor

Tremor which only occurs to any significant extent during the performance of highly skilled activities such as writing, playing a musical instrument or using a jeweller's screwdriver.

Some patients report tremor only during the execution of a specific task, such as when writing, or when standing still. In this case it is of paramount importance if at all possible to watch the patient during the activity in question.

Isometric tremor

Tremor which occurs when a voluntary muscle contraction is opposed by a rigid stationary object.

Tremor severity

Most, if not all, tremors vary continuously according to posture and activity. The impact of tremor on patients' quality of life may therefore not be obvious from a cursory examination, nor from electrophysiological measures such as accelerometry. One approach which has been validated by both inter- and intra-rater reliability uses a combination of clinical estimation of tremor severity in several body parts.[3]

Physiological tremor

Everyone has some degree of 'physiological' tremor. For most of us, this presents little difficulty. It may be accentuated, however, by a variety of everyday influences including anxiety and fatigue and it may then cause minor disability. The mechanism of this apparently 'normal' tremor is thought to be a complex interaction between diverse mechanical and neuromuscular factors, such as the beating of our heart and synchronization of motor neuron firing by muscle spindle feedback.[4]

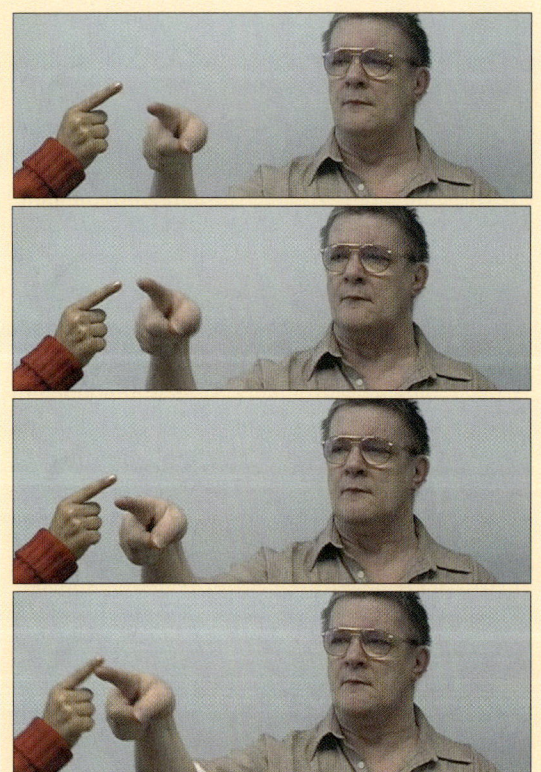

CD 5.3. Intention tremor.

Essential tremor

Although this commonest kind of tremor is sometimes regarded as an innocuous entity, it can at its worst be a severe and disabling condition. It is geographically widespread and more common in older subjects. Many affected patients have a fairly strong family history of the same disorder. Oliver Cromwell is said to have suffered from a familial tremor of the right hand (his signature is reproduced in a manuscript published in 1949 by Macdonald Critchley).[5]

Clinical features
Essential tremor is a monosymptomatic disorder comprising a postural tremor which is usually unaffected by movement and is absent at rest. If other symptoms or signs are found, then either the diagnosis of essential tremor is incorrect, or a second diagnosis must be made. Signs of parkinsonism and cerebellar disease are absent. Writing is often 'scruffy', but micrographia is not seen.

The most typical phenotype is a mild symmetrical postural tremor of the arms. In a study of hereditary essential tremor, tremor of the legs, head, facial muscles, voice, jaw and tongue were all seen, but never in isolation.[6] The tremor frequency is usually 4–10 Hz. It usually stops during sleep.

Many patients are responsive to alcohol; alcohol consumption is so common that most patients are able to say at the time of presentation whether they have noticed a response to alcohol.

Epidemiology
Community based studies in Scandinavia,[7] India,[8] USA[9,10] and Italy[11] suggest that the overall prevalence of essential tremor is 300–1700 per 100 000. It is more common in those over 40 (0.5–7%) and particularly in those aged over 70 (8–12%). Around 20% have an age of onset under 30. There is no definite difference in incidence between the sexes.

Genetics
Many patients report a strong family history. In those who do, an autosomal dominant pattern of inheritance is usual. In many families the penetrance appears complete by the age of 65.[6] In some families all affected members share a similar degree of alcohol responsiveness; but in 20% of families there is a heterogeneity in

this respect. The sex of the affected parent has no influence on the severity of tremor or the degree of disability experienced by an affected child.[6]

Patients with essential tremor do not have the DYT1 gene (at 9q32–34)[12] found in some families with idiopathic generalized dystonia.[13]

Differential diagnosis
The commonest differential diagnosis (and therefore the commonest misdiagnosis) is Parkinson's disease. In most cases the latter condition can be distinguished by the presence of bradykinesia and/or rigidity and classical teaching is that neither occur in essential tremor. In truth there has been some debate in the literature regarding the possibility that Parkinson's disease and essential tremor are different expressions of the same disorder, but this is not a commonly held view. In one review of 678 patients with essential tremor, 6.1% had concomitant Parkinson's disease (a greater percentage than would be expected by chance), 6.9% had coexisting dystonia and 1.8% had myoclonus.[14]

Patients with a postural tremor clinically similar to essential tremor may also exhibit features of dystonia such as torticollis. It is known that some patients with idiopathic generalized dystonia show postural tremor as their only clinical manifestation.[15]

Pathophysiology
The cause of essential tremor remains unknown. Pathological studies have shown no consistent abnormalities.[16] Positron emission tomography (PET) scan studies sensitive to changes in cerebral blood flow show a bilateral increase in cerebellar (hemisphere and vermis) activation during postural arm tremor. Activity in contralateral striatum, thalamus and sensorimotor cortex is also increased. This compares with passive wrist oscillation during which only *ipsilateral* cerebellar activity is increased. Even at rest (no tremor) cerebellar blood flow is higher in essential tremor patients than in control subjects.[17,18]

In primates, harmaline (a reversible monoamine oxidase inhibitor) has been used together with lesions of either the superior cerebellar peduncle, the central tegmental tract, the olivocerebellar pathways or the lateral cerebellar nuclei, to generate a 4–8 Hz postural tremor which is similar in many ways to essential tremor in humans.[19]

Drug treatment

The three most useful agents for treating essential tremor are alcohol, beta blockers, and primidone. Each has its own advantages and disadvantages.

Alcohol

In my experience patients with essential tremor fall into two groups. There are those who have already found that alcohol suppresses their tremor (a subset of whom treat themselves with liberal, if not excessive doses). And there are those to whom the suggestion that they might *try* the effect of a modest alcoholic drink is a complete anathema. Despite the marked symptomatic effect in some patients, alcoholism seems no more common in essential tremor patients than in the general population.[20]

In those who are alcohol responsive (about 50–75%), most experience a marked rebound of tremor severity once the beneficial effect of a 'dose' of alcohol has worn off.

Ingesting 2–3 units of alcohol leads to a bilateral reduction in cerebellar blood flow in controls and patients with essential tremor. In these patients, there is also an *increase* in blood flow in the inferior olivary nucleus,[21] suggesting that alcohol-induced suppression of essential tremor is mediated via a reduction of cerebellar synaptic overactivity resulting in increased afferent input to the inferior olivary nuclei.

Propranolol

Beta blockers, particularly propranolol, are widely used in the treatment of essential tremor. Interestingly, however, many patients are prescribed only a very small dose (20–40 mg daily) which may have no effect at all. Yet patients continue with such medication, sometimes indefinitely. Dose–response curves for individual patients show a marked variation in the sensitivity of essential tremor to propranolol; some patients showing complete suppression at 80 mg a day, yet others derive no benefit from as much as 800 mg.[22] Although a few patients respond well to doses in the 30–60 mg range,[23] the important message is that if patients do *not* derive optimal benefit from a small dose, then it should be increased to at least 320 mg daily (by 40–80 mg increments) or until either maximal benefit is reached or side-effects intervene. If patients are able to tolerate

propranolol (and many cannot, because of worsening airways obstruction, nightmares or any of the other well-known side-effects of propranolol) then between a half and three-quarters find it useful. The slow release preparation allows less frequent tablet taking and works well in this context. Once daily dosage (in the morning) is usually best.

Quite how beta blockers suppress essential tremor is unknown. Propranolol reduces the amplitude of the tremor, rather than the frequency. Atenolol (which is a predominantly cardioselective beta blocker, with maximal action at β_1 receptor sites) has little effect on essential tremor, whereas sotalol (which is a peripherally active non-selective beta blocker with poor penetration into the brain) *is* active.[24] From these data, it has been inferred that the effect of propranolol is via peripheral β_2 blockade.

Primidone

The beneficial effect of primidone in essential tremor was first noticed by chance in a patient who had both essential tremor and epilepsy.[25] It is undoubtedly effective in many of the patients who are able to tolerate the sedative effect of the drug. Because it is so sedating, I often prescribe it in liquid formulation so that patients can very slowly build up the dose from a smaller starting dose (50 mg) than can easily be achieved using tablets. Once patients are on 250 mg or more, I switch over to the tablets. Whereas propranolol is best taken in the morning, primidone is best taken at night.

As with propranolol, the mechanism of action of primidone is unknown. Neither of the two known 'active' metabolites (phenobarbitone and phenylethylmalonamide) suppress tremor.

Other drugs

A variety of other drugs have been used in the treatment of essential tremor. Some have been subjected to controlled trials with benefit reported. None have yet become standard treatment.

Alprazolam

This benzodiazepine drug is generally used for the short-term treatment of moderate to severe anxiety states. It has been shown in a single placebo controlled trial to reduce essential tremor.[26] The extent to which this or other benzodiazepine drugs act indirectly by suppressing anxiety (which itself worsens tremor) rather than by a fundamental effect on the tremor itself is unclear.

Flunarizine

In one open trial, flunarizine (a selective calcium-channel blocker used in the treatment of migraine and vertigo) at a dose of 10 mg daily was effective in suppressing essential tremor in some patients, though a third developed side-effects (dystonia, parkinsonism, weight gain and depression) and in another third the beneficial effect was not sustained.[27] Other authors reported that flunarizine was more likely to worsen essential tremor, than improve it.[28]

Nicardipine

A single oral dose of 30 mg nicardipine (also a calcium-channel blocker) has been shown in a placebo-controlled study to reduce tremor amplitude.[29] It is not known whether this beneficial effect is sustained, although at 1 month in a cross-over trial some beneficial activity remained (though the benefit from propranolol was non-significantly greater).[30]

Methazolamide

Initial enthusiasm for the use of this carbonic anhydrase inhibitor in the treatment of essential tremor[31] was largely quelled when a double-blind placebo-controlled trial showed no benefit.[32]

Dystonic tremor

Patients with dystonia frequently have tremor as a component of their movement disorder.[33] In spasmodic torticollis, for example, there is often a mixture of twisting abnormal posture and variable jerky tremor (CD 5.4). In families who carry the gene for idiopathic generalized dystonia, some obligate gene carriers have tremor, but *no* other evidence of dystonia. In these patients it is usual to diagnose the tremor as 'dystonic tremor'. But how would these same patients be diagnosed it they presented *without* a family history of dystonia? Most, I suggest, would be mislabelled as suffering with essential tremor.

There is a considerable literature on the possible relationship between dystonia and peripheral trauma.

Some patients who develop dystonia after trauma have tremor also.[34] It may be, therefore, that dystonic tremor (without other manifestations of dystonia) can occur as a post-traumatic syndrome.

Distinguishing between essential tremor and dystonic tremor

Dystonic tremor is usually postural, localized, and irregular in amplitude and periodicity.[35] Myoclonus is a frequent accompaniment. The overall appearance is often of a 'jerky' tremor (CD 5.5).

Armed with this information, is it possible to make a diagnosis of *dystonic* tremor in a patient, based on the clinical features of the tremor alone? In honesty, this distinction can be very difficult.

Some patients who present with, for example, hand tremor, have asymptomatic dystonia affecting another body part. Quite a common scenario is for a patient to present with a symptomatic hand tremor, but to be unaware of mild torticollis. In such patients, the distant dystonia allows proper classification of the tremor. But when patients have no personal signs of dystonia, or family history of the

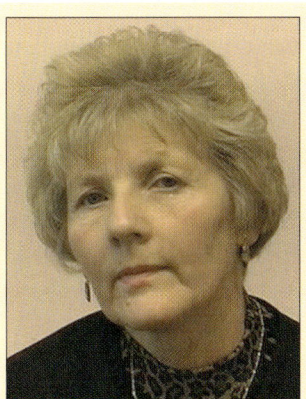

CD 5.4. Torticollis with neck tremor.

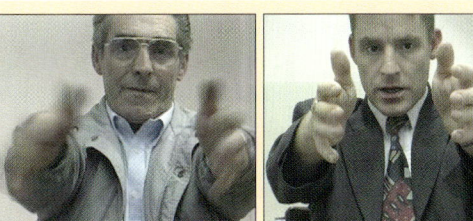

CD 5.5. Dystonic tremor in two generations.

same, it may be impossible to decide whether they have essential tremor or dystonic tremor. If attempted drug treatment for one condition (such as beta blockers for essential tremor) fails, it is reasonable to try therapy aimed at the other (such as an anticholinergic agent for dystonia).

Since essential tremor is a common disorder, we should also bear in mind the likelihood that essential tremor and dystonia will occur together in some patients, quite by chance. Even so, essential tremor is not so common as to explain all of the incidence of tremor in dystonia.[33]

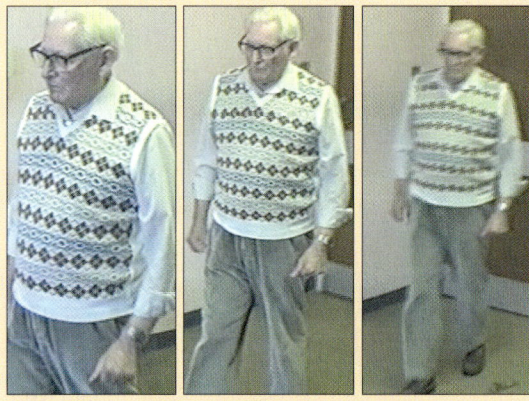

CD 5.6. Pill rolling tremor.

The tremor(s) of Parkinson's disease

Patients who have a resting tremor are likely to be diagnosed as having Parkinson's disease, and in most cases this is correct. But not all patients with Parkinson's disease have a resting tremor, and furthermore some patients have both a resting tremor and a postural tremor whilst others have a postural tremor *only*, at least early in the disease.

Parkinsonian rest tremor

The most characteristic tremor of Parkinson's disease is a pill-rolling 4–6 Hz rest tremor. The phrase 'pill-rolling' refers to the opposing movements of the thumb and index finger, reminiscent of a pharmacist rolling pills by hand in a bygone age (CD 5.6). It is often the presenting symptom in Parkinson's disease.[36]

The hands are most commonly affected (the only site in which pill-rolling is a fair description) but the chin and lips, the trunk and the legs are all commonly affected. It is very *unusual* for the neck to be affected. The tremor is abolished on movement, such as when performing the finger–nose test. Walking, on the other hand, may exacerbate hand tremor to a marked degree (CD 5.7); commonly there is a coincident loss of arm swing. Anxiety worsens the tremor (as it does most symptoms). The tremor is absent during sleep. In some cases a marked resting tremor stops when the arms are lifted and held outstretched, only to return again within a few seconds. This is referred to as re-emergent rest tremor (CD 5.8) and should be distinguished from the more common postural tremor of this condition (see below).

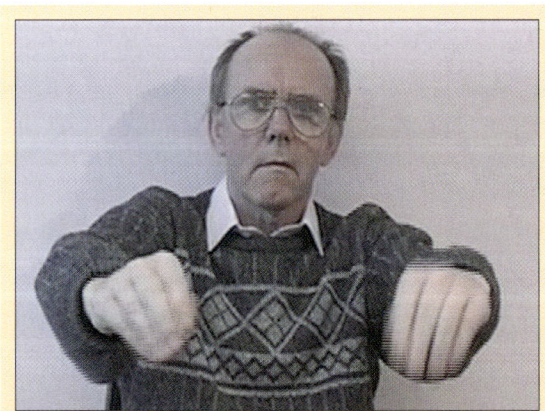

CD 5.7. The effect of walking on parkinsonian rest tremor.

CD 5.8. Re-emergent rest tremor.

As with the other limb signs of Parkinson's disease, the tremor is usually asymmetrical, and it may remain purely unilateral for years. In the early stages it may be intermittent; only evident, for example, when under some kind of duress. Rarely it actually become *less* severe as the disease progresses.[37]

Even though rest tremor is so characteristic of the condition that James Parkinson named it the 'shaking palsy', there has been disagreement about whether patients can truly have long-term Parkinson's disease without ever having a rest tremor. Experts agree that tremor need not be present at the time of diagnosis. Some say that up to 15% 'never' develop tremor,[38] whereas other believe that most, if not all, patients show rest tremor at some stage in their illness.[39] It is possible, of course, that the treatment patients with Parkinson's disease are given for initial bradykinesia and rigidity might mask a mild or moderate resting tremor which would otherwise have been evident if treatment had not been given. The same caveat must be held against the observation of patients with long-term 'pure' hemiparkinsonism. PET scans using fluorodopa may show bilateral disease in apparently unilaterally affected patients even in early disease, and it is not uncommon for hitherto asymptomatic limbs to show obvious signs when medication has to be discontinued for some reason.

Drug treatment

In some patients with Parkinson's disease, tremor is their most disabling symptom. In others, it is obvious but of little practical nuisance or functional significance and such patients should not be treated aggressively in an effort to abolish their tremor for the sake of it. When treatment for tremor is required, several agents have shown to be effective.

Many, but not all, authors have observed a greater effect of anticholinergic drugs on tremor than on rigidity (and, in turn, a greater effect on rigidity than on bradykinesia). Both trihexphenidyl (8 mg daily) and levodopa (300 mg daily with carbidopa 75 mg) were shown to suppress tremor by a mean of 50% in a controlled clinical trial of previously drug naïve patients.[40] Some patients preferred the tremor-suppressing effect of levodopa, whilst others preferred the anticholinergic (trihexphenidyl).

When anticholinergic drugs are used, there is some evidence to suggest that small doses give as much benefit as larger ones. Even in patients who report little obvious improvement on anticholinergics, the tremor often becomes very much more severe when attempts are made to withdraw the drug. Because anticholinergics are widely believed to suppress tremor more than they relieve rigidity and bradykinesia, some doctors suppose that anticholinergic drugs are a more effective agent against tremor than levodopa. The principal difference in efficacy between the two is that levodopa is better than anticholinergics at treating bradykinesia and rigidity. Levodopa may also be (and this has been observed in many studies, but not all) a more effective drug in suppressing tremor. In some of the early studies it was found that tremor initially *worsened* on levodopa, with a reduction in symptom severity with increasing doses. In part, this may have been due to peripheral adrenergic stimulation as the earliest work in this sphere used levodopa without concurrent administration of a peripheral decarboxylase inhibitor.

Amantadine (200 mg daily) has a small (less than 25%) beneficial effect in tremor reduction.[40] Propranolol, when given as an adjunct to levodopa, improves rest tremor in some patients.[41]

Dopamine agonists have a beneficial effect upon tremor, though they tend not to be as powerful as levodopa. All are effective when used as an adjunct to levodopa.

Postural tremor in Parkinson's disease

The postural tremor seen often in Parkinson's disease is faster than the typical rest tremor, the mean frequency being 6 Hz. The postural tremor may precede other symptoms of Parkinson's disease and when this occurs a misdiagnosis of essential tremor is not uncommon.

Drug treatment

The postural tremor of Parkinson's disease responds in some patients to beta blockers[41,42] and to alcohol. Rarely, it may worsen with levodopa, but more commonly it is improved by levodopa, though the degree of improvement may be less than the improvement in resting tremor.[43] Primidone, which is helpful in essential tremor, lacks efficacy in parkinsonian postural tremor.

Is there a relationship between Parkinson's disease and essential tremor?

In considering the relationship between these conditions we must explain several observations.

(i) The incidence of Parkinson's disease in patients with essential tremor is greater than can reasonably be explained by chance alone and has recently been estimated at around 6%[14] (previous higher estimates of up to 20% of essential tremor patients having incidental Parkinson's disease[44] have been criticized on methodological grounds[45]).

(ii) The pathology of the two conditions is very different. Patients with Parkinson's disease have Lewy bodies as do a significant number of patients without evidence of parkinsonism in life (incidental Lewy bodies; subjects widely assumed to have preclinical Parkinson's disease). Yet even 'incidental' Lewy bodies have not been found in the few patients with essential tremor who have come to postmortem.[16]

(iii) PET scans using fluorodopa as ligand show grossly impaired tracer uptake in Parkinson's disease, and have also shown low uptake in some patients in an apparently preparkinsonian state.[46,47] Uptake of the same tracer is normal in patients with essential tremor.[48]

(iv) Patients with Parkinson's disease may have a postural tremor.[43] The postural tremor may begin several years before any other sign of Parkinson's disease; some patients with Parkinson's disease are therefore likely to be misdiagnosed as having essential tremor in the early stages.

(v) If essential tremor were really a precursor of Parkinson's disease, then some signs such as impairment of the sense of smell, which are common in early Parkinson's disease, might be expected to be common amongst patients with essential tremor. But this is not the case.[49]

Piecing these observations together, it seems likely that essential tremor and Parkinson's disease are indeed two quite separate pathophysiological entities. The apparently frequent occurrence of Parkinson's disease in patients with essential tremor may be partly explained by misdiagnosis of the original postural tremor. There may be yet other factors, such as a shared genetic predisposition, which are as yet unrecognized.

Primary writing tremor

The commonest neurological disorder which occurs only on writing is writer's cramp, a focal dystonia. Some patients with writer's cramp develop tremor as well as dystonia. But other patients present with tremor on writing, *without* any evidence of dystonia. This is referred to as writing tremor.

The clinical features are mainly a pronation-supination movement with a frequency of 5–7 Hz. Although it is usually tremor on writing which brings the condition to medical attention, some patients develop a similar tremor in other circumstances, such as using a knife, holding a cup,[50] or swinging a golf club.[51] In patients with tremor limited to writing, it may begin either on adopting the hand position used for writing, or only after writing has begun.[52] Some affected patients also have a postural tremor.[53]

One critical question is whether isolated primary writing tremor is due to dystonia, is a variant of essential tremor, or is a separate clinical entity. The jury is still out on this issue; both data and opinion conflict. Some patients have a positive family history of writing tremor, other forms of tremor, or dystonia. PET studies using oxygen-15 labelled water have shown similar abnormal bilateral cerebellar activation to that seen in patients with essential tremor[54] (Fig. 5.1).

Anticholinergic agents are effective in some patients,[53,55] suggesting a link with dystonia, whilst others respond better to propranolol, primidone, or alcohol,[52] typical of essential tremor. A small number of patients have been treated successfully by stereotactic thalamotomy (lesion site in nucleus ventralis intermedius).[56] Lisuride was effective in one reported patient.[57]

Very rarely, unilateral writing tremor may follow a discrete frontal cortical infarct.[58]

Head tremor

As with primary writing tremor, head tremor can occur in patients who have other evidence of dystonia or

PRIMARY WRITING TREMOR

Sagittal

Coronal

72

R

0

0

32

c v c

64

VPC VAC

−104

68

VPC VAC

SPM
projections

0

c

v

c

64

R

Transverse

Figure 5.1. PET activation scan in writing tremor. Increased activation in vermis (v) and both cerebellar hemispheres (c). (Courtesy of A. Wills.)

essential tremor. In these circumstances, the differential diagnosis may be relatively easy. But there are also patients who have only head tremor, in which case accurate diagnosis can be more difficult. The one condition which should *not* be diagnosed in patients with head tremor is Parkinson's disease. Although jaw and facial tremors are well recognized, head tremor is extremely rare in that condition.

The easiest way to describe the direction of head movement is according to gesture; so a 'yes–yes' tremor is a nodding (vertical, pitch) movement (CD 5.9),

whereas a 'no–no' tremor is a side-to-side (horizontal, yaw) tremor (CD 5.10). In many patients these two combine to produce a complex multidirectional movement; even so, it may be possible on simple inspection to discern the dominant direction of movement.

Not infrequently, head tremors are asymptomatic. I have several times regretted pointing out to a patient who is complaining about a hand tremor that they have a head tremor too! Other patients are greatly disturbed by even the slightest involuntary head movement.

Head tremor in essential tremor

Essential tremor is the commonest identified cause of head tremor. Some patients have a positive family history, whereas others do not. Some patients with essential tremor have an intermittent head tremor which is usually in the 'yes–yes' direction. Less commonly the head is continuously tremulous (except when fully supported at rest) in which case both 'yes–yes' and 'no–no' components are seen.[6] When due to essential tremor, the frequency is usually greater than 7 Hz.

Head tremor in dystonia

Head tremor occurs as a common component of cervical dystonia. It may be the first manifestation of dystonia.[59] Patients may even first have torticollis, then go into spontaneous remission, and then relapse with head tremor.[60] The peak tremor frequency is 5 Hz. Dystonic head tremors are more 'jerky' and disorganized in appearance than those due to essential tremor, and it is more often evident that activity or posture affects the movement severity.[61] Sometimes a sensory trick is effective in stopping a dystonic neck tremor.

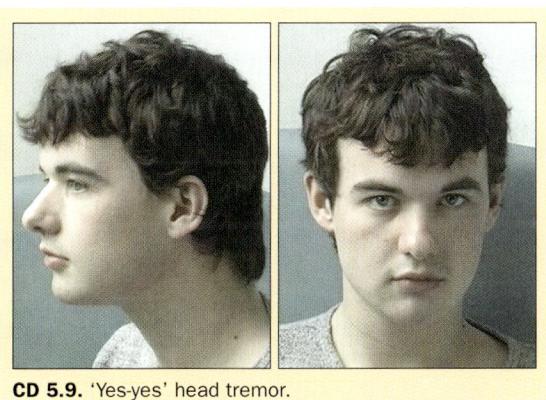

CD 5.9. 'Yes-yes' head tremor.

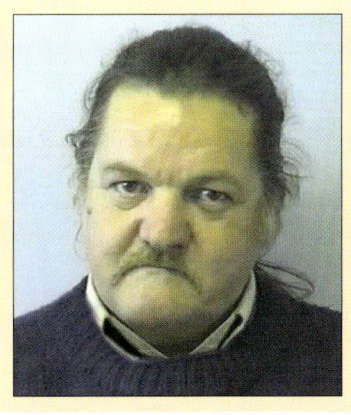

CD 5.10. 'No-no' head tremor.

Head tremor in cerebellar disease

Conditions in which the cerebellum and/or brain-stem–cerebellar connections are affected, such as multiple sclerosis, can cause severe head tremor. Rarely, thalamic, midbrain[62] or cerebellar[63] infarction may be responsible.[62]

Treating head tremors

Propranolol in large doses (160–320 mg/day) and primidone in small doses are sometimes effective treatment[64,65] in head tremor due to essential tremor, though the beneficial effect of propranolol may not be sustained[66] and some patients with dystonic tremor report some benefit too.

Anticholinergic drugs may help dystonic head tremor.

Botulinum toxin has been shown in a placebo controlled trial to be effective in isolated head tremor.[67]

Isoniazid and acetylcholine precursors have been reported to benefit some patients with cerebellar head tremors, but the results of these agents are usually disappointing.

Primary orthostatic tremor
(CD 5.11)

Heilman was the first to describe patients with tremor of the legs and trunk present only when standing.[68]

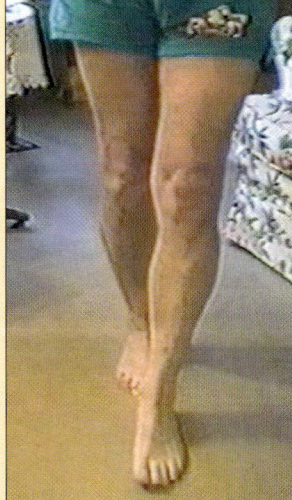

CD 5.11. Orthostatic tremor.

Two were successfully treated with clonazepam. In a general sense other conditions such as Parkinson's disease and essential tremor can cause a tremor or other involuntary leg movements in the *ortho* (upright) *static* (still) position, but the term orthostatic tremor is generally reserved for the specific condition as first described by Heilman.

This tremor is characteristically very fast (14–16 Hz) so that muscle contraction is partially fused and for this reason the subjective experience for the patient varies from a jelly-like sensation of the legs to a feeling of gross unsteadiness or apparent shaking of the whole body. The tremor is too fast to produce a visible oscillation; rather it can more easily be felt by palpation as a rippling movement of the quadriceps. If the muscles of the thigh and calf (particularly quadriceps and hamstrings) are listened to using a stethoscope, a repetitive thumping sound may be heard at either 15–16 Hz or at harmonics of this frequency. This sound has been likened to the noise of a distant helicopter.[69] In some patients the frequency may drop to 7–8 Hz and then the amplitude of muscle movement increases. As soon as patients begin to walk, both the tremor and their feelings of unsteadiness pass. When they stand still again, the symptoms reappear within a few seconds. The arms are generally much less affected than the legs, though some patients have a postural tremor of the outstretched arms of either 8 or 16 Hz. Interestingly, if a patient is asked to crouch on all fours, an otherwise absent 16 Hz arm tremor may be seen. The tremor is present only when weight-bearing; if an affected patient remains in the upright posture, but is lifted up so that his or her feet are no longer in contact with the floor, then the tremor stops.

PET scanning using oxygen-15 labelled water to measure cerebral blood flow, shows abnormal bilateral cerebellar and contralateral lentiform and thalamic blood flow during postural arm tremor in affected patients[70] (Fig. 5.2) (though scans in the upright position are not, of course, possible).

Drug treatment

Modest benefit may be gained from either primidone or clonazepam. Both drugs taken together may be the best option.[71] Alcohol and beta blockers are usually ineffective.

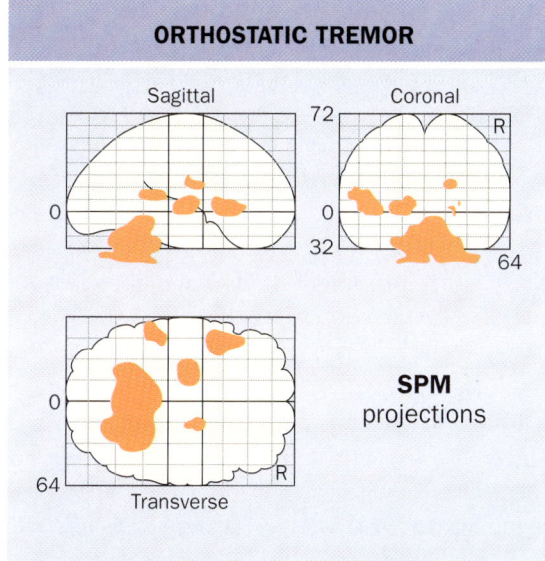

Figure 5.2. PET activation scan in orthostatic tremor. Increased cerebellar, thalamic and lentiform blood flow during postural arm tremor. (Courtesy of A. Wills.)

Cerebellar and midbrain tremors

The commonest kind of tremor associated with dysfunction of the cerebellum and its connections is a kinetic tremor. As the limb approaches a target, its progress is disrupted by jerky movements causing a deviation from the intended direction (CD 5.12). Such tremor may begin at the start of movement. When it is most obvious as the limb approaches the target, it is called an *intention* tremor, and this is the pattern of tremor most characteristic of cerebellar lesions. The amplitude and frequency are variable, the latter being generally low (3–5 Hz).

Clinically the tremor appears most 'wild' when the proximal muscles are affected in addition to distal muscles. For this reason, a patient's posture (lying versus sitting, for example) may define the degree of tremor seen during movement.

Some patients with cerebellar disease also have a more modest postural tremor.

Electrophysiologically, patients with cerebellar tremor have a reaction time which is 60–80 ms longer than normal. Whereas normal human movements are accomplished by an initial agonist burst followed by an antagonist burst and then a second agonist burst, in cerebellar disease not only is the initial agonist burst delayed and prolonged, but the timing of the antagonist and second agonist bursts are temporally smeared and may be superimposed on to the first agonist burst.[72]

Towards the end of an intended movement, if there is a delay in contraction of the antagonist muscle, this leads to an overshoot beyond the target. There follows an increased contraction of the antagonist, causing overshoot in the opposite direction. Continuing erroneous 'corrections' cause the characteristic intention tremor, worsening as the target is approached.

Midbrain (often called 'rubral') tremor refers to the tremor caused by a lesion affecting the cerebellar outflow pathways, or the immediate environment of the red nucleus. There may be a resting tremor, which worsens on trying to maintain a steady posture and is then further and dramatically enhanced on attempting controlled movement. The kinetic tremor is fairly slow (2–5 Hz). Other signs of midbrain disease, such as an occulomotor nerve palsy or hemiparesis, are common.

Cerebellar lesions causing tremor include the demyelinating plaques of multiple sclerosis, infarction, and a host of degenerative disorders (including primary cerebellar degenerations). Lesions in the midbrain are often infarction or haemorrhage, sometimes demyelinating and rarely infective or secondary to trauma.

Drug treatment

Although several drugs have been advocated in the treatment of cerebellar tremor, none are so efficacious as to be more than occasionally helpful. Perhaps best known is the effect of isoniazid which has been shown to provide useful tremor relief in some studies, particularly in patients with severe cerebellar tremor due to multiple sclerosis.[73,74] Isoniazid has also been tried in some patients with otherwise refractory severe essential

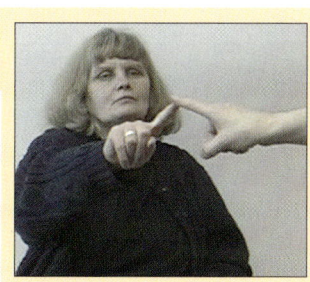

CD 5.12. Cerebellar tremor.

tremor, mostly without benefit.[75] Long-term administration of isoniazid and (separately) propranolol to patients with cerebellar tremor due to either multiple sclerosis or primary cerebellar degeneration in a controlled trial showed no benefit.[76]

Alternative means of helping patients with cerebellar tremor have utilized the observation that adding weights to an affected limb may to some extent dampen the tremor.[77] Efforts to alleviate cerebellar tremor by neurosurgical means have yet to gain widespread support, though some encouraging results have been reported.[78]

Palatal tremor

Rhythmic contractions of the soft palate have variously been called palatal myoclonus, palatal tremor, brainstem myorrhythmia and palatal nystagmus. The term palatal tremor is used here because of the rhythmical nature of the disorder. The principal disadvantage of this nomenclature is that the term palatal myoclonus has been favoured in the past.

History and neuropathology

Palatal tremor was first described in the 1860s and from the early 20th century it has been recognized that many patients develop olivary hypertrophy (for review see Deuschl et al.[79]). Rarely, magnetic resonance imaging (MRI) performed prior to the onset of palatal tremor, has shown bilateral enlargement of the olives.[80] Noting the olivary hypertrophy, Guillain and Mollaret proposed a causal lesion within the triangular relationship joining the red nucleus and ipsilateral inferior olive, and the contralateral dentate nucleus (subsequently known as the 'Guillain–Mollaret triangle'). Two sides of this triangle remain valid; lesions seemingly responsible for palatal tremor have been described in the route from the dentate to the contralateral olive via the superior cerebellar peduncle, red nucleus, and the central tegmental tract. A somatotopic relationship between the dentate and contralateral olive has also been shown.[81]

Because even normal olivary cells can yield spontaneous rhythmical synchronous discharges, and because PET scans using fluorodeoxyglucose as tracer have suggested olivary hypermetabolism,[82] the hypertrophied inferior olive has been considered to be the pacemaker in this condition.

The commonest identified cause of palatal tremor is cerebrovascular disease but a wide range of other disease processes have been reported, including neoplasia, trauma, and inflammation (Fig. 5.3). Uncommonly responsible conditions include multiple sclerosis, Behçet's disease,[83] Krabbe's disease,[84] dialysis encephalopathy[85] and herpes zoster.[86] In more than a quarter of reported patients there are *no* signs of any other condition[79] and imaging studies are normal. Such patients are referred to as having 'idiopathic' palatal tremor.

Clinical features

The mean age at onset in the symptomatic group is 49, while the idiopathic patients are typically younger, having a mean age at onset of 30. Because the diseases most commonly responsible for symptomatic palatal tremor are more common in men (stroke and head injury) the symptomatic form of the disorder is also more common in men (approximately 2:1), whereas there is no sexual preponderance in patients with essential palatal tremor.

There is usually synchronized movement of the soft palate and pharynx (CD 5.13), but other brainstem innervated muscles may be affected too, including the external ocular muscles and the diaphragm. When the eyes are involved they show pendular nystagmus. Complaints of oscillopsia are uncommon. The frequency of movement is most often 100–150 per minute, though exceptionally there may be as few as 20[87] or as many as 600[88] movements per minute. In 80% the movements are bilateral and symmetrical.

The palatal movement itself may be asymptomatic, in which case it is the involvement of other muscles which draws the condition to the patient's attention. When the tensor veli palatini muscle is involved (as it very often is in patients with essential palatal tremor), this causes a clicking sound as the inner end of the eustachian tube opens and closes with each movement. Rarely, ear clicks are due to movement of the *levator veli palatini* muscle.[89]

While patients are awake, the movements are continuous, except when interrupted by voluntary muscle contraction. The movements classically continue during sleep, although the frequency and amplitude of movement may vary according to sleep stage.[90] It is usual for the condition to be lifelong,

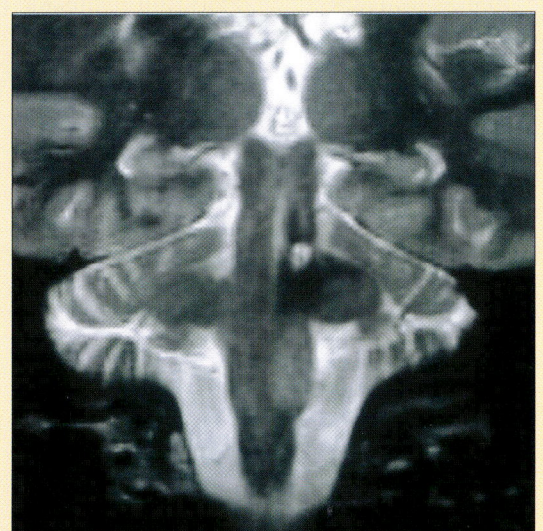

Figure 5.3. MRI scan of olivary hypertrophy in a patient with a pontine cavernous haemangioma. (Courtesy of N. McConachie.)

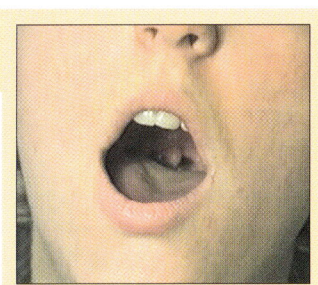

CD 5.13. Palatal tremor (myoclonus).

once it has started. Symptomatic palatal tremor persists even during narcotic anaesthesia, whereas essential palatal tremor stops.[79]

Treatment
In most cases, drug treatment is unhelpful, though there have been a few reports of patients who have improved with, for example, 5-hydroxytryptophan,[86] carbamazepine,[91] trihexphenidyl,[92] clonazepam,[93] sodium valproate,[94] or baclofen.[95]

Some patients find the ear clicks extremely annoying. Several surgical treatments have been tried. Sometimes cutting the levator palatini or tensor palatini muscle, or weakening the responsible muscle using botulinum toxin injections,[89,96] is helpful.

Vocal tremor

Unlike the movement of other body parts, phonation is itself a means of generating a regular oscillation. Vocal tremor is therefore not a tremor of the cords, but rather a tremulous superimposition on normal speech production, with modulation in the fundamental frequency, frequency spectrum and amplitude. These are the same parameters which vary in normal vibrato singing.

The normal rhythm and tonal variation of speech can be interrupted by a wide variety of tremulous disorders. Up to 20% of patients with essential tremor develop a quavering intonation, most obvious during the pronunciation of sustained vowel sounds. It can even be the presenting symptom of the condition.[97,98] Involvement of the voice is equally common irrespective of the age of onset or presence of a positive family history.[99] Vocal tremor also occurs in dystonia, though adductor and abductor spasms are more common. Patients with cerebellar ataxia may also have a tremulous voice.[100]

When Parkinson's disease affects speech, it more commonly causes difficulty with phonation than articulation. Some develop a mild vocal tremor, most obvious with sustained vowels.[101]

Tremor in neuropathy

Tremor is a common symptom of some kinds of peripheral neuropathy, particularly hereditary motor and sensory neuropathy, chronic inflammatory demyelinating polyneuropathy (CIDP) and benign IgM demyelinating paraproteinaemic neuropathy (Fig. 5.4). Tremor has also been reported alongside peripheral neuropathy in a wide variety of other conditions, although in many cases, such as in drug toxicity and vitamin E deficiency, there are associated CNS changes which may be responsible for the neuropathy.

Tremor in IgM paraproteinaemic neuropathy
Up to 90% of patients with this late onset chronic sensorimotor neuropathy have upper limb tremor.[102] A smaller number of patients with IgM and IgA

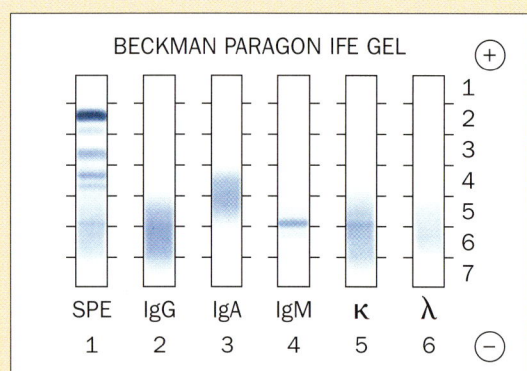

Figure 5.4. Urine protein electrophoresis. Banding pattern indicates IgM κ paraprotein. (Courtesy of N. Kalsheker.)

neuropathy are similarly affected.[103] Motor nerve conduction velocity is very slow, presumed due to the deposition of antimyelin antibody on the myelin sheaths.[104] The tremor is mainly evident on posture and on action (CD 5.14), but there is marked variation in severity between patients. Rarely a 'pill-rolling' tremor typical of the kind seen in Parkinson's disease has been reported.[102] It is usual for sensory loss and weakness to precede the tremor, and this may explain why some authors have found far fewer cases with tremor than others. In some series the degree of tremor has been found to correlate with the loss of upper limb joint position sense,[102] but in other patients this sensory modality is entirely normal.[105] Although the natural course of the neuropathy is a slow progression over 2–5 years with subsequent stabilization,[102] treatment using steroids, cytotoxic agents and immunoglobulin may be effective and in at least some patients the tremor improves also.[106]

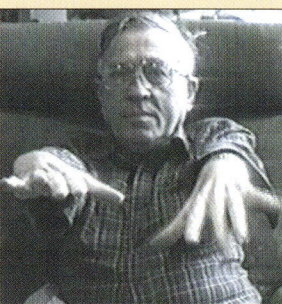

CD 5.14. Tremor in IgM paraproteinopathy.

Propranolol has also been found to reduce tremor in some cases.[106]

Tremor in CIDP

Although probably less common than in IgM paraproteinaemic neuropathy, tremor is a recognized feature of some patients with CIDP.[107,108] Both the tremor frequency and severity vary, but in most cases it is most obvious on posture and action. The neuropathy often responds to corticosteroid treatment, to cytotoxic agents, to plasma exchange or to immunoglobulin therapy; when it does, the tremor usually improves also.[106] Tremor may also (rarely) accompany recurrent Guillain–Barré syndrome.[109]

Tremor in hereditary motor and sensory neuropathy

Patients with Type I hereditary motor and sensory neuropathy (HMSN) may have tremor too. This has been called the Roussy–Lévy syndrome, although evidence that it is a separate clinical entity is lacking.[110] Less often, tremor occurs in patients with Type II (axonal) HMSN.[111] Some patients report benefit from propranolol.[107]

The mechanism of tremor in peripheral neuropathy

Because of the variety of neuropathic conditions which may be associated with tremor, and the lack of consistent relationship between the extent of motor or sensory impairment and tremor severity, it has been suggested that tremor in this context is simply an enhancement of physiological tremor due to minimal weakness.[112] Patients with paraproteinaemic neuropathy do not have overt CNS disease. Detailed neurophysiological studies in patients with benign IgM paraproteinaemic neuropathy have shown triphasic EMG in agonist-antagonist-agonist muscles; but the timing is prolonged and the second agonist burst delayed. Perhaps delayed and distorted cerebellar afferent input is responsible for resetting the intact cerebellum to produce the mis-timed second agonist burst, ultimately leading (through mis-timed corrective movements) to tremor production.[105] Others have argued that an *abnormal* central tremor generator is likely,[107] acting together with a peripheral component, most likely the slowing of sensory conduction.

Tremor due to trauma

Children are more likely than adults to develop tremor after serious head injury (perhaps because they are more likely to survive the kind of injury which gives rise to tremor). Up to 45% of severely head-injured children are said to develop a tremor over the following 18 months.[113]

Most patients who suffer tremor after severe head trauma do so because of injury to the midbrain; hence a midbrain tremor (i.e. a resting tremor, which worsens on posture and is further and dramatically enhanced on attempting movement) is usual, affecting both proximal and distal muscles at a frequency of 1.5–3 Hz.[114] In some patients the tremor appears particularly jerky, with an apparently myoclonic component,[115] though EMG analysis shows the jerks are actually due to sudden increments in the amplitude of the EMG bursts producing the tremor.[116] Many of these patients have other neurological evidence of severe brain trauma, including hemiparesis which typically precedes the tremor. This kind of tremor sometimes responds to treatment with anticholinergic or dopaminergic agents, carbamazepine, or glutethamide.[114,117,118]

Rarely, a postural and kinetic tremor may follow minor head trauma. As with more serious injury, the tremor may be both postural and kinetic, often with myoclonic-like jerking. Clonazepam and propranolol have been shown to help some patients in this context.[119]

Epidemiological studies lend little definitive support to the suggestion that idiopathic Parkinson's disease follows head injury,[120] though there have been occasional reports of a parkinsonian syndrome developing *without Lewy bodies* in patients after head trauma sufficient to cause a skull fracture.[121]

The longer the delay between trauma and the onset of tremor, the more difficult it is to be sure of the causal relationship. Nevertheless, it appears that the onset of genuine post-traumatic tremor may be delayed for many weeks after the original insult. Rarely, patients develop a cerebellar syndrome with a comprehensive set of cerebellar signs (including an intention tremor) as long as 2 years after head injury. Perhaps such a long interval indicates that this syndrome is due to the development of postsynaptic supersensitivity in involved brainstem or thalamic pathways.[122]

Injury to the limbs is even more rarely followed by tremor than injury to the head. But just as there are a number of reports of dystonia beginning in a limb which has suffered recent trauma, so also has tremor been described following limb trauma. It may be that an increase in afferent input to the spinal cord (including substance P containing neurons) acts via the sympathetic nervous system to excite anterior horn cells, hence inducing tremor (or other forms of involuntary movement).[123]

Aside from the direct effects of physical injury, patients may suffer an anxiety-related tremor as a component of the post-traumatic stress disorder, whether or not it follows any kind of injury to the head. Such a tremor may be intermittent and induced by particular subsequent stimuli (such as noise).[124]

Post-traumatic kinetic tremor may respond to stereotactic procedures which target the thalamus[115] and zona incerta; but persisting side-effects are common.[125] The improvement in tremor severity may be less than expected in patients with Parkinson's disease.[126] Thalamic stimulation of the ventralis intermedius nucleus has also been shown to be effective.[127]

Drug-induced tremor

Drugs are a common cause of tremor (see Chapter 11).

References

1. Elble R J, Koller W C. Tremor. Baltimore: Johns Hopkins, 1990

2. Koller W, Findley L J, de Witt P et al. Classification and definition of tremor. World Neurology, 1993

3. Bain P G, Findley L J, Atchison P et al. Assessing tremor severity. J Neurol Neurosurg Psychiat 1993; 56: 868–873

4. Marsden C D. Origins of normal and pathological tremor. In: Findley L J, Capildeo R (eds) Movement disorders: Tremor. New York: Oxford University Press, 1984: 37–84

5. Critchley M. Observations on essential (heredofamilial) tremor. Brain 1949; 72: 113–139

6. Bain P G, Findley L J, Thompson P D et al. A study of hereditary essential tremor. Brain 1994; 117: 805–824

7. Larsson T, Sjögren T. Essential tremor: A clinical and genetic population study. Acta Psychiat Scand 1960; 36 (Suppl. 144): 1–176

8. Bharucha N E, Bharucha E P, Bharucha A E et al. Prevalence of essential tremor in the Parsi community of Bombay, India. Arch Neurol 1988; 45: 907–908

9. Haerer A F, Anderson D W, Schoenberg B S. Prevalence of essential tremor: Results from the Copiah County study. Arch Neurol 1982; 39: 750–751

10. Rajput A H, Offord K P, Beard C M, Kurland L T. Essential tremor in Rochester, Minnesota: A 45 year study. J Neurol Neurosurg Psychiat 1984; 47: 466–470

11. Salemi G, Savettieri G, Rocca W A et al. Prevalence of essential tremor: A door-to-door survey in Terrasini, Italy. Neurology 1994; 44: 61–64

12. Ichinose H, Ohye T, Takahashi E I et al. Hereditary progressive dystonia with marked diurnal fluctuation caused by mutations in the GTP cyclohydrolase I gene. Nature Gen 1994; 8: 236–242

13. Dürr A, Stevanin G, Jedynak C P et al. Familial essential tremor and idiopathic torsion dystonia are different genetic entities. Neurology 1993; 43: 2212–2214

14. Koller W C, Busenbark K, Miner K, Essential Tremor Study Group. The relationship of essential tremor to other movement disorders: Report on 678 patients. Ann Neurol 1994; 35: 717–723

15. Fletcher N A, Harding A E, Marsden C D. A genetic study of idiopathic torsion dystonia in the United Kingdom. Brain 1990; 113: 379–395

16. Rajput A H, Rozdilsky B, Ang L, Rajput A. Clinicopathologic observations in essential tremor: Report of six cases. Neurology 1991; 41: 1422–1424

17. Colebatch J G, Findley L J, Frackowiak R S J et al. Preliminary report: Activation of the cerebellum in essential tremor. Lancet 1990; 336: 1028–1030

18. Jenkins I H, Bain P G, Colebatch J G et al. A positron emission tomography study of essential tremor: Evidence for overactivity of cerebellar connections. Ann Neurol 1993; 34: 82–90

19. Poirier L J, Sourkes T L, Bouvier G, Boucher R, Carabin S. Striatal amines, experimental tremor and the effect of harmaline in the monkey. Brain 1966; 89: 37–52

20. Koller W C. Alcoholism in essential tremor. Neurology 1983; 33: 1074

21. Boecker H, Wills A J, Ceballos-Baumann A et al. The effect of alcohol on alcohol-responsive essential tremor: A positron emission tomographic study. Ann Neurol 1996; 39: 650–658

22. Koller W C. Dose–response relationship of propranolol in the treatment of essential tremor. Arch Neurol 1986; 43: 42–43

23. Larsen T A, Calne D B. Essential tremor. Clin Neuropharmacol 1983; 6: 185–206

24. Jefferson D, Jenner P, Marsden C D. β-Adrenoceptor antagonists in essential tremor. J Neurol Neurosurg Psychiat 1979; 42: 904–909

25. O'Brien M D, Upton A R, Toseland P A. Benign familial tremor treated with primidone. Br Med J 1981; 282: 178

26. Huber S J, Paulson G W. Efficacy of alprazolam for essential tremor. Neurology 1988; 38: 241–243

27. Biary N, Al Deeb S M, Bahou Y. Long-term therapy of essential tremor with flunarizine. Eur Neurol 1995; 35: 217–219

28. Curran T, Lang A E. Flunarizine in essential tremor. Clin Neuropharmacol 1993; 16: 460–463

29. Garcia Ruiz P J, De Yebenez P J G, Jimenez-Jimenez F J. Effect of nicardipine on essential tremor: Brief report. Clin Neuropharmacol 1993; 16: 456–459

30. Jimenez-Jimenez F J, Garcia Ruiz P J, Cabrera Valdivia F. Nicardipine versus propranolol in essential tremor. Acta Neurol Scand 1994; 49: 184–188

31. Muenter M D, Daube J R, Caviness J N, Miller P M. Treatment of essential tremor with methazolamide. Mayo Clin Proc 1991; 66: 991–997

32. Busenbark K, Pahwa R, Hubble J et al. Double-blind controlled study of methazolamide in the treatment of essential tremor. Neurology 1993; 43: 1045–1047

33. Dubinsky R M, Gray C S, Koller W C. Essential tremor and dystonia. Neurology 1993; 43: 2382–2384

34. Jankovic J, Van der Linden C. Dystonia and tremor induced by peripheral trauma: Predisposing factors. J Neurol Neurosurg Psychiat 1988; 51: 1512–1519

35. Jedynak C P, Bonnet A M, Agid Y. Tremor and idiopathic dystonia. Mov Disord 1991; 6: 230–236

36. Hoehn M M, Yahr M D. Parkinsonism: Onset, progression, and mortality. Neurology 1967; 17: 427–442

37. Stern G. Prognosis in Parkinson's disease. In: Marsden C D, Fahn S (eds) Movement disorders 2. London: Butterworth & Co, 1987: 91–98

38. Jankovic J. Pathophysiology and clinical assessment of motor symptoms in Parkinson's disease. In: Koller W C (ed) Handbook of Parkinson's disease. New York: Marcel Dekker, 1987: 99–126

39. Rajput A H, Rozdilsky B, Ang L. Occurrence of resting tremor in Parkinson's disease. Neurology 1991; 41: 1298–1299

40. Koller W C. Pharmacologic treatment of parkinsonian tremor. Arch Neurol 1986; 43: 126–127

41. Koller W C, Herbster G. Adjuvant therapy of parkinsonian tremor. Arch Neurol 1987; 44: 921–923

42. Owen D A L, Marsden C D. Effect of adrenergic beta-blockade on parkinsonian tremor. Lancet 1965; 2: 1259–1262

43. Koller W C, Overfield B V, Baxter R. Tremors in early Parkinson's disease. Clin Neuropharmacol 1989; 12: 293–297

44. Lou J J, Jankovic J. Essential tremor: Clinical correlates in 350 patients. Neurology 1991; 41: 234–238

45. Lang A E, Quinn N P, Marsden C D. Essential tremor (letter). Neurology 1992; 42: 1432–1433

46. Calne D B, Langston J W, Martin W R W et al. Positron emission tomography after MPTP: Observations relating to the cause of Parkinson's disease. Nature 1985; 317: 246–248

47. Sawle G V, Wroe S J, Lees A J et al. The identification of presymptomatic parkinsonism: Clinical and [18F]Dopa PET studies in an Irish kindred. Ann Neurol 1992; 32: 609–617

48. Brooks D J, Playford E D, Ibanez V et al. Isolated tremor and disruption of the nigrostriatal dopaminergic system. Neurology 1992; 42: 1554–1560

49. Busenbark K, Huber S, Greer G et al. Olfactory function in essential tremor. Neurology 1992; 42: 1631–1632

50. Rothwell J C, Traub M M, Marsden C D. Primary writing tremor. J Neurol Neurosurg Psychiat 1979; 42: 1106–1114

51. Kachi T, Rothwell J C, Cowan J M A, Marsden C D. Writing tremor: Its relationship to benign essential tremor. J Neurol Neurosurg Psychiat 1985; 48: 545–550

52. Bain P G, Findley L J, Britton T C et al. Primary writing tremor. Brain 1995; 118: 1461–1472

53. Klawans H L, Glantz R, Tanner C M, Goetz C G. Primary writing tremor: A selective action tremor. Neurology 1982; 32: 203–206

54. Wills A J, Jenkins I H, Thompson P D et al. A positron emission tomography study of cerebral activation associated with essential and writing tremor. Arch Neurol 1995; 52: 299–305

55. Ravits J, Hallett M, Baker M, Wilkins D. Primary writing tremor and myoclonic writer's cramp. Neurology 1985; 35: 1387–1391

56. Ohye C, Miyazaki M, Hirai T et al. Primary writing tremor treated by stereotactic selective thalamotomy. J Neurol Neurosurg Psychiat 1982; 45: 988–997

57. Torun S, Erdinc O. Suppression of primary writing tremor by lisuride. A case report. Eur J Neurol 1996; 3: 71–74

58. Kim J S, Lee M C. Writing tremor after discrete cortical infarction. Stroke 1994; 25: 2280–2282

59. Rivest J, Marsden C D. Trunk and head tremor as isolated manifestations of dystonia. Mov Dis 1990; 5: 60–65

60. Factor S A. Head tremor after a remission of spasmodic torticollis. Mov Dis 1990; 5: 353–354

61. Mossman S, Cleeves L, Findley L. The influence of head position upon head tremor (2). J Neurol Neurosurg Psychiat 1992; 55: 1209–1210

62. Otto S, Buttner T, Schols L et al. Head tremor due to bilateral thalamic and midbrain infarction [1]. J Neurol 1995; 242: 608–610

63. Finsterer J, Muellbacher W, Mamoli B. Yes/yes head tremor without appendicular tremor after bilateral cerebellar infarction. J Neurol Sci 1996; 139: 242–245

64. Koller W C. Propranolol therapy for essential tremor of the head. Neurology 1984; 34: 1077–1079

65. Findley L J, Cleeves L, Calzetti S. Primidone in essential tremor of the hands and head: A double blind controlled clinical study. J Neurol Neurosurg Psychiat 1985; 48: 911–915

66. Calzetti S, Sasso E, Negrotti A et al. Effect of propranolol in head tremor: Quantitative study following single-dose and sustained drug administration. Clin Neuropharmacol 1992; 15: 470–476

67. Pahwa R, Busenbark K, Swanson-Hyland E F et al. Botulinum toxin treatment of essential head tremor. Neurology 1995; 45: 822–824

68. Heilman K M. Orthostatic tremor. Arch Neurol 1984; 41: 880–881

69. Brown P. New clinical sign for orthostatic tremor. Lancet 1995; 346: 306–307

70. Wills A J, Thompson P D, Findley L J, Brooks D J. A positron emission tomography study of primary orthostatic tremor. Neurology 1996; 46: 747–752

71. Poersch M. Orthostatic tremor: Combined treatment with primidone and clonazepam. Mov Dis 1996; 9: 467

72. Rondot P, Bathien N. Cerebellar tremors: Physiological basis and treatment. In: Findley L J, Koller W C (eds) Handbook of tremor disorders. New York: Marcel Dekker Inc., 1995: 371–385

73. Hallett M, Lindsey J W, Adelstein B D, Riley P O. Controlled trial of isoniazid therapy for severe postural cerebellar tremor in multiple sclerosis. Neurology 1985; 35: 1374–1377

74. Morrow J, McDowell H, Ritchie C, Patterson V. Isoniazid and action tremor in multiple sclerosis. J Neurol Neurosurg Psychiat 1985; 48: 282–283

75. Hallett M, Ravits J, Dubinsky R M et al. A double blind trial of isoniazid for essential tremor and other action tremors. Mov Dis 1991; 6: 253–256

76. Koller W C. Pharmacologic trials in the treatment of cerebellar tremor. Arch Neurol 1984; 41: 280–281

77. Langton Hewer R, Cooper R, Morgan M H. An investigation into the value of treating intention tremor by weighting the affected limb. Brain 1972; 95: 579–590

78. Narabayashi H. Surgical approach to tremor. In: Marsden C D, Fahn S (eds) Movement disorders. London: Butterworth Scientific, 1982: 292–299

79. Deuschl G, Mischke G, Schenck E et al. Symptomatic and essential rhythmic palatal myoclonus. Brain 1990; 113: 1645–1672

80. Yokota T, Tsukagoshi H. Olivary hypertrophy precedes the appearance of palatal myoclonus. J Neurol 1991; 238: 408

81. Lapresle J, Ben Hamida M. The dentato-olivary pathway. Arch Neurol 1970; 22: 135–143

82. Dubinsky R M, Hallett M, Di Chiro G et al. Increased glucose metabolism in the medulla of patients with palatal myoclonus. Neurology 1991; 41: 557–562

83. Shuttleworth E C, Voto S, Sahar D. Palatal myoclonus in Behçet's disease. Arch Intern Med 1985; 145: 949–950

84. Yamanouchi H, Kasai H, Sakuragawa N, Kurokawa T. Palatal myoclonus in Krabbe disease. Brain Dev 1991; 13: 355–358

85. Snider W D, DeMaria A A Jr, Mann J D. Diazepam and dialysis encephalopathy. Neurology 1979; 29: 414–415

86. Williams A, Goodenberger D, Calne D B. Palatal myoclonus following herpes zoster ameliorated by 5-hydroxytryptophan and carbidopa. Neurology 1978; 28: 358–359

87. Alajouanine Th, Thurel R, Wolfromm R. Myoclonies rythmiques du voile, de la glotte et du diaphragme, survant par accès périodiques et se traduisant par du hoquet. Revue Neurologique 1944; 76: 96–97

88. Frank H, Chantraine A, Melon J, Mouchette R. Le syndrome clonique du voile du palais (5 observations). Etude clinique, électromyographique et cinématographique. Revue Neurologique 1965; 113: 46–56

89. Jamieson D R S, Mann C, O'Reilly B, Thomas A M. Ear clicks in palatal tremor caused by activity of the levator veli palatini. Neurology 1996; 46: 1168–1169

90. Kayed K, Sjaastad O, Magnussen I, Marvik R. Palatal myoclonus during sleep. Sleep 1983; 6: 130–136

91. Sakai T, Shiraishi S, Murakami S. Palatal myoclonus responding to carbamazepine. Ann Neurol 1981; 9: 199–200

92. Jabbari B, Gunderson C H. Palatal myoclonus responding to trihexphenidyl. Ann Neurol 1983; 14: 951

93. Bakheit A, Behan P O. Palatal myoclonus successfully treated with clonazepam. J Neurol Neurosurg Psychiat 1990; 53: 806

94. Borggreve F, Hageman G. A case of idiopathic palatal myoclonus: Treatment with sodium valproate. Eur Neurol 1991; 31: 403–404

95. Brown P. Myoclonus: A practical guide to drug therapy. CNS Drugs 1995; 3: 22–29

96. Varney S M, Demetroulakos J L, Fletcher M H et al. Palatal myoclonus: Treatment with clostridium botulinum toxin injection. Otolaryngology – Head and Neck Surgery 1996; 114: 317–320

97. Brown J R, Simonson J. Organic voice tremor: A tremor of phonation. Neurology 1963; 13: 520–525

98. Tomoda H, Kuroda Y, Shibasaki H, Shin T. A case of essential tremor presenting with marked voice tremor. Clin Neurol 1985; 25: 16–20

99. Lou J S, Jankovic J. Essential tremor: Clinical correlates in 350 patients. Neurology 1991; 41: 234–238

100. Ackermann H, Ziegler W. Cerebellar voice tremor: An acoustic analysis. J Neurol Neurosurg Psychiat 1991; 54: 74–76

101. Stewart C, Winfield L, Hunt A et al. Speech dysfunction in early Parkinson's disease. Mov Dis 1995; 10: 562–565

102. Smith I S. The natural history of chronic demyelinating neuropathy associated with benign IgM paraproteinaemia: A clinical and neurophysiological study. Brain 1994; 117: 949–957

103. Yeung K B, Thomas P K, King R H M et al. The clinical spectrum of peripheral neuropathies associated with benign monoclonal IgM, IgG and IgA paraproteinaemia: Comparative clinical, immunological and nerve biopsy findings. J Neurol 1991; 238: 383–391

104. Smith I S, Kahn S N, Lacey B W et al. Chronic demyelinating neuropathy associated with benign IgM paraproteinaemia. Brain 1983; 106: 169–195

105. Bain P G, Britton T C, Jenkins I H et al. Tremor associated with benign IgM paraproteinaemic neuropathy. Brain 1996; 119: 789–799

106. Dalakas M C, Teravainen H, Engel W K. Tremor as a feature of chronic relapsing and dysgammaglobulinemic polyneuropathies. Incidence and management. Arch Neurol 1984; 41: 711–714

107. Smith I S. Tremor in peripheral neuropathy. In: Findley L J, Koller W C (eds) Handbook of tremor disorders. New York: Marcel Dekker, 1995: 443–454

108. Dalakas M C, Engel W K. Chronic relapsing (dysimmune) polyneuropathy: Pathogenesis and treatment. Ann Neurol 1981; 9 (Suppl.): 134–145

109. Grand-Maison F, Feasby T E, Hahn A F, Koopman W J. Recurrent Guillain–Barre syndrome. Clinical and laboratory features. Brain 1992; 115: 1093–1106

110. Barbieri F, Filla A, Ragno M et al. Evidence that Charcot–Marie–Tooth disease with tremor coincides with the Roussy–Levy syndrome. Can J Neurol Sci 1984; 11: 534–540

111. Harding A E, Thomas P K. The clinical features of hereditary motor and sensory neuropathy types I and II. Brain 1980; 103: 259–280

112. Said G, Bathien N, Cesaro P. Peripheral neuropathies and tremor. Neurology 1982; 32: 480–485

113. Johnson S L J, Hall D M B. Post-traumatic tremor in head injured children. Arch Dis Childhood 1992; 67: 227–228

114. Samie M R, Selhorst J B, Koller W C. Post-traumatic midbrain tremors. Neurology 1990; 40: 62–66

115. Andrew J, Fowler C J, Harrison M J G. Tremor after head injury and its treatment by stereotaxic surgery. J Neurol Neurosurg Psychiat 1982; 45: 815–819

116. Obeso J A, Narbona J. Post-traumatic tremor and myoclonic jerking. J Neurol Neurosurg Psychiat 1983; 46: 788

117. Harmon R L, Long D F, Shirtz J. Treatment of post-traumatic midbrain resting-kinetic tremor with combined levodopa/carbidopa and carbamazepine. Brain Inj 1991; 5: 213–218

118. Aisen M L, Holzer M, Rosen M et al. Glutethimide treatment of disabling action tremor in patients with multiple sclerosis and traumatic brain injury. Arch Neurol 1991; 48: 513–515

119. Biary N, Cleeves L, Findley L, Koller W. Post-traumatic tremor. Neurology 1989; 39: 103–106

120. Factor S A, Weiner W J. Prior history of head trauma in Parkinson's disease. Mov Dis 1991; 6: 225–229

121. Bruetsch W L, DeArmond M. The parkinsonian syndrome due to trauma. A clinicoanatomical study of a case. J Nerv Ment Dis 1935; 81: 531–543

122. Louis E D, Lynch T, Ford B et al. Delayed-onset cerebellar syndrome. Arch Neurol 1996; 53: 450–454

123. Curran T G, Lang A E. Trauma and tremor. In: Findley L J, Koller W C (eds) Handbook of tremor disorders. New York: Marcel Dekker, 1995: 411–428

124. Walters A S, Hening W A. Noise-induced psychogenic tremor associated with post-traumatic stress disorder. Mov Dis 1992; 7: 333–338

125. Krauss J K, Mohadjer M, Nobbe F, Mundinger F. The treatment of posttraumatic tremor by stereotactic surgery. Symptomatic and functional outcome in a series of 35 patients. J Neurosurg 1994; 80: 810–819

126. Jankovic J, Cardoso F, Grossman R G et al. Outcome after stereotactic thalamotomy for parkinsonian, essential, and other types of tremor. Neurosurgery 1995; 37: 680–687

127. Broggi G, Brock S, Franzini A, Geminiani G. A case of posttraumatic tremor treated by chronic stimulation of the thalamus. Mov Dis 1993; 8: 206–208

chapter 6

Dystonia

Guy Sawle

Dystonia is perhaps the least recognized and poorest understood of the common movement disorders. Patients with dystonia are varied in the extreme and to the casual observer there might seem little connection between an elderly patient who cannot keep their eyes open, and a child with generalized torsion dystonia. Yet these patients share a common kind of involuntary movement.

More than any other kind of movement disorder, patients with focal dystonias have been considered to be mad. It is still not uncommon to see a patient with obvious dystonia who has already been referred to and seen by a psychiatric colleague. Some have been treated for depression or other psychopathology. Many others have been simply left to their own devices on the assumption that nothing useful can be done.

Oppenheimer is credited with having been the first to coin the word 'dystonia' in 1911. He used the term to refer to variability of muscle tone between hypotonia and spasm, changes in tone sometimes being due to activity. He was describing a syndrome which had been reported some 3 years earlier by Schwalbe who had described a family of three affected siblings with what he had called 'chronic cramp syndrome with hysterical symptoms'. Schwalbe thought the problem was a psychological one, whilst Oppenheimer considered it to be a physical disease. So in a way, very little has changed; two doctors looking at the same patient with dystonia may still disagree. A neurologist should recognize the illness as an organic movement disorder, while other practitioners may yet assume that the disorder has an entirely psychological basis.

The more difficult problem in movement disorder practice today is in the interpretation of patients whose movements look odd, even for dystonia, yet who just *might* have organic dystonia.

Since Oppenheimer's description, there have been many efforts to define exactly what is meant by dystonia. A workable, sensible, and contemporary definition is *A syndrome dominated by sustained muscle contractions, frequently causing twisting and repetitive movements, or abnormal postures*.[1]

Is dystonia a symptom, sign, syndrome or a disease?

Despite this eloquent definition, we must still grapple with the reality that 'dystonia' is used to mean different things in different circumstances. The classical idiopathic generalized condition with onset usually in childhood, formerly referred to as dystonia musculorum deformans, is now typically referred to as idiopathic generalized dystonia. But this is often abbreviated to 'dystonia'; so dystonia can mean a specific disease.

Next, dystonia can mean a clinical syndrome, since a patient may have an illness where the only or the dominant clinical manifestation is dystonia, yet where there is clearly another recognizable and diagnosable cause, such as Wilson's disease or a basal ganglia stroke.

Thirdly, dystonia is used to describe a particular kind of involuntary movement which may of course be seen in the company of other physical signs too; so we may say that a patient with Parkinson's disease has dystonia affecting one leg on waking in the morning. Or we might say that a particular patient has a mixture of chorea, myoclonus and dystonia in order to disentangle the various threads of abnormal movements seen in an effort to better understand their genesis, likely aetiology and possible treatment.

In summary, the single word dystonia may be used in a context-specific way to refer to either a clinical sign, a syndrome, or a particular disease. In this chapter, I consider chiefly those conditions in which the clinical picture is dominated by dystonia. This includes both dystonic syndromes and idiopathic torsion dystonia.

Dystonic movements

In all kinds of usage of the word dystonia, we refer directly or by implication to the manifestation of dystonic movement. The relevant part of the definition above is '*sustained muscle contractions, frequently causing twisting and repetitive movements, or abnormal postures*'. Dystonic movements may affect almost any muscle, either at rest or on action.

Very often the abnormality only becomes evident on moving, and in this case it is referred to as 'action dystonia'. In fact the abnormality may occur *only* on the performance of a particular action such as writing, in which case it is said to be 'task specific'. The observation that patients may develop severe dystonic posturing of the hand when writing and yet may be able to play the piano to a high standard is nowadays recognized as evidence of this task specificity. Yet to the uninitiated this apparent contradiction can still be a foil to the recognition of dystonia as an organic condition.

Sometimes dystonia occurs in a body part during movement of another part (such as dystonia of the left hand when writing with the right hand). This is referred to as 'overflow'. Dystonic movements may of course occur at rest, and patients may also develop sustained dystonic postures. Usually the movements are worsened when patients are anxious or tired. The movements may continue into light (stage I) sleep and follow brief awakenings from stage II sleep, but are generally absent in stage III and IV and REM sleep.[2]

If the spasms are intermittent, rather than sustained, then they may appear jerky in which case the dystonia can appear 'myoclonic'. Some patients with dystonia have tremor and a broad range of frequencies are seen. Whilst many patients have dystonia *and* tremor, others who clearly carry the dystonia gene have tremor *only*. In this case the appearance of the tremor may be similar to that of essential tremor and in an isolated case, precise clinical diagnosis can be difficult. Dystonic tremor is considered in Chapter 5.

Some patients discover sensory tricks, which are manoeuvres that involve cutaneous sensory or proprioceptive feedback to reduce their dystonia. For example, a patient with torticollis may be able to keep their head comparatively straight by touching their chin gently with a finger (CD 6.1), a newspaper, or even a rolled-up umbrella. A variety of 'tricks' have been described; such as patients who are able to inhibit blepharospasm by singing.[3]

Classification

The classification of dystonia can appear initially rather complicated, since it may be easily divided up either according to age of onset, to the part of the body affected, or to the aetiology. Each of these divisions is useful, however, and all are inter-related.

Age of onset

By an arbitrary division of human aging, dystonia coming on in the first 12 years is referred to as *childhood onset*, in the thirteenth to the twentieth year as *adolescent onset* and thereafter *adult onset*. The usefulness of this classification is that age of onset is the single most accurate prognostic factor — childhood onset disease having a worse prognosis, usually with more widespread disease and more serious disability.

Distribution

Dystonia may be generalized or confined to only a part of the body. When confined to one part only, it is referred to as *focal* (e.g. blepharospasm, if the eyelids are affected in isolation). There are three 'intermediate' grades, comprising segmental, multifocal and hemidystonia. *Segmental* dystonia refers to two or more contiguous areas being affected, such as one arm plus the neck. *Multifocal* dystonia refers to two non-contiguous areas being affected, such as one arm and the opposite leg. *Hemidystonia* affects the whole of one side of the body. This is of particular importance, because the chance of finding a structural brain lesion as the cause of dystonia is very much higher in patients with hemidystonia than in patients with other patterns of involvement.[4,5] Lastly, dystonia may be *generalized*.

Aetiology

In some patients, dystonic movements are symptomatic of another identifiable disease. Most simply, hemidystonia may occur as a result of a structural lesion (such as a tumour, haemorrhage, or infarction) affecting the basal ganglia, usually the putamen.

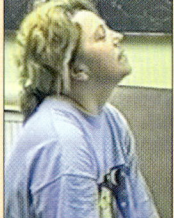
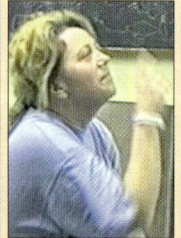
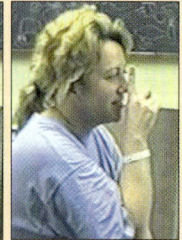

CD 6.1. Geste in cervical dystonia.

More generalized dystonia may be due to a systemic disease with a predilection for the basal ganglia such as Wilson's disease, or it may be due to one of a variety of degenerative disorders. In other patients, there is no clear evidence of an underlying illness; dystonia seems to be the primary condition. In this case the disease is traditionally referred to as *idiopathic* and the disorder may appear clinically to be familial or sporadic.

Idiopathic generalized dystonia

In the classification terms listed above, this condition is typically of childhood onset, it is generalized, and it is idiopathic. So 'idiopathic generalized dystonia' is a fairly satisfactory and non-controversial name. In many ways it is an improvement over some of the terms formerly used to describe the same condition. 'Dystonia musculorum deformans' was one such term. Although it painted a picture in the physician's mind, it was rejected by patients as sounding derogatory and I think it is proper that this term has now largely been dropped. 'Torsion dystonia' has also been used to refer to the same condition. This phrase is less unpleasant than dystonia musculorum deformans, and it remains in use, although because of possible confusion with the syndrome of dystonia, rather than the specific idiopathic generalized condition, 'idiopathic generalized dystonia' may be preferable.

Clinical features

Idiopathic generalized dystonia usually begins in childhood with dystonia of one leg. Initially, the leg inverts and plantar flexes only on walking (action dystonia), but later dystonic spasms occur during other activities and at rest, and other body parts become involved too. This period of progressive deterioration may span five or ten years.

Minute by minute, there may be considerable variation in the severity of the spasms. Patients with idiopathic generalized dystonia may be able to move around surprisingly well, despite what appear as severe and intrusive intermittent and/or continuous spasms.

When the muscles are not in spasm, then the muscle tone is normal. Patients are not weak and nor are they parkinsonian. They may, however, be tremulous.

There is poor correlation between the age of onset among family members, particularly between parent and offspring.[6]

Which patients with focal dystonia will progress to idiopathic generalized dystonia?

As will be appreciated, patients who are destined to develop idiopathic generalized dystonia will actually fulfil different criteria in the aforementioned classification in early disease. In other words, although they later develop idiopathic generalized dystonia, they start off with idiopathic *focal* dystonia. So which patients with focal dystonia are destined to develop generalized disease, and whose symptoms will remain localized to the site of origin?

Significance of site of onset

The closer to the ground the dystonia begins, the more likely the patient is to go on to develop generalized dystonia. In patients whose symptoms begin in the legs, 90% go on to develop symptoms in other body parts, whereas only a third of those whose symptoms begin in the neck develop symptoms elsewhere. Likewise, patients with onset in the lower limbs are more than three times as likely to end up with dystonia affecting all four limbs, than are patients whose symptoms start in the arms.[7]

Significance of age

Of patients with onset before age ten, 85% develop generalized disease, compared with only 59% of those aged ten or over at onset. Site of onset and age at onset are associated; when analysed together for predictive value on the time to spread to another body part, only site of onset is significant.[7]

Genetics

It has long been recognized that the Ashkenazi Jewish population has a higher incidence of generalized dystonia than either the Sephardic Jews or non-Jewish populations. Most reported cases are sporadic, although there are occasional instances of parent and child being affected.[8] For a time, it was proposed that this was due to 'pseudodominance', the situation where (with a high gene frequency in an inbred community) an affected individual marries a carrier,[9] although the condition is now thought to be due to a dominant gene, with very variable penetrance.

In British and French families (both Jewish and non-Jewish) there is a linkage to 9q34 in a subset of families, though there is also clear evidence of genetic heterogeneity.[10] A gene in the same region is implicated in the Ashkenazi Jewish population in the USA[11] (Fig. 6.1). This gene at 9q34, referred to as DYT1, cannot be the cause of all autosomal dominant idiopathic generalized dystonia, since the same region has been *excluded* in an Australian kindred[12] and a large non-Jewish North American family.[13]

Further investigation of the 9q34 region in Ashkenazi Jews with dystonia reveals a marked difference amongst those with dystonia who are carriers or non-carriers of a DYT1-associated haplotype. Amongst carriers of this haplotype, 94% have limb onset (arm and leg being affected first in equal proportions) with only a few percent having onset in the neck or larynx. In non-carriers of the DYT1-associated haplotype, around 80% have onset in the neck, larynx or other cranial muscles, and the remainder have onset in the arms. Onset in the legs appears not to occur in this group.[14] In Ashkenazi Jews with occupational hand dystonia, *no* consistent DYT1 haplotype has been determined.[15] Why is idiopathic generalized dystonia more common amongst the Ashkenazi Jewish population? On the basis of these studies, it is believed that this is the effect of a founder mutation in the DYT1 gene, estimated to have occurred around 350 years ago.[14,16]

In the context of other widespread and profound neurological deficits, dystonia has also been reported to arise from other known genetic defects including deletion of 18q.[17,18]

Genetic studies are made more difficult when the range of onset in a single affected family is very broad. Such is the case in focal dystonia (such as nine members from two generations of a single family with onset at age 8–71 years, mean 37)[19] (Fig. 6.2).

Rarely, focal dystonia (such as adult onset cervical dystonia) may present as an autosomal dominant condition;[20] these patients do not share the same DYT1 haplotype as patients with idiopathic generalized dystonia.

In a genetic study of idiopathic focal dystonia (torticollis, other focal cranial dystonia and writer's cramp) in

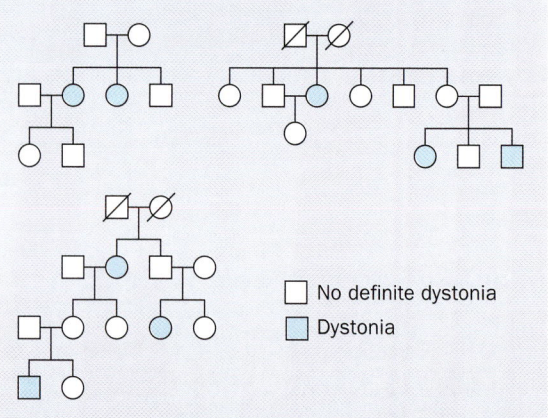

GENETICS OF IDIOPATHIC GENERALIZED DYSTONIA

☐ No definite dystonia
☐ Dystonia

Figure 6.1. Pedigrees of Ashkenazi Jewish families with idiopathic generalized dystonia [11].

the United Kingdom, a quarter of the index cases had relatives with dystonia. The authors suggested that a single autosomal dominant gene might be responsible for most inherited dystonia, irrespective of distribution or severity.[21]

Trauma and idiopathic dystonia

There can be few neurological conditions in which sufferers do not wonder whether a prior history of trauma might be relevant. Doctors have wondered whether local trauma might in some way precipitate dystonia for a long time; in fact Gowers described a patient who developed writer's cramp while recovering from a thumb injury more than 100 years ago.[22] Patients with limb dystonia very often report a prior injury to the affected limb.

Some patients who suffer neck injuries subsequently go on to develop dystonia (Fig. 6.3a,b; CD 6.2).[23] Electrical trauma to an extremity has also been reported to result in dystonia of the electrocuted limb, days to months after the event.[24] Such patients have developed a fixed dystonic posture at rest and some cases have shown additional action dystonia or signs of reflex sympathetic dystrophy .

Dystonia following head trauma is usually associated with brain lesions and is considered below (secondary dystonia).

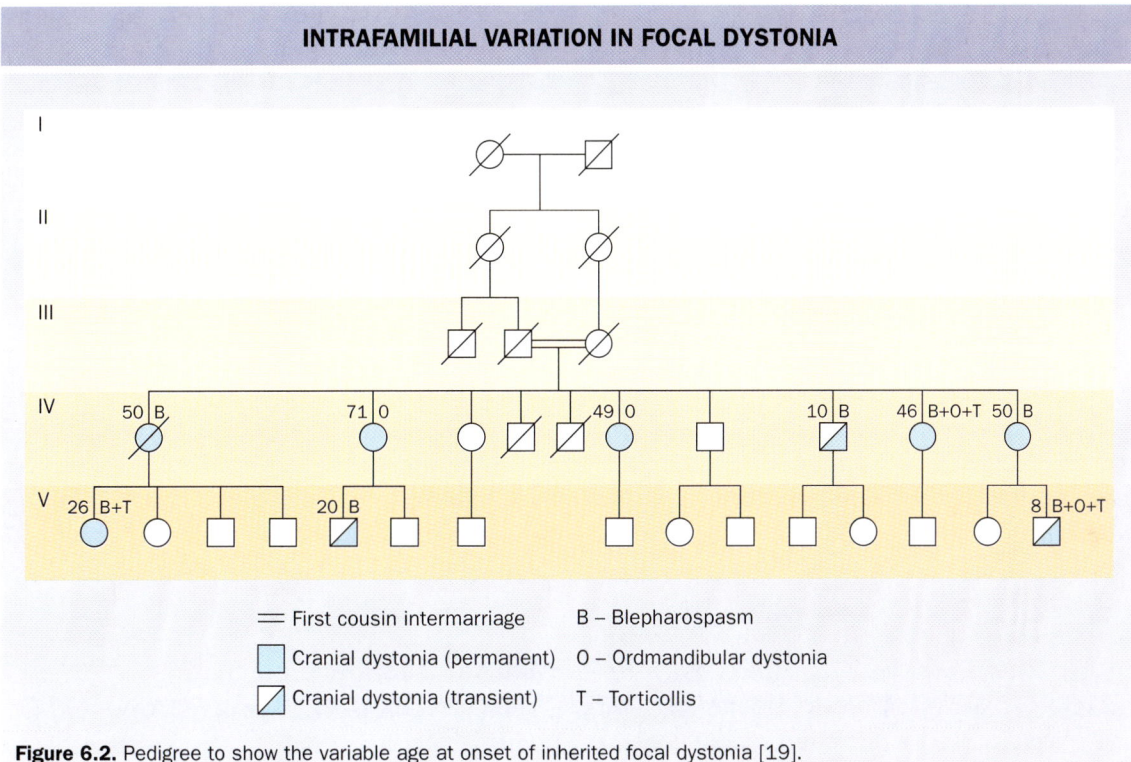

INTRAFAMILIAL VARIATION IN FOCAL DYSTONIA

== First cousin intermarriage   B – Blepharospasm

☐ Cranial dystonia (permanent)   O – Ordmandibular dystonia

⧄ Cranial dystonia (transient)   T – Torticollis

Figure 6.2. Pedigree to show the variable age at onset of inherited focal dystonia [19].

Since considerable numbers of patients with apparently trauma-induced dystonia have affected relatives,[25] it seems reasonable to suppose that peripheral injuries in some way influence basal ganglia function in order to precipitate dystonia in carriers of the dystonia gene. We do not know whether gene carriers are more likely to develop dystonia if subjected to trauma than if they are able to avoid it.

Imaging

Dominantly inherited dystonia with basal ganglia calcification has been described.[26] Rarely, computed tomography (CT) may show putaminal lesions,[27] typically in hemidystonia.

Positron emission tomography (PET) studies using fluorodopa have shown reduced putamen uptake in some cases,[28] but not in others. The significance of this observation is uncertain. Patients with low fluorodopa uptake are not more likely to respond to levodopa than those in whom uptake is normal. During a free-choice joystick activation task in patients with idiopathic generalized dystonia,

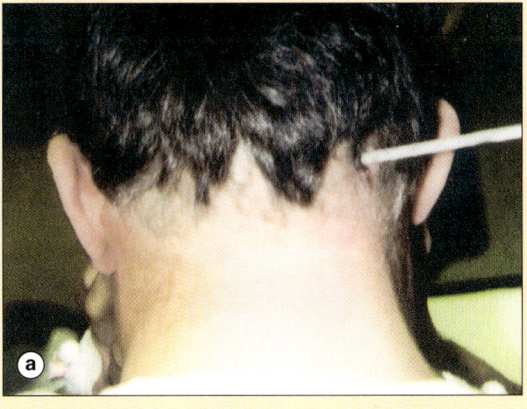

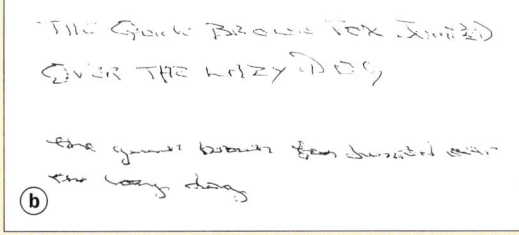

Figure 6.3. (a) Patient impaled on a metal spike. The spike has stopped just short of emerging behind his ear. (b) Handwriting sample following neck injury.

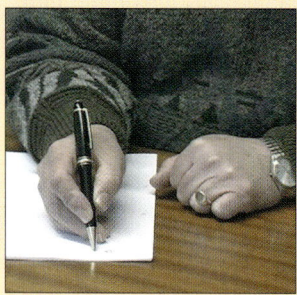

CD 6.2. Dystonia following neck injury. (Same patient as in Figure 6.3a,b.)

regional cerebral blood flow (measured by PET with oxygen-15 labelled water) has been shown to be impaired in the caudal supplementary motor area, bilateral sensorimotor cortex, posterior cingulate and mesial parietal cortex; yet increased in contralateral premotor cortex, rostral supplementary motor area, Brodmann area 8 (frontal eye fields), anterior cingulate, ipsilateral dorsolateral prefrontal cortex and bilateral lentiform nuclei. The proposed interpretation of this complex schema is inappropriate overactivity within striatofrontal projections, together with impaired activation of motor executive areas.[29]

In fluorodeoxyglucose PET scans, lentiform and thalamic metabolism appear to be dissociated, with relative metabolic *over*activity in the lentiform nucleus and the premotor cortices. It is suggested that the hyperkinetic movements in dystonia arise through excessive activity in the direct putamenopallidal inhibitory pathway.[30]

Vibrotactile stimulation of the hand produces a diminished regional blood flow response in sensorimotor cortex in patients with unilateral dystonia.[31] The abnormal response is seen in both hemispheres, even in patients with unilateral dystonia. It has been suggested that this finding indicates an abnormality of central sensorimotor processing. In some cases, such stimulation precipitates dystonic spasms in affected hands.

Pathology

Little is known of the pathological basis of idiopathic generalized dystonia. Two patients examined at postmortem showed no structural abnormalities in basal ganglia, cerebral cortex, higher brainstem nuclei, dorsal raphe or locus ceruleus. Choline acetyltransferase and gamma-aminobutyric acid (GABA) levels were normal in cortex and basal ganglia. Noradrenaline levels were low in the hypothalamus, mamillary body, subthalamic nucleus and locus ceruleus, but high in the septum, thalamus, colliculi, red nucleus and dorsal raphe. Serotonin levels, on the other hand, were decreased in the dorsal raphe and increased in the globus pallidus, subthalamic nucleus, and locus ceruleus. Dopamine was reduced in the accumbens and (in one of two cases) in the striatum. 5-hydroxyindoleacetic acid was increased in the globus pallidus, subthalamic nucleus and raphe.[27,32]

Only a handful of patients with cranial dystonia have come to postmortem. In more than half, histopathological examination of the brain has been entirely normal,[33] whilst some other cases who developed reversible parkinsonism when treated with dopamine antagonists have subsequently shown the typical features of Parkinson's disease.[34]

Medical Treatment

Whilst many drugs have been advocated in the treatment of dystonia (and the multiplicity of tested agents may reflect the poor efficacy of most), oral anticholinergics and botulinum toxin injections are the most widely and effectively used agents. Several of the commonly used drugs are listed briefly below. Specific treatment protocols for focal dystonias are listed together with the relevant clinical descriptions.

Anticholinergics

In the USA trihexphenidyl,[35] and in the UK benzhexol, have been shown to provide symptomatic relief in both children and adults. Treatment using these agents is generally more successful in children than in adults, because they are better able to tolerate the large doses often needed for symptomatic relief.

Tetrabenazine

Although less effective than in the treatment of chorea, tetrabenazine has been shown to suppress dystonia.[36]

Alcohol

Both intravenous and oral alcohol have been shown to temporarily improve dystonia in some patients,[37,38] though the degree of improvement is not usually as striking as that seen in patients with essential tremor, or hereditary essential myoclonus.

Levodopa

The magnitude of clinical response to levodopa in patients with dopa-responsive dystonia (page 108) is dramatic. A patient who has lived for decades by crawling around their home and who has only been out by wheelchair can be transformed over a period of weeks to full upright mobility with good enough function to begin dancing lessons. Just as the only sure way not to miss Wilson's disease in a young dystonic/parkinsonian patient is to check the copper studies in all patients where the diagnosis is even remotely possible, so the conventional way to avoid missing the diagnosis of dopa-responsive dystonia is to treat a broad range of dystonic patients with levodopa. If patients do not respond to levodopa 200 mg three times daily for several weeks, then they probably do not have dopa-responsive dystonia. Some patients with other kinds of dystonia also show some response to levodopa or dopamine agonists, although any improvement is typically modest[39,40] and some patients actually get worse on levodopa rather than better.

Antihistamine

Diphenhydramine, a histamine H1 antagonist with both sedative and anticholinergic properties, has been reported to benefit some patients with idiopathic trunkal dystonia when given either intravenously (50 mg) or orally (up to 500 mg/day).[41] The authors considered that the drug appeared most useful in patients who experienced lightning jerks. Previous experience with intravenous chlorpheniramine showed no benefit.[42]

Botulinum toxin

Judicious injections of botulinum toxin can, through the induction of selective weakness, lead to marked symptomatic benefit in dystonia. The spectrum of dystonic disorders which are considered appropriate for botulinum toxin therapy is constantly rising.

Clearly botulinum toxin cannot be used as a systemic treatment, and it is not a practical treatment for generalized dystonia. It is used chiefly in patients with focal dystonia as described below. In some patients with idiopathic generalized dystonia, aspects of their dystonia (such as blepharospasm) may be successfully alleviated by appropriate injections of botulinum toxin.

Baclofen

As with other drugs used to treat dystonia, better results have been reported from using baclofen in children rather than adults. Up to a third of children have been reported to respond 'dramatically', whilst no more than one in five adults shows even a modest response.[43] A continuous intrathecal infusion of baclofen may provide symptomatic relief in patients for whom oral therapy has been unhelpful.[44–46]

Treating severe dystonia

In patients with severe disabling dystonia, several drugs in combination may provide useful benefit. The combination of an anticholinergic together with pimozide and tetrabenazine has been shown to be an effective approach in adults.[47] In this approach tetrabenazine is started first, aiming for a dose of 75 mg daily (in three divided doses). Next, pimozide is added and the dose increased (in the range 6–25 mg daily) until either the dystonia abates, or else parkinsonism or other side-effects intervene. Next, benzhexol is added (6–30 mg daily), both to control the antidopamine side-effects from the first two agents, and also in an effort to gain further symptomatic control. The merit of this approach is that patients with otherwise untreatable severely disabling disease may be given some respite; the disadvantage is that such aggressive dopamine agonist treatment may lead ultimately to tardive movement disorders. For this reason, high-dose anticholinergic treatment is preferred in the first instance in younger patients.

Surgical treatment

In broad terms, there are two kinds of operations used to treat dystonia. There are procedures in which the surgical target is either the peripheral nerves and/or muscles which execute the dystonic movement. And there are central procedures such as thalamotomy which aim to disrupt central circuitry believed to be involved in the genesis and maintenance of dystonia.

Peripheral surgery for dystonia

The introduction of botulinum toxin has led to a great reduction in the number of such procedures performed. In former years, many patients with torticollis had operations such as cervical rhizotomy (intradural section of the anterior cervical roots at C1–C3 bilaterally), posterior ramisectomy (dividing the dorsal rami outside the dura), or even microvascular decompression of the spinal accessory nerve.[48,49] Complications of these procedures included a feeling that the head and neck had become 'disconnected', neck weakness and dysphagia. These procedures are now very rare; such has been the effectiveness of treatment with botulinum toxin.

Patients with blepharospasm were also formerly treated with a variety of surgical operations, including selective destruction of branches of the facial nerve, and even removal of much of the orbicularis oculi muscle.

Despite such drastic treatments, the blepharospasm returned in many patients, just as torticollis returned in many cases after initially successful surgery. It is assumed that the central mechanisms which determine the (abnormal and unwanted) head posture or eye closure simply recruit other muscles or nerves to execute their will. Similarly, patients in whom peripheral tendon transplants are performed for leg dystonia may enjoy short-lived benefit. But later, many find that their abnormal postures and movements return, now being executed by other muscles from those originally responsible.

Central surgery for dystonia

Although peripheral surgery for dystonia is now much less common, there has been no reduction of interest in central procedures such as thalamotomy and basal ganglia stimulation.

In one retrospective review, 8 of 17 dystonic patients were reported to show moderate improvement immediately after single or bilateral staged thalamotomy. Six maintained their improvement, and two other patients improved during the follow-up period (mean, 37.6 months). The authors noted better long-term outcome in patients with secondary dystonia than in patients with primary dystonia.[50]

Elsewhere, 54 patients with dystonia who underwent thalamotomy were studied prospectively. Twenty-five had torsion dystonia and 29 had secondary dystonia. Fifty-nine percent showed a greater than 25% improvement in symptom severity, while 23% were slightly improved and 16% showed no change or a worsening of symptoms.[51]

The most common side-effects of thalamotomy are contralateral weakness and dysarthria. The latter is far more common when bilateral lesions are necessary; so thalamotomy is best reserved for patients with severe hemidystonia who have proven refractory to other medical treatments.

Studies of pallidotomy and basal ganglia stimulation in dystonia are ongoing.

Task-specific and other focal dystonias

In many patients, focal dystonia is part of the spectrum of generalized dystonia, as a 'forme fruste' of idiopathic generalized dystonia. Nevertheless, it is common for such a task-specific or focal presentation to persist without generalization, particularly in patients who first develop symptoms in adult life.

Task-specific dystonias typically affect the individual's most complex, detailed, or over-learned motor act. For most of us, the most dextrous task we perform is writing, whereas for those who play sport or musical instruments, this may be their most complex motor skill. The issue of repetitive limb use may also be significant; most patients who develop lateralized limb dystonia do so on their motor dominant side.[52]

Writer's cramp

The commonest task-specific dystonia is writer's cramp (CD 6.3) (Fig. 6.4). Patients report a progressive difficulty with writing, even though they may be able to perform other manual activities, some of which may appear to require equal or even greater manual dexterity than writing (CD 6.4). When they start to write, patients often find they are involuntarily gripping the pen harder and harder. This increased muscular activity may spread up the arm, leading to involuntary flexion at the wrist and commonly elevation of the ipsilateral elbow and shoulder. In a minority of patients there is more focal muscle involvement, such as unwanted extension of the index finger during writing (CD 6.5).

Some patients are able to learn to write with their other hand. Some of these patients are lucky, but many go on to develop writer's cramp on that side too; it is

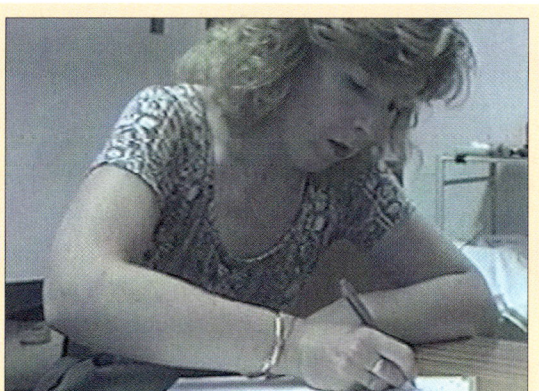

CD 6.3. Writer's cramp: wrist dors: dorsiflexion and elevating elbow.

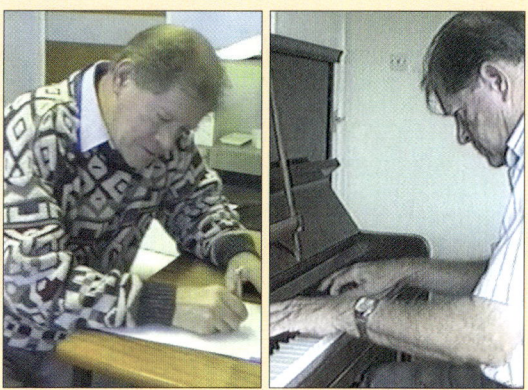

CD 6.4. The same patient writing, and playing the piano.

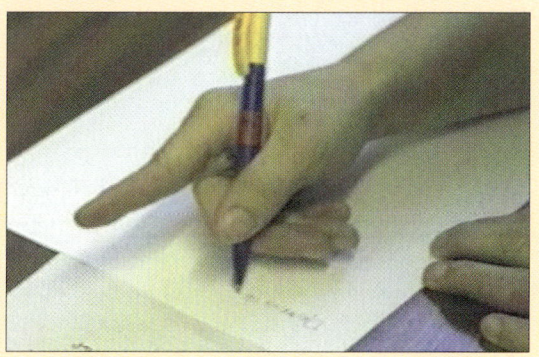

CD 6.5. Writer's cramp: extension of index finger.

Figure 6.4. Handwriting in writer's cramp.

wise to advise patients of this possibility before they embark on what can be an arduous task of learning to write with their non-dominant hand. Other patients derive benefit from adopting a different grip — perhaps holding their pen in a whole-hand grip, rather than their usual writing position. Switching to a fat-bodied pen may help.

For perhaps the majority of patients, however, none of these approaches proves sufficient to enable them to write as well as they need in order to carry on as normal. If they can learn to use a word processor or typewriter instead, that is better, as it is unusual for the dystonia to come to affect that activity also.

Focal hand dystonia is not associated with serious psychopathology.[53]

Some patients with writer's cramp benefit from injections of botulinum toxin,[54] particularly those in whom relatively few muscles seem to contribute to the dystonic contraction.

Sports dystonia
The yips
Golfers have complained for years that they suffer with a variety of jerks, tremors and spasms, particularly when putting. A questionnaire distributed to over 1000 golfers revealed a 28% reported incidence amongst the 42% of responders.[55]

Musician's dystonia
Pianists may develop dystonic hand posturing only when playing the piano. Likewise a variety of other musicians complain of highly and precisely task-specific dystonic movements only when playing their instrument. A French horn player developed a dystonic spasm of the embouchure (pursed lips) which was brought on by lifting his instrument to his mouth in preparation for playing. The effect was to add an unwelcome vibrato to the sound of his instrument. If he held the instrument left-handed and brought it up to his mouth, then there was no problem, except that he could not play his instrument left-handed. Dystonic hand cramps have been reported in (for example) pianists, drummers, violinists and bagpipe players.[53]

Focal dystonia
Blepharospasm

Involuntary eye closure may occur as the sole manifestation of dystonia. Blepharospasm is more common in women than men (sex ratio 1.8:1)[56] with onset typically in the sixth decade. Approximately 10% have a positive family history for dystonia. In many patients, involvement spreads beyond the upper face;[7] but half of these have spasms limited to the muscles of facial expression. In around 20% of patients symptoms ultimately spread beyond the cranial muscles, usually within a few months of onset.

More than half of affected patients recall other ocular symptoms in the weeks and months prior to the onset of blepharospasm.[56] In some cases there is clear-cut evidence of ocular disease, in others the symptoms are less clearly due to independent ocular disease and may be themselves the first symptoms of the impending dystonia (such as excessive blinking).

The symptoms are usually worsened by bright lights (in half), watching television (around half), reading (around one-third), stress (in about 40%) and driving (in about a third).[56] Patients are typically worse when they are out and about, particularly on a bright sunny day, than when at home. They may notice an improvement after sleep, when relaxed, when concentrating, on looking down, or on particular facial movements. Not uncommonly, patients report that their eyes stay open when they visit their doctor who may be perplexed by their story. They walk out of the consulting room feeling somewhat sheepish, and their eyes slam shut again before they leave the building.

Two-thirds of patients are rendered functionally blind; indeed patients may be registered blind, even if they have normal visual acuity when their eyes are open.

The response of blepharospasm to drug treatment is poor, only around 20% responding to anticholinergics and far fewer responding to any other oral medication. Botulinum toxin injections are now the treatment of choice. Previously surgical treatments, such as avulsion of the facial nerve (the so-called 'spaghetti operation') were favoured treatments (although the problem recurred in up to three-quarters of so treated patients), and some patients had their orbicularis oculi muscles all but removed, sometimes on more than one occasion. Other procedures tried in the past include alcohol injections into orbicularis oculi, thermolytic lesions of the facial nerves, blepharoplasty, and stereotactic thalamotomy.

Blepharospasm versus 'apraxia of lid opening'

Many patients with blepharospasm show obvious active contractions of the orbicularis oculi which prevent eye opening. The eyes are not only failing to open, they are being actively squeezed shut. In other cases, however, there may appear to be little to see by way of active muscle contraction; patients simply report that they cannot open their eyes. This latter condition has been called an 'apraxia of eyelid opening',[57] and 'levator inhibition'.[58] Electrophysiological investigation of such patients reveals that there actually *is* abnormal muscle contraction, but it is limited to the pre-tarsal portion of the orbicularis oculi[59] (Fig. 6.5) and on this basis it has been suggested that the terms 'apraxia of lid opening' and 'levator inhibition' should be dropped in favour of 'focal eyelid dystonia'.[60]

Focal eyelid dystonia occurs occasionally as a lone symptom; such patients report transient inability to open their eyes. The symptoms may be triggered by activities such as looking up, bright light, watching television, or driving a car. The resulting marked frontalis contraction without obvious orbicularis oculi spasm may be asymmetric and some patients discover a sensory trick, such as pressure in the temporal region to keep their eyes open.[60]

Focal eyelid dystonia also occurs in patients with otherwise typical blepharospasm, being a common cause of failure to respond to conventional botulinum toxin injections. It may also occur in other conditions, and has been particularly associated with progressive supranuclear palsy, in which condition it typically begins several years after clinical disease onset. Patients with oromandibular dystonia and some with Parkinson's disease are also affected.[59,60] Very rarely, 'apraxia of eyelid opening' (as then described) has been reported as a temporary phenomenon in association with right parietal lobe infarction.[61]

Injections of botulinum toxin into the outer and inner aspects of the superior and inferior sulcus palpebralis help some patients (see below); a few others may derive benefit from low-dose trihexphenidyl or lid crutches.[60]

Cranial dystonia

Various combinations of oral, lingual and mandibular dystonia and blepharospasm are referred to as cranial dystonia. Common synonyms are 'Meige syndrome' and 'Brueghel's syndrome' (after the Flemish painter) (Fig. 6.6).

Permanent spasm with trismus and paroxysms triggered by various sensory stimuli may occur. Electrophysiological examination shows extensive co-contraction of the masseters during attempted jaw opening.

A patient who suffered involuntary tongue protrusion during speaking noticed that the abnormal movements were abolished if she placed a small piece of tissue paper on the tip of her tongue.[62] This is an example of a sensory trick.

A patient with longstanding blepharospasm (treated with botulinum toxin injections) developed lingual dystonia (CD 6.6). She discovered that her tongue movements were lessened if she chewed gum; furthermore, so long as she chewed gum, she found her eyes stayed open also.

Laryngeal dystonia

Dystonia of the larynx can affect either the adductor, or the abductor muscles. When the *ab*ductors are affected (posterior cricoarytenoid ± cricothyroid muscles), the cords are held apart during attempted phonation, with the effect that the patient is only able to speak in a whisper. When it is the *ad*ductors that are affected, then the cords may slam shut during phonation, so that the voice develops a 'strangled' sound to it, as the flow of air is intermittently cut off during speech (CD 6.7). Both kinds of dysphonia can respond to injections of botulinum toxin.[63]

Patients with dystonia beginning in the larynx rarely (around 15%)[7] develop more widespread dystonia.

Cervical dystonia (torticollis)

It is believed that the term 'torty colly' originated in the 16th century,[64] although the same disorder was undoubtedly known in ancient times, when it was referred to as 'caput obstipum'.[65] There are, of course, causes of abnormal neck posture other than dystonia. These include a wide range of congenital and acquired disorders,[66] including musculoskeletal conditions, which are generally referred to as 'wry

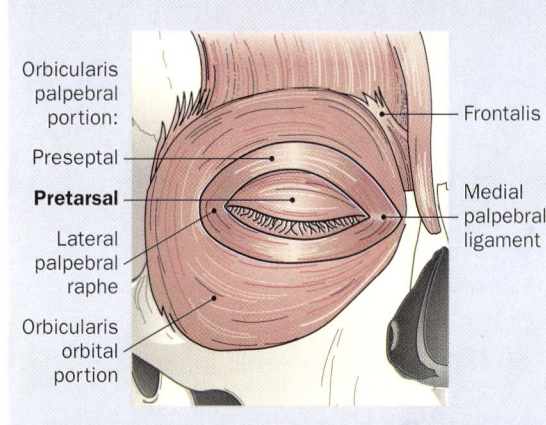

MUSCLES INVOLVED IN BLEPHAROSPASM

Orbicularis palpebral portion:
Preseptal
Pretarsal
Lateral palpebral raphe
Orbicularis orbital portion
Frontalis
Medial palpebral ligament

Figure 6.5. Anatomy of the orbicularis oculi muscle.

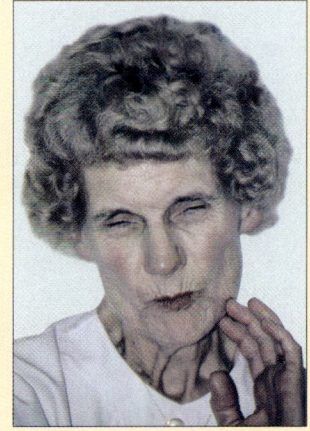

Figure 6.6. Cranial dystonia.

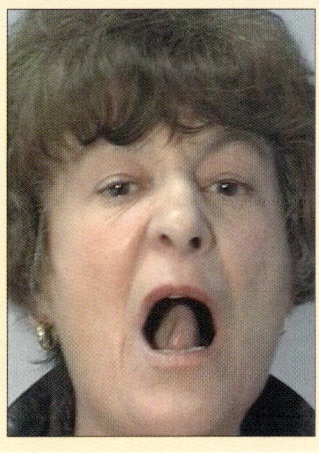

CD 6.6. Lingual dystonia.

103

neck'. Torticollis is sometimes used in a rather indiscriminant way to refer to abnormal neck postures from almost any cause, and so in the context of movement disorder practice, it is probably best to refer to 'cervical dystonia', when we mean torticollis due to dystonia.

As with other forms of dystonia, torticollis has been mistakenly thought to be due to psychological factors. Patients with torticollis do show more evidence of depression than, for example, patients with cervical spondylosis.[67] After treatment with botulinum toxin in which 85% of patients (and 88% of relatives) reported improvement in head position and neck pain, scores for depression and disability improved significantly.[68] Modest improvements in 'body concept' were also noted. All of these changes were reversed once the toxin wore off, suggesting that the depression and resulting psychological disability is the result of the torticollis, and not vice versa.

Based on epidemiological investigation covering the years 1960–1979, the incidence of cervical dystonia has been estimated at 1.2 per 100 000 person years in Rochester, Minnesota,[69] with a female:male age-adjusted incidence ratio of 3.6:1. Prepubertal onset of cranial dystonia is rare. From adolescence to the fifth decade, the incidence rises for both sexes, with a subsequent fall to baseline by the eighth decade.[70]

Most patients suffer progressive symptoms over 2–5 years, after which the condition reaches a plateau. Approximately 10–20% enter a period of remission. Some relapse later,[71] but others remain symptom-free for decades.[69] In 25–30% of patients, dystonia spreads beyond the neck,[7,71] usually to the lower face, jaw, or arm. Many patients with cervical dystonia report pain as a main symptom[72] (this is unlike most other kinds of focal dystonia).

The head movements observed include rotation (CD 6.8) and tilt. Many patients have a combination of rotation to left or right together with either antecollis or retrocollis. It is typical for the movement to be more obvious and/or severe when walking than when sitting or lying at rest. Two-thirds of patients have jerky movements or forced transient spasms in addition to an underlying abnormal neck posture.[72]

In some studies, an increased frequency of thyroid disease has been noted in patients with cervical dystonia,[70] particularly in women.

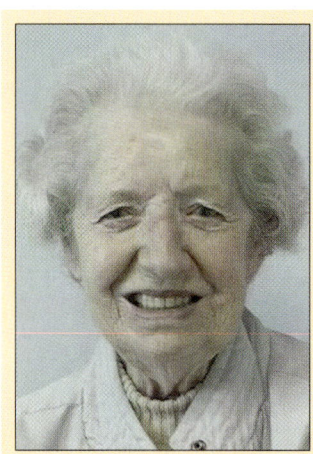

CD 6.7. Laryngeal dystonia.

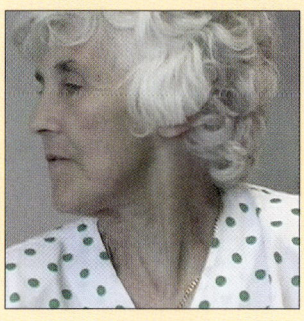

CD 6.8. Torticollis.

When patients describe vertigo, they may refer to their 'head spinning'. Put crudely, we know that our balance mechanism has both efferent (head position) and afferent (mechanoreceptor) connections to our neck. So it is perhaps hardly surprising that attention has turned to the possibility that torticollis is either causally related to vestibular dysfunction, or else might be modified by manipulating vestibular control mechanisms. Neuro-otological study of patients with cervical dystonia reveals a directional preponderance of vestibular nystagmus opposite to the direction of the torticollis; this fits with the notion that patients have a tonic imbalance in both the neck and the extraocular muscles, tending to drive them both in the *same* direction. It appears, therefore, that there is a breakdown in the mechanisms responsible for signalling head posture.[73]

In a prospective randomized double-blind trial, - botulinum toxin injections have been shown to provide superior efficacy and less frequent side-effects than trihexphenidyl.[74] Both pain and neck posture improve.[75]

Axial dystonia

Although spinal dystonia is usually cervical, in some patients the involuntary movements involve the dorsal and lumbar spine too, and these patients are said to have axial dystonia. The movements may be of very large amplitude, and can render patients almost unable to stand or sit comfortably (CD 6.9).

Botulinum toxin therapy of focal dystonia

Injections of botulinum toxin are presently considered to be the treatment of choice for a variety of focal neurological disorders[76] (not all of which applications are necessarily recognized by the various regulatory authorities, such as the Food and Drug Administration).

Clostridium botulinum produces a variety of neuroparalytic toxins (A, B, C_1, D, E, F and G) of which type A has been most extensively used for therapeutic purposes. It is obtained from *C. botulinum* culture and the resulting toxin dispensed into vials, potency being measured in 'mouse units' (u), a single mouse unit being the amount of toxin found to kill half of a group of mice (i.e. the LD_{50}). For clinical use the freeze-dried toxin must first be reconstituted with normal saline and then administered by injection.

There are presently two principal suppliers of botulinum toxin for clinical use. Botox is distributed by Allergan Pharmaceuticals (USA), whilst Dysport is produced at Porton Down (UK). There is a 16-fold difference in mouse unit potency per nanogram of powder. In clinical use, however, 1 unit of Botox has an efficacy approximately equivalent to 3–4 units of Dysport.

Based on monkey data, the human LD_{50} for intramuscular Botox would be 2500–3000 mouse units.

Mechanism of action

Botulinum toxin acts by binding to peripheral nerve receptors followed by internalization. Types A, C and E next interfere with the docking and fusion of synaptic vesicles with the presynaptic plasma membrane, whereas types D and F destroy the presynaptic vesicle.[77] Toxin injected into muscle is known to be transported centrally into the spinal cord, although the practical significance of this is not known.

It generally takes 1–3 days after intramuscular injection for muscular weakness and subsequent atrophy to

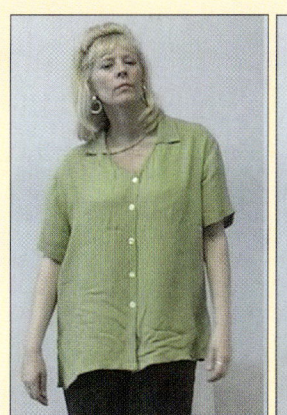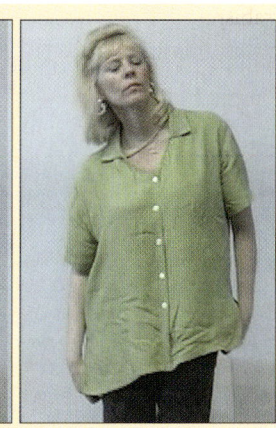

CD 6.9. Axial dystonia.

begin. Maximal weakness typically occurs around 1 week after injection. Rarely patients notice the onset of muscle weakening as late as 2 weeks after injection. The duration of effect is variable. In most cases, benefit declines to an extent sufficient to justify repeat injection in around 3 months.

Contraindications

Even though only a minute quantity of toxin enters the circulation after intramuscular injection, it is assumed that patients with disorders of neuromuscular transmission (myasthenia gravis, Eaton–Lambert syndrome) may be at risk of harm and these conditions are considered a relative contraindication against botulinum toxin therapy. The same applies to patients with motor neuron disease or those receiving drugs known to affect neuromuscular transmission (such as aminoglycoside antibiotics).

There are few available data on the use of botulinum toxin in human pregnancy and during lactation. In the handful of cases mentioned in the medical literature, there have been no obvious adverse effects on the fetus.[78]

Anaphylaxis has not been reported. Skin rashes may occur after injection, though they also occur after injection of placebo and it may be a component of the vehicle, rather than the toxin itself.

Clinical use of botulinum toxin

The range of disorders in which botulinum toxin has been tried is constantly expanding. The first reported clinical application was in the treatment of childhood strabismus.[79] Dystonic and other forms of involuntary movements have attracted most attention in neurology, though the use of botulinum toxin in spasticity (such as following stroke or in the context of multiple sclerosis) is currently increasing. Outside of neurology and ophthalmology, botulinum toxin has also been tried in, for example, disorders of intestinal contraction as well as in cosmetic surgery. The principal current uses of botulinum toxin in dystonia are as follows.

Blepharospasm

Both neurologists and ophthalmologists have come to consider botulinum toxin as the treatment of choice in blepharospasm. Most clinical trials in this context have been open,[80,81] though small double-blind placebo controlled trials have also shown benefit.[82]

The success rate of botulinum toxin injections for blepharospasm is around 80–90%. This includes causes of blepharospasm other than idiopathic dystonia, such as drug-induced blepharospasm (neuroleptics, levodopa) and blepharospasm following birth injury.

Different centres have developed different treatment protocols. Most use multiple (typically 3–7) injections around each eye. The precise sites chosen vary. As with all botulinum toxin treatments, it is customary to begin with a small total dose (such as 25 units of Botox, or 120 units of Dysport) per eye. Patients who fail to respond to this dose may derive benefit from twice or three times the dose.

The most common side-effect is ptosis which occurs in 10% or more patients. Rarely, however, is the degree of ptosis sufficient to impair visual function. Other common side-effects include bruising, excess tearing, and dry eyes. Exposure keratitis, pain at the injection site, ectropion, entropion, conjunctivitis and diplopia have also been reported. When side-effects occur, they are usually transient, typically lasting less than 2 weeks.

Not all patients respond satisfactorily to botulinum toxin. In some cases the dose used is simply too low. Other causes for treatment failure include an enhanced Bell's phenomenon, or persistent blinking after injection despite reduction of the sustained contractions.

Some patients who are initially diagnosed as suffering with blepharospasm but fail to respond to initial botulinum toxin injections have apraxia of eyelid opening, or focal eyelid dystonia (see above). Injections of botulinum toxin into the outer and inner aspects of the superior and inferior sulcus palpebralis (the junction of the preseptal and pretarsal part of the palpebral orbicularis oculi) have been reported to help in more than 80% of such patients.

Hemifacial spasm (see also Chapter 14)

Although not strictly a kind of dystonia at all, the treatment of hemifacial spasm with botulinum toxin is so similar to the treatment of blepharospasm, that mention here is appropriate. Reported success rates are around 90%. Patients with hemifacial spasm usually respond to smaller doses of toxin than patients with blepharospasm (presumably because they have peripheral nerve damage). Many physicians inject only the periorbital muscles, though some also inject the lower facial muscles. Doing so greatly increases the risk of facial drooping. Otherwise, the side-effect profile is similar to that for treating blepharospasm, except that patients may more readily notice minor degrees of ptosis, because unlike most patients with blepharospasm, they have a normal (contralateral) side for comparison.

Lower facial mandibular and lingual dystonia

Botulinum toxin therapy generally works less well for lower facial dystonia than blepharospasm or hemifacial spasm. These disorders may be profoundly disabling, however, and drug treatments are not usually helpful. Cautious botulinum toxin injection may be one of the best possibilities for giving symptomatic relief. Because of the rather variable results of lower facial/jaw injections, several authors have advocated injection via a hollow EMG needle with simultaneous electrophysiological recording in order to identify the target site.

In patients with jaw-closing dystonia, botulinum toxin provides partial relief from symptoms in the majority of patients.[76,83] Results are less good in patients with jaw-opening dystonia. The most common side-effect after injecting the jaw muscles is dysphagia. This is a particularly common problem if the lateral pterygoid muscles are injected and so these muscles are best avoided.

Patients with oromandibular dystonia may derive some benefit from botulinum toxin, although the reported results have mostly been rather disappointing in comparison to its use in other sites.[84]

Lingual dystonia can be treated with botulinum toxin, but side-effects are very common, including dysphagia and even aspiration pneumonia.

Laryngeal dystonia

Patients with *ad*ductor dysphonia may be effectively treated using injection of small quantities of botulinum toxin via a concentric EMG needle placed in the thyroarytenoid muscle complex. Locating the correct site for injection demands training in the anatomy and physiology of the larynx. Laryngeal EMG procedures sometimes induce laryngeal stridor, and for this reason the treatment should only take place within an environment equipped to deal with this complication. In expert hands, patients treated in open studies typically report a dramatic response to treatment, such as a '75–100% improvement' in speech quality. In more scientific terms, the treatment significantly decreases the standard deviation of the fundamental frequency of a speech sample, indicating that treated patients enjoy a reduction in the variation in pitch of their speech.[85] Patients who have previously been treated surgically by recurrent laryngeal nerve section may also derive benefit, although the reported results are a little less good than in surgically naïve patients.

It is presently unclear whether it is better to inject a very small dose (1.25–4 units of Botox) into both vocal folds,[85] or a slightly larger dose (5–30 units Botox) into one side.[86] The injections may be performed perorally or percutaneously.[87]

Patients may experience transient breathy hypophonia or hoarseness after injection. Mild aspiration is common, but pneumonia (a theoretical possibility) seems not to occur.

Patients with *ab*ductor dysphonia may also derive benefit from botulinum toxin injection, although fewer such patients have been reported in the literature. In this case the target muscle is the posterior cricoarytenoid.[88] The intention when treating abductor dysphonia is to bring the cords closer together. Injecting a single side may suffice; if not, patients may require a contralateral injection. The penalty of overweakening the target muscle is stridor, and mild (particularly exercise-induced) stridor is a common transient side-effect.

Cervical dystonia

Botulinum toxin injection is accepted as a safe and efficacious modality for the treatment of cervical dystonia (CD 6.10).[76] There have been a large number of publications describing benefit in the majority of patients.[82,89–91] The pain of cervical dystonia responds at least as well to botulinum toxin as the involuntary movements.

The detail of which particular muscles contribute to the disease of cervical dystonia can vary greatly according to the task in hand, the time of day, and from one patient to another. Because of this variability, each time patients are treated they should be examined carefully to tailor the sites for injection and the dose of toxin used.

In patients who have mainly rotation, typical sites for injection include (in a patient turning to the right) the (left) sternomastoid and the (right) splenius capitis and (right) trapezius. Patients who have retrocollis typically need injections into both trapezii and splenius capitis muscles. With tilt to one side, the muscles injected (all ipsilaterally) are the sternomastoid, splenius capitis, levator scapulae and trapezius. Many patients have neck movements which cannot be summarized in such terse terminology; complex and varying patterns of turning, tilt, flexion and extension are seen, and the above patterns of injections must be adapted accordingly.

Typical doses used are 100–200 mouse units of Botox (divided between several muscles). Some physicians use multiple small injections, for example dividing a dose of around 50 units between 8–10 sites along the length of the sternomastoid. Others use fewer injection sites per muscle. In most cases it is not necessary to use EMG to localize the contracting muscles, although it may be helpful in patients where palpation fails to give the required information, and, in at least one study, the magnitude of benefit was found to be better with EMG assistance than without.[92]

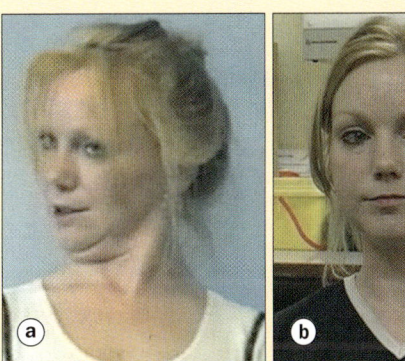
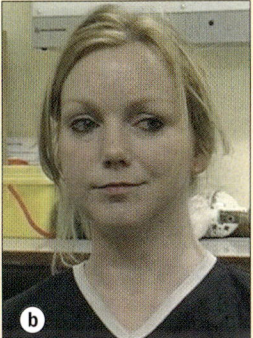

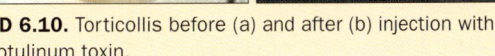
CD 6.10. Torticollis before (a) and after (b) injection with botulinum toxin.

The commonest side-effect is dysphagia.[93] Mostly this is mild, but occasional patients may need to modify their diet for a period, and very rarely patients have required temporary nasogastric feeding. Because of proximity to the swallowing mechanism, injections into the sternomastoid are more likely to cause dysphagia than at some other sites.

Hand dystonia

The use of botulinum toxin in focal hand dystonia has been less universally helpful, though some authors have reported considerable success with persisting benefit after repeat injections over a period of several years.[94]

Subgroups of patients with limb focal dystonia benefit from botulinum toxin injections. In writer's cramp, the patients who benefit most are those in whom it is easy to identify a small number of muscles contributing to the abnormal posture. For example patients who develop 'isolated' index finger extension during writing are easier to treat (and usually derive greater benefit) than those in whom multiple muscles are involved with finger flexion, wrist extension and shoulder/elbow elevation. Part of the problem is that in order to stop the involuntary movements the muscles may have to be weakened to such an extent that normal function is significantly impaired. In an effort to lessen side-effects due to limb weakness, it is usual to begin with very small doses and to titrate the dose upwards over the course of a series of several injections. EMG may be used to identify the affected muscles and to ensure injection into the correct site. Despite the above reservations, botulinum toxin injections for limb dystonia may give definite, reproducible, and sustained benefit over years.[95–97]

Dopa-responsive dystonia

Around 5–10% of patients with inherited dystonia show a dramatic response to levodopa. This condition is inherited as an autosomal dominant condition and it has been shown to be due to a variety of defects in the guanosine triphosphate (GTP) cyclohydrolase I gene.[98–101] Variation in the ratio of mutant/normal mRNA encoding GTP cyclohydrolase I may vary amongst members of a single family who share the same genetic mutation, yet have different clinical characteristics.[100]

Terminology

Patients with the condition which we now call dopa-responsive dystonia have been reported in the neurological literature under a number of diagnostic labels, such as hereditary parkinsonism–dystonia, fluctuating dystonia, dopa-sensitive progressive dystonia of childhood, Segawa's syndrome, and hereditary dystonia–parkinsonism syndrome of juvenile onset. The term dopa-responsive dystonia is now preferred because it emphasizes the central unifying features of dystonia and levodopa responsiveness.[102]

One of the greatest challenges in reading the neurological literature lies in deciding whether patients initially reported under a particular diagnostic label would still be best classified in the same way. It is likely that patients with dopa-responsive dystonia have been reported as examples of a variety of other conditions; but equally, some patients with other conditions have been reported as (or discussed in subsequent reviews as suffering from) dopa-responsive dystonia. Let the reader beware.

Biochemistry

The rate-limiting step in the dopamine synthetic pathway is the hydroxylation of tyrosine to dihydroxyphenylalanine (dopa) by tyrosine hydroxylase (TH). This is followed by decarboxylation (by aromatic amino acid decarboxylase) of dopa to dopamine (Fig. 6.7). TH requires molecular oxygen and reduced tetrahydrobiopterin as cofactors (tetrahydrobiopterin is also required for tryptophan hydroxylase activity in serotonin production). In the brain, tetrahydrobiopterin is synthesized *de novo* from GTP via dihydroneopterin triphosphate.[103] The enzyme responsible for the catalysis of GTP to dihydroneopterin triphosphate is *GTP cyclohydrolase*, and *this* is the enzyme which is deficient in dopa-responsive dystonia. So dopa-responsive dystonia is due to an enzyme deficiency which leads to reduced dopa synthesis from tyrosine.

Clinical features

There are a number of clinical pointers to this condition. Firstly, onset is usually in childhood, typically between 9 months and 16 years of age. In most patients symptoms begin in the legs and 'toe walking' is common (though it should be remembered that many otherwise normal children walk on their toes up to around the age

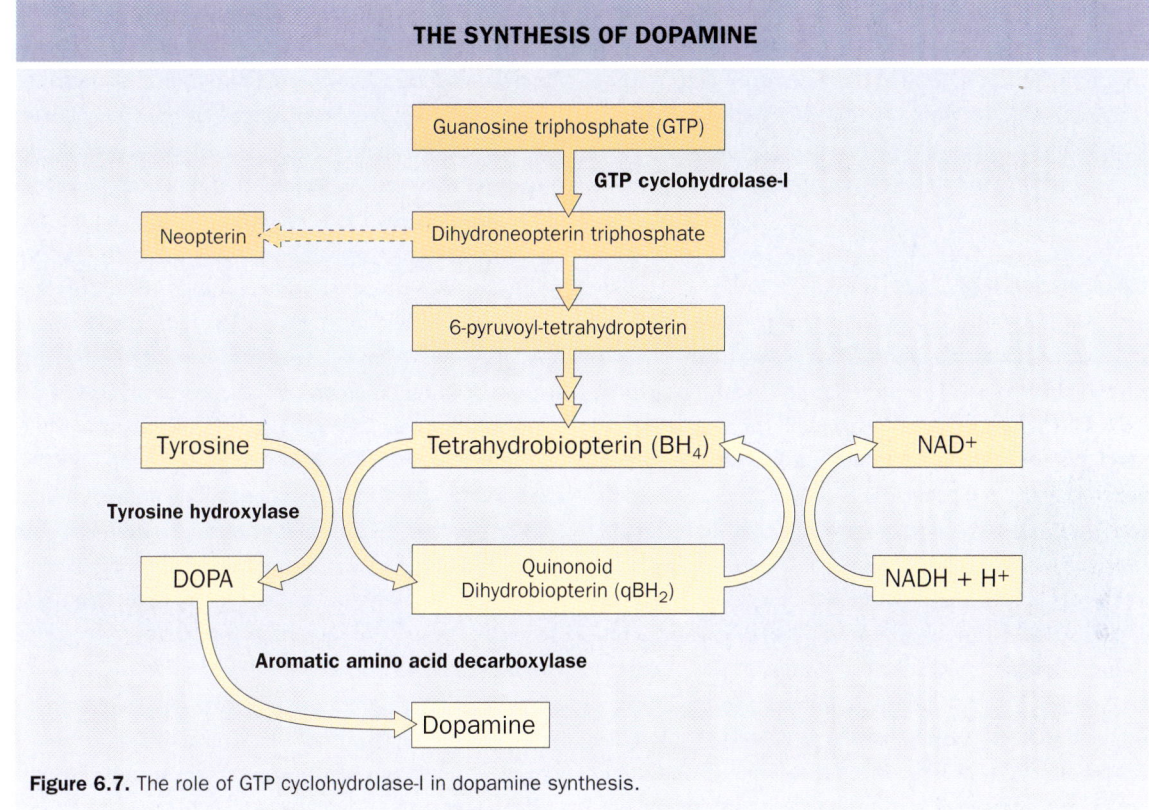

THE SYNTHESIS OF DOPAMINE

Figure 6.7. The role of GTP cyclohydrolase-I in dopamine synthesis.

of 2 years). Standing and walking can lead to either an increased lumbar lordosis, or a crouched posture. Falls, largely due to postural instability, are common.

There is often a mixture of dystonia and parkinsonism, although either may dominate the clinical picture. When tremor is present early on it is usually postural, though a typical parkinsonian rest tremor may be seen later. Cog-wheel rigidity, bradykinesia and hypomimia all occur.

Response to levodopa
It hardly needs stating that patients with dopa-responsive dystonia respond to levodopa. In many cases only a small dose is required, and occasional patients do not even need to take the medication every day. Nevertheless, there are other patients who respond only after chronic treatment and a 'trial of levodopa' in this context means taking up to 200 mg levodopa (plus decarboxylase inhibitor) three times daily for at least a several week period. Unlike patients with Parkinson's disease, those with dopa-responsive dystonia continue to show an essentially undimmed response to levodopa throughout

their lives. As young patients grow up they may require a bigger dose, but adults typically derive the same response from the same dose of drug for many years. Some patients develop a little chorea when first treated with levodopa, but this generally settles over a few weeks. A minority of patients who present with a phenotypically similar condition in childhood do experience wearing-off after a few months or years of treatment and it is likely that these patients have juvenile-onset parkinsonism, rather than dopa-responsive dystonia.[102]

Response to other drugs
Patients may also respond to anticholinergic drugs and some respond to carbamazepine (which acts as a weak dopamine reuptake inhibitor, but also increases noradrenergic firing in the locus coeruleus; the latter may be relevant to the dystonia in dopa-responsive dystonia).

Diurnal fluctuations
Apart from their dramatic response to levodopa, many patients also describe diurnal variation in symptom severity. They may be able to walk almost normally in

the morning and yet they succumb to a progressive worsening of symptoms as the day passes. Although a common clinical feature in dopa-responsive dystonia, it is a mistake to think of this as a pathognomonic symptom since up to a quarter of patients do not report such variability in their symptoms, and up to a fifth of patients with idiopathic generalized dystonia do.

Differential diagnosis

The two principal differential diagnoses are idiopathic generalized dystonia and juvenile parkinsonism. In those patients who present chiefly with dystonia, pointers to dopa-responsive dystonia rather than idiopathic generalized dystonia include symptom onset below the age of 6 years, bradykinesia, rigidity (which is usually increased on activation), hyper-reflexia and the marked and sustained response to levodopa. Onset in the arm or axial structures is rare in dopa-responsive dystonia but occurs in more than half of patients with idiopathic generalized dystonia.

Patients with juvenile parkinsonism rarely present before the age of 8 years. In other respects the differential diagnosis may be difficult in the early stages and, since both patient groups respond well to levodopa, it may not be until response fluctuations and other complications of levodopa treatment emerge in those with juvenile parkinsonism that the diagnosis becomes clearer. Positron emission tomography using [18F]fluorodopa as tracer may be able to distinguish between dopa-responsive dystonia and juvenile parkinsonism much earlier. Why is this important? Because patients with parkinsonism and early onset typically suffer capricious and severe response fluctuations and treatment complications on levodopa, whereas patients with dopa-responsive dystonia enjoy a smooth and prolonged response. So patients with dopa-responsive dystonia will benefit from early levodopa therapy, while patients with juvenile parkinsonism are best treated with other agents (such as anticholinergics and dopamine agonists) in the first instance.

Alternative presentations

In families where one or more patients have typical dopa-responsive dystonia, attention has been focused on older relatives who have presented over the age of 50 years with a tremor-dominant parkinsonian syndrome which would otherwise have been assumed to be due to 'benign' Parkinson's disease but in whom [18F]dopa PET scans have shown normal striatal tracer uptake.[104,105] This is very much *against* the diagnosis of idiopathic Parkinson's disease as an explanation for these patients' symptoms and it has been suggested that their illness may instead be an alternative manifestation of dopa-responsive dystonia.[105] In support of this assertion, these patients have been noted to have a sustained and smooth levodopa response over many years.

Dystonic foot posturing beginning in adult life has also been observed in otherwise unaffected relatives of patients with typical dopa-responsive dystonia and it is assumed that this also may be a phenotypic variant of the disease.[104,105] Some asymptomatic family members also show subtle signs of parkinsonism (including bradykinesia and rigidity) or dystonia (including unusual arm or writing postures and intermittent equinovarus posturing at rest).[104] Such signs are assumed to be the minimal clinical expression of disease in dopa-responsive dystonia.

Investigations

Dopa-responsive dystonia remains a clinical diagnosis in which the physician's skills together with an observation of levodopa response are paramount. Efforts have nevertheless been made to explore the place of laboratory investigations though it is fair to say that the impetus for these studies was initially in order to better understand the pathophysiology of the disease, rather than to formulate a diagnostic test.

CSF biochemistry

CSF tetrahydrobiopterin (a tyrosine hydroxylase cofactor) may be reduced.[106]

Positron emission tomography

Several patients with dopa-responsive dystonia have been scanned using PET with fluorodopa as tracer. Intrinsic dopamine production is via hydroxylation of tyrosine to dopa and then decarboxylation of dopa to dopamine. Whilst dopa-responsive dystonia is due to a defect in the initial hydroxylation phase of this process, fluorodopa PET scanning measures the rate of the second (decarboxylation) step as experienced by exogenously synthesized (fluoro-)dopa. In Parkinson's disease the nigrostriatal neurons are missing and fluorodopa uptake is impaired. In dopa-responsive dystonia fluorodopa uptake has been reported to be either normal,[105] or near normal,[107] but certainly much better preserved than in Parkinson's disease (Fig. 6.8). Patients with young-onset dystonia/parkinsonism may be one of the few patient groups in whom a fluorodopa scan could reasonably be said to be justified on clinical grounds.[108]

Pathology

Only one patient with dopa-responsive dystonia has come to postmortem and been subject to detailed neuropathological and neurochemical study.[109] Symptom onset in the girl in question was at age 5 years. By the age of 8 she had generalized dystonia and levodopa treatment was started. She responded well to levodopa and led a normal life. She died in a car accident 11 years later.

Pathological examination revealed normal dopaminergic substantia nigra cell body density, TH immunoreactivity and TH protein level, but subnormal melanin and dopamine, also a reduction of dopamine, TH activity, TH protein and [³H]GBR 12935 binding in the striatum.

The combination of striatal dopamine deficit with reduced TH activity and TH protein would be consistent with nerve terminal loss. [³H]GBR 12935 binds to dopamine nerve terminals and in this case binding was at the lower end of the normal range.

Importantly, no structural abnormality of the nigral cell bodies or their striatal projections were identified, even though melanin content and dopamine levels were reduced. Lewy bodies were not seen.

Paroxysmal dystonia

A minority of patients with dystonia have episodic symptoms between which they are entirely normal.

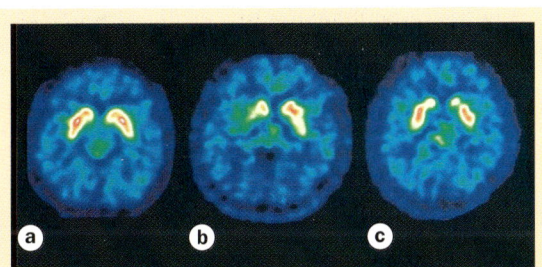

Figure 6.8. Fluorodopa uptake in dopa-responsive dystonia. Tracer uptake is close to normal. (a) Normal; (b) Parkinson's disease; (c) dopa-responsive dystonia.

Several varieties of 'attacks' are recognized. They may have a flavour of chorea rather than pure dystonia and there is uncertainty over whether they should properly be classified as a kind of dystonia, or an unusual form of epilepsy.

Paroxysmal kinesogenic choreoathetosis

This condition is inherited in an autosomal dominant pattern. Each attack is brief, lasting only seconds or at the most minutes. The attacks are classically brought on by movement, particularly by sudden movement, such as rising quickly from a chair. The movements themselves can be either choreic, dystonic, or a mixture of both. Patients may have many attacks in the space of a single day. There is no disturbance of conscious level. Many patients respond dramatically to carbamazepine, with complete abolition of their attacks on even a small daily dose.

Paroxysmal non-kinesogenic dystonia

As might be inferred from the title, this condition is non-kinesogenic, and the movements are more definitely dystonic in appearance. It also differs from its kinesogenic cousin in that the attacks are usually very much longer (minutes to hours), they are less frequent, and do not respond so well to anticonvulsants. Some patients are better when taking clonazepam.

Secondary dystonia

A wide range of causes of secondary dystonia have been recognized. Broadly, they may be split into common conditions like stroke and tumour, which usually present in other ways, but which rarely cause dystonia if they happen to give rise to a lesion in a particular anatomical site, and less common diseases in which dystonia is a more typical feature, even though the disease may be rare. Secondary dystonia is probably more common as a rare presentation of common diseases, than as a classical presentation of a rare disorder.

Clinical clues to symptomatic dystonia

A variety of points in the clinical history or the physical examination may give rise to the suspicion that a patient has secondary, rather than primary, dystonia. In some cases an abnormal perinatal history or delayed early milestones may provide a clue, or there may have been an obvious precipitating illness (such as a stroke or episode of encephalitis). Patients with idiopathic dystonia do not suffer seizures, nor intellectual impairment, nor defects of vision or hearing.

Idiopathic dystonia does not affect eye movements, and the optic fundi should be normal. Parkinsonism, loss of postural reflexes, pyramidal, cerebellar or sensory signs do not occur. Hepatomegaly suggests a secondary cause.

The character of the dystonia itself may also give a clue. Hemidystonia is very commonly secondary. Also fixed postures are more common in secondary dystonia. Leg involvement is unusual in adult idiopathic dystonia and rapid progression to multifocal or generalized involvement in adult life suggests a secondary cause.

Focal brain lesions

A variety of disease processes can cause dystonia if they lead to a lesion in an appropriate site. The most commonly reported sites, and a variety of aetiologies for such lesions, are given below.

Basal ganglia

Rarely a tumour involving the putamen may give rise to hemidystonia, such as in an 8-year-old boy where an 18-month history of left hemidystonia was found to be due to an astrocytoma.[110] Also, a patient with laterocollis who was initially responsive to trihexphenidyl was later shown to have a basal ganglia glioma. As the tumour grew further and a hemiparesis developed, the laterocollis lessened.[111]

In another study using CT imaging, three-quarters of 22 patients with hemidystonia had either contralateral basal ganglia lesions, or a history of hemiparesis (or both).[5] In an MRI study, poststroke patients with hemidystonic spasms all had lesions in the striatopallidal complex (involving the putamen posteriorly to the anterior commisure and extending variably into the dorsolateral part of the caudate, the posterior limb of the internal capsule, or the lateral segment of the globus pallidus), whilst poststroke patients with 'myoclonic dystonia' had lesions in the contralateral (ventral intermediate and ventral caudal) thalamus.[112]

Very rarely, patients with torticollis may have infarcted their contralateral putamen.[113,114] Other traumatic basal ganglia lesions have been reported in

patients with torticollis.[115,116] Generalized dystonia may be the presenting neurological manifestation of human immunodeficiency virus infection with bilateral putaminal lucencies seen on CT and may also rarely be seen following childhood encephalitis (Fig. 6.9).[117] A patient with multiple sclerosis had lesions in the right caudate and lentiform, and developed involuntary ocular deviation, blepharospasm, torticollis and chorea of the right arm and head during relapses precipitated by intercurrent infections.[118] In patients who have suffered either severe or mild head injury, dystonia occurring months to years later may be a manifestation of (presumably trauma-related) contralateral basal ganglia lesions.[119,120]

Brainstem

Blepharospasm is only very rarely due to an identifiable focal lesion; one such patient had an angioma in the rostral brainstem.[121] Patients with central pontine myelinolysis may develop dystonia.[122,123] An MR scan in a single patient with hemidystonia and torticollis following severe head trauma in childhood showed a lesion extending from the subthalamic region to the superior cerebellar peduncle.[119]

Spinal cord

Hand dystonia has been described in patients with definite multiple sclerosis in whom MRI showed lesions in the cervical cord, but no involvement of either the basal ganglia or thalamus.[124] A patient with a cervical ependymoma presented with gait ataxia, leg weakness and torticollis.[125] The patient had intermittent spasmodic neck movements, and showed intermittent touching of his face and nose (a sensory 'trick'). A patient of mine aged in his 30s has dystonia affecting

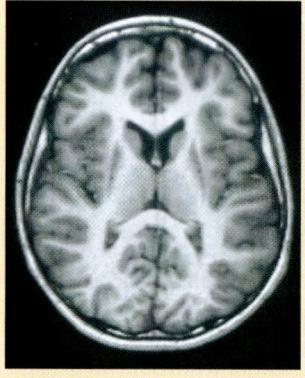

Figure 6.9. Dystonia following childhood encephalitis. Bilateral basal ganglia signal change on MRI. (Courtesy of N. McConachie.)

his right arm only; he also has mild mirror movements affecting his hands (CD 6.11). He had a cervical myelomeningocoele repaired as a baby (Fig. 6.10), but other brain imaging has all been normal. His dystonia may be due to his cervical lesion.

Metabolic disorders

Dystonia has been reported in a variety of illnesses associated with a known metabolic defect. See Chapter 3 for a description of Wilson's disease, and Chapter 12 for those conditions most common in childhood.

Other specific causes

A small number of recognized causes of secondary dystonia remain. Dystonia due to drugs is considered in Chapter 11. Transient dystonia has been reported as a complication of varicella infection.[126]

Head trauma

There are a small number of well-documented patients in whom head trauma (usually in the first or second decade of life) has led to dystonia.[127] Most,

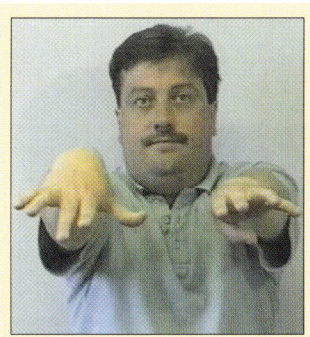

CD 6.11. Dystonia associated with cervical cord lesion.

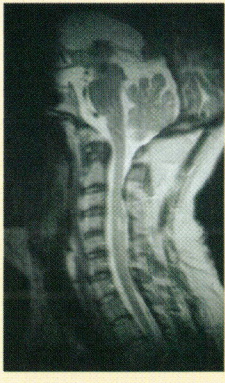

Figure 6.10. Syrinx following repair of cervical meningocoele in a patient with arm dystonia (same patient as CD 6.11).

but not all, patients had severe head injuries with prolonged coma initially complicated by hemiplegia which later gave way to a hemidystonic syndrome. Imaging studies have generally shown basal ganglia lesions. Even more rarely, patients who have suffered apparently minor trauma (such as falling off a bicycle, without any loss of consciousness) have subsequently developed hemidystonia.[128] Again, most have been shown to have basal ganglia lesions (of presumed traumatic aetiology). The interval between the time of trauma and the onset of dystonia may be several years, making it difficult to be certain that the trauma has been truly causative.

Investigations in dystonia

Given the broad spectrum of diseases which can cause dystonia either in childhood or adult life, but bearing in mind that most of these diseases are rare, and that most adults with dystonia have the genetically determined idiopathic disorder, to what extent should patients with dystonia undergo laboratory, electrophysiological or imaging investigations? Table 6.1 gives suggested investigations for assessing patients with apparently idiopathic dystonia with onset in childhood/adolescence or adult life, and when there is a suspicion of secondary dystonia irrespective of age. Some of the recommended investigations are invasive (such as bone marrow, muscle and skin biopsy) and should only be performed after careful consideration of the results of simpler investigations. As with parkinsonism, all patients with onset before age 50 years should have serum copper studies and a slit lamp examination of Descemet's membrane in a search for evidence of Wilson's disease.

Late complications

Patients with torticollis, whether or not in the context of generalized dystonia, may develop secondary neurological damage, including cervical myelopathy, due to cervical spondylosis. Anterior cervical fusion is the preferred treatment.[129] Carpal tunnel syndrome has also been reported in patients with idiopathic generalized dystonia, presumably as a result of prolonged and repetitive flexion posturing at the wrist.[130]

● **Table 6.1.** The investigation of patients with dystonia. (Adapted with permission from Marsden C D, Quinn N P. The dystonias. Br Med J 1990; 300: 138–144.)

	Idiopathic dystonia		Symptomatic dystonia (onset at any age)
	Onset in childhood or adolescence	Onset in adult life	
Blood			
Ceruloplasmin concentration	+	+*	+
Syphilis serology	+	+	+
Blood count erythrocyte sedimentation rate	+	+	+
Acanthocytes	+		+
Antinuclear antibodies	+		+
Segmental multiple analyser with computer (SMAC)	+	+	+
Creatine phosphokinase activity			+
Uric acid concentration			+
Amino acid concentration			+
White cell lysomal enzymes			+
Hypoxanthine-guanine phosphoribosyltransferase activity			+
α-fetoprotein concentration			+
Urine			
Amino acid concentration			+
24-hour excretion of copper			+
Oligosaccharide concentration			+
Mucopolysaccharide concentration			+
Organic acid concentration			+
Examination of cerebrospinal fluid	+		+
Biopsy			
Bone marrow			+
Muscle			+
Skin			+
Other			
Slit lamp examination of eyes	+	+*	+
Computed tomography or magnetic resonance imaging of brain	+	+	+
Electromyopathy or nerve conduction	+		+
Electroencephalography	+		+
Electroretinography			+
Evoked potentials	+		+

*Wilson's disease should be excluded in all those with onset at or before age 50 years.

References

1. Fahn S, Marsden C D, Calne D B. Classification and investigation of dystonia. In: Marsden C D, Fahn S (eds) Movement disorders 2. London: Butterworths, 1987: 332–358

2. Fish D R, Sawyers D, Allen P J et al. The effect of sleep on the dyskinetic movements in Parkinson's disease, Gilles de la Tourette syndrome, Huntington's disease, and torsion dystonia. Arch Neurol 1991; 48: 210–214

3. Weiner W J, Nora L M. 'Trick' movements in facial dystonia. J Clin Psych 1984; 45: 519–521

4. Marsden C D, Obeso J A, Zaranz J J, Lang A E. The anatomical basis of symptomatic hemidystonia. Brain 1985; 108: 461–483

5. Pettigrew L C, Jankovic J. Hemidystonia: a report of 22 patients and a review of the literature. J Neurol Neurosurg Psychiat 1985; 48: 650–657

6. Fletcher N A, Harding A E, Marsden C D. Intrafamilial correlation in idiopathic torsion dystonia. Mov Dis 1991; 6: 310–314

7. Greene P, Kang U J, Fahn S. Spread of symptoms in idiopathic torsion dystonia. Mov Dis 1995; 10: 143–152

8. Korczyn A D, Kahana E, Zilber N et al. Torsion dystonia in Israel. Ann Neurol 1980; 8: 387–391

9. Eldridge R. Inheritance of torsion dystonia in Jews. Ann Neurol 1981; 10: 203–204

10. Warner T T, Fletcher N A, Davis M B et al. Linkage analysis in British and French families with idiopathic torsion dystonia. Brain 1993; 116: 739–744

11. Kramer P L, de Leon D, Ozelius L et al. Dystonia gene in Ashkenazi Jewish population is located on chromosome 9q32–34. Ann Neurol 1990; 27: 114–120

12. Ahmad F, Davis M B, Waddy H M et al. Evidence for locus heterogeneity in autosomal dominant torsion dystonia. Genomics 1993; 15: 9–12

13. Bressman S B, Heiman G A, Nygaard T G et al. A study of idiopathic torsion dystonia in a non-Jewish family: Evidence for genetic heterogeneity. Neurology 1994; 44: 283–287

14. Bressman S B, de Leon D, Kramer P L et al. Dystonia in Ashkenazi Jews: Clinical characterization of a founder mutation. Ann Neurol 1994; 36: 771–777

15. Gasser T, Bove C M, Ozelius L J et al. Haplotype analysis at the DYT1 locus in Ashkenazi Jewish patients with occupational hand dystonia. Mov Dis 1996; 11: 163–166

16. Risch N, de Leon D, Ozelius L et al. Genetic analysis of idiopathic torsion dystonia in Ashkenazi Jews and their recent descent from a small founder population. Nature Gen 1995; 9: 152–159

17. Gordon M F, Bressman S, Brin M F et al. Dystonia in a patient with deletion of 18q. Mov Dis 1995; 10: 496–499

18. Kakinuma S, Sasabe F, Negoro K et al. 18p-syndrome with bilateral pyramidal tract signs, dystonia of the lower extremities and concentric visual field defect. Clin Neurol 1994; 34: 474–478

19. Micheli S, Fernández-Pardal M, Quesada P et al. Variable onset of adult inherited focal dystonia: A problem for genetic studies. Mov Dis 1994; 9: 64–68

20. Uitti R J, Maraganore D M. Adult onset familial cervical dystonia: Report of a family including monozygotic twins. Mov Dis 1993; 8: 489–494

21. Waddy H M, Fletcher N A, Harding A E, Marsden C D. A genetic study of idiopathic dystonias. Ann Neurol 1991; 29: 320–324

22. Gowers W R. A manual of diseases of the nervous system. London: Churchill, 1888: 656

23. Goldman S, Ahlskog J E. Posttraumatic cervical dystonia. Mayo Clinic Proc 1993; 68: 443–448

24. Tarsy D, Sudarsky L, Charness M E. Limb dystonia following electrical injury. Mov Dis 1996; 9: 230–232

25. Fletcher N A, Harding A E, Marsden C D. The relationship between trauma and idiopathic torsion dystonia. J Neurol Neurosurg Psychiat 1991; 54: 713–717

26. Larsen T A, Dunn H G, Jan J E, Calne D B. Dystonia and calcification of the basal ganglia. Neurology 1985; 35: 533–537

27. Fross R D, Martin W R W, Li D et al. Lesions of the putamen: Their relevance to dystonia. Neurology 1987; 37: 1125–1129

28. Playford E D, Fletcher N A, Sawle G V et al. Striatal [^{18}F]dopa uptake in familial idiopathic dystonia. Brain 1993; 116: 1191–1199

29. Ceballos Baumann A O, Passingham R E, Warner T et al. Overactive prefrontal and underactive motor cortical areas in idiopathic dystonia. Ann Neurol 1995; 37: 363–372

30. Eidelberg D, Moeller J R, Ishikawa T et al. The metabolic topography of idiopathic torsion dystonia. Brain 1995; 118: 1473–1484

31. Tempel L W, Perlmutter J S. Abnormal vibration-induced cerebral blood flow responses in idiopathic dystonia. Brain 1990; 113: 691–707

32. Hornykiewicz O, Kish S J, Becker L E et al. Brain neurotransmitters in dystonia musculorum deformans. N Engl J Med 1986; 315: 347–353

33. Bhatia K, Daniel S E, Marsden C D. Orofacial dystonia and rest tremor in a patient with normal brain pathology. Mov Dis 1993; 8: 361–362

34. Rajput A H, Rozdilsky B, Hornykiewicz O et al. Reversible drug-induced parkinsonism: Clinico-pathological study of two cases. Arch Neurol 1982; 39: 644–646

35. Burke R E, Fahn S, Marsden C D. Torsion dystonia: A double-blind prospective trial of high-dosage trihexphenidyl. Neurology 1986; 36: 160–164

36. Jankovic J, Orman J. Tetrabenazine therapy of dystonia, chorea, tics, and other dyskinesias. Neurology 1988; 38: 391–394

37. Biary N, Koller W. Effect of alcohol on dystonia. Neurology 1985; 35: 239–240

38. Gudin M, Vaamonde J, Rodriguez M, Obeso J A. Alcohol sensitive dystonia. Mov Dis 1993; 8: 122–123

39. Lang A E. Dopamine agonists in the treatment of dystonia. Clin Neuropharmacol 1985; 8: 38

40. Stahl S M, Berger P A. Bromocriptine, physostigmine, and neurotransmitter mechanisms in the dystonias. Neurology 1982; 32: 889

41. Truong D D, Sandroni P, Van den Noort S, Matsumoto R R. Diphenhydramine is effective in the treatment of idiopathic dystonia. Arch Neurol 1995; 52: 405–407

42. Lang A E, Sheehy M P, Marsden C D. Anticholinergics in adult-onset focal dystonia. Can J Neurol Sci 1982; 9: 313–319

43. Greene P. Baclofen in the treatment of dystonia. Clin Neuropharmacol 1992; 15: 276–288

44. Albright A L, Barry M J, Fasick P et al. Continuous intrathecal baclofen infusion for symptomatic generalised dystonia. Neurosurgery 1996; 38: 934–939

45. Paret G, Tirosh R, Ben Zeev B et al. Intrathecal baclofen for severe torsion dystonia in a child. Acta Paed 1996; 85: 635–637

46. Narayan R K, Loubser P G, Jankovic J et al. Intrathecal baclofen for intractable axial dystonia. Neurology 1991; 41: 1141–1142

47. Marsden C D, Marion M-H, Quinn N. The treatment of severe dystonia in children and adults. J Neurol Neurosurg Psychiat 1984; 47: 1166–1173

48. Maccabe J J. Surgical treatment of spasmodic torticollis. In: Marsden C D, Fahn S (eds) Movement disorders. London: Butterworth Scientific, 1982: 308–314

49. Bertrand C. Peripheral versus central surgical approach for the treatment of spasmodic torticollis. In: Marsden C D, Fahn S (eds) Movement disorders. London: Butterworth Scientific, 1982: 315–318

50. Cardoso F, Jankovic J, Grossman R, Hamilton W. Outcome after stereotactic thalamotomy for dystonia and hemiballismus. Neurosurgery 1995; 36: 501–508

51. Yamashiro K, Tasker RR. Stereotactic thalamotomy for dystonic patients. Stereotactic Funct Neurosurg 1993; 60: 81–85

52. Inzelberg R, Zilber N, Kahana E, Korczyn A D. Laterality of onset in idiopathic torsion dystonia. Mov Dis 1993; 8: 327–330

53. Grafman J, Cohen L G, Hallett M. Is focal hand dystonia associated with psychopathology? Mov Dis 1991; 6: 29–35

54. Rivest J, Lees A J, Marsden C D. Writer's cramp: Treatment with botulinum toxin. Mov Dis 1991; 6: 55–59

55. McDaniel K D, Cummings J L, Shain S. The 'yips': A focal dystonia of golfers. Neurology 1989; 39: 192–195

56. Grandas F, Elston J, Quinn N, Marsden C D. Blepharospasm: A review of 264 patients. J Neurol Neurosurg Psychiatr 1988; 51: 767–772

57. Goldstein J E, Cogan D G. Apraxia of lid opening. Arch Ophthalmol 1965; 73: 155–159

58. Lepore P E, Duvoisin R C. Apraxia of lid opening: An involuntary levator inhibition. Neurology 1985; 35: 423–427

59. Elston J S. A new variant of blepharospasm. J Neurol Neurosurg Psychiat 1992; 55: 369–371

60. Krack P, Marion M H. 'Apraxia of lid opening', a focal eyelid dystonia: Clinical study of 32 patients. Mov Dis 1994; 9: 610–615

61. Johnston J C, Rosenbaum D M, Picone C M, Grotta J C. Apraxia of eyelid opening secondary to right hemisphere infarction. Ann Neurol 1989; 25: 622–624

62. Blunt S B, Fuller G, Kennard C. Orolingual dystonia with 'tip of the tongue' geste. Mov Dis 1994; 9: 466

63. Blitzer A, Brin M F. Laryngeal dystonia: A series with botulinum toxin therapy. Ann Otol Rhinol Laryngol 1991; 100: 85–89

64. Tibbetts R W. Spasmodic torticollis. J Psychosom Res 1971; 15: 461–469

65. Anon. Spasmodic torticollis. Lancet 1978; 2: 301–302

66. Suchowersky O, Calne D B. Non-dystonia causes of torticollis. In: Fahn S et al (eds) Advances in neurology, Vol 50: Dystonia 2. New York: Raven Press, 1988: 501–508

67. Jahanshahi M, Marsden C D. Depression in torticollis: A controlled study. Psychol Med 1988; 18: 925–933

68. Jahanshahi M, Marsden C D. Psychological functioning before and after treatment of torticollis with botulinum toxin. J Neurol Neurosurg Psychiat 1992; 55: 229–231

69. Claypool D W, Duane D D, Ilstrup D M, Melton L J III. Epidemiology and outcome of cervical dystonia (spasmodic torticollis) in Rochester, Minnesota. Mov Dis 1995; 10: 608–614

70. Duane D D. Spasmodic torticollis: Clinical and biologic features and their implications for focal dystonia. In: Fahn S et al (eds) Advances in neurology, Vol 50: Dystonia 2. New York: Raven Press, 1988: 473–492

71. Jahanshahi M, Marion M-H, Marsden C D. Natural history of adult-onset idiopathic torticollis. Arch Neurol 1990; 47: 548–552

72. Chan J, Brin M F, Fahn S. Idiopathic cervical dystonia: Clinical characteristics. Mov Dis 1991; 6: 119–126

73. Bronstein A M, Rudge P. The vestibular system in abnormal head postures and in spasmodic torticollis. In: Fahn S et al (eds) Advances in neurology, Vol 50: Dystonia 2. New York: Raven Press, 1988: 493–500

74. Brans J W M, Lindeboom R, Snoek J W et al. Botulinum toxin versus trihexphenidyl in cervical dystonia: A prospective, randomized, double-blind controlled trial. Neurology 1996; 46: 1066–1072

75. Blackie J D, Lees A J. Botulinum toxin injection in spasmodic torticollis. J Neurol Neurosurg Psychiat 1990; 53: 640–643

76. Therapeutics and Technology Assessment Subcommittee of the American Academy of Neurology. Assessment: The clinical usefulness of botulinum toxin-A in treating neurologic disorders. Neurology 1990; 40: 1332–1336

77. Jankovic J. Use of botulinum toxin in neurology. In: Kennard C (ed) Recent advances in clinical neurology 8. Edinburgh: Churchill Livingstone, 1995: 89–110

78. Greene P, Fahn S, Brin M F, Blitzer A. Botulinum toxin therapy. In: Marsden C D, Fahn S (eds) Movement disorders 3. Oxford: Butterworth Heinemann, 1994: 477–502

79. Scott A B. Botulinum toxin injection into extraocular muscles as an alternative to strabismus surgery. Ophthalmology 1980; 87: 1044–1049

80. Elston J S. The management of blepharospasm and hemifacial spasm. J Neurol 1992; 239: 5–8

81. Kennedy R H, Bartley G B, Flanagan J C, Waller R R. Treatment of blepharospasm with botulinum toxin. Mayo Clin Proc 1989; 64: 1085–1090

82. Jankovic J, Orman J. Botulinum A toxin for cranial–cervical dystonia: A double-blind, placebo-controlled study. Neurology 1987; 37: 616–623

83. Langueny A, Deliac M M, Julien J et al. Jaw closing spasm — a form of focal dystonia? An electrophysiological study. J Neurol Neurosurg Psychiat 1989; 52: 652–655

84. Hermanowicz N, Truong DD. Treatment of oromandibular dystonia with botulinum toxin. Laryngoscope 1991; 101: 1216–1218

85. Whurr R, Lorch M, Fontana H, Brookes G, Lees A, Marsden C D. The use of botulinum toxin in the treatment of adductor spasmodic dysphonia. J Neurol Neurosurg Psychiatr 1993; 56: 526–530

86. Jankowic J, Schwartz K, Donovan D T. Botulinum toxin treatment of cranial–cervical dystonia, spasmodic dysphonia, other focal dystonias and hemifacial spasm. J Neurol Neurosurg Psychiat 1990; 53: 633–639

87. Castellanos P F, Gates G A, Esselman G et al. Anatomic considerations in botulinum toxin type A therapy for spasmodic dysphonia. Laryngoscope 1994; 104: 656–662

88. Blitzer A, Brin M F, Stewart C et al. Abductor laryngeal dystonia: A series treated with botulinum toxin. Laryngoscope 1992; 102: 163–167

89. Jankovic J, Schwartz K. Botulinum toxin injections for cervical dystonia. Neurology 1990; 40: 277–280

90. Lees A J, Turjanski N, Rivest J et al. Treatment of cervical dystonia, hand spasms, and laryngeal dystonia with botulinum toxin. J Neurol 1992; 239: 1–4

91. Greene P, Kang U, Fahn S et al. Double-blind, placebo-controlled trial of botulinum toxin injections for the treatment of spasmodic torticollis. Neurology 1990; 40: 1213–1218

92. Comella C L, Buchman A S, Tanner C M et al. Botulinum toxin injection for spasmodic torticollis: Increased magnitude of benefit with electromyographic assistance. Neurology 1992; 42: 878–882

93. Comella C L, Tanner C M, De Foor-Hill L, Smith C. Dysphagia after botulinum toxin injections for spasmodic torticollis: clinical and radiologic findings. Neurology 1992; 42: 1307–1310

94. Karp B I, Cole R A, Cohen L G et al. Long-term botulinum toxin treatment of focal hand dystonia. Neurology 1994; 44: 70–76

95. Cohen L G, Hallett M, Geller B D, Hochberg F. Treatment of focal dystonias of the hand with botulinum toxin injections. J Neurol Neurosurg Psychiat 1989; 52: 355–363

96. Jankovic J, Schwartz K. The use of botulinum toxin in the treatment of hand dystonias. J Hand Surg 1993; 30: 295–296

97. Pullman S L, Greene P, Fahn S, Pedersen S F. Approach to the treatment of limb disorders with botulinum toxin A. Arch Neurol 1996; 53: 617–624

98. Ichinose H, Ohye T, Takahashi E I et al. Hereditary progressive dystonia with marked diurnal fluctuation caused by mutations in the GTP cyclohydrolase I gene. Nature Gen 1994; 8: 236–242

99. Bandmann O, Nygaard T G, Surtees R et al. Dopa-responsive dystonia in British patients: New mutations of the GTP-cyclohydrolase I gene and evidence for genetic heterogeneity. Hum Molec Gen 1996; 5: 403–406

100. Hirano M, Tamaru Y, Ito H et al. Mutant GTP cyclohydrolase I mRNA levels contribute to dopa-responsive dystonia onset. Ann Neurol 1996; 40: 796–798

101. Beyer K, LaoVilladoniga J I, VecinoBilbao B et al. A novel point mutation in the GTP cyclohydrolase I gene in a Spanish family with hereditary progressive and dopa responsive dystonia [4]. J Neurol Neurosurg Psychiat 1997; 62: 420–421

102. Nygaard T G, Marsden C D, Fahn S. Dopa-responsive dystonia: Long term treatment, response and prognosis. Neurology 1991; 41: 174–181

103. Levine R A, Miller L P, Lovenberg W. Tetrahydrobiopterin in striatum: Localization in dopamine nerve terminals and role in catecholamine synthesis. Science 1981; 214: 919–921

104. Nygaard T G, Trugman J M, de Yebenes J G, Fahn S. Dopa-responsive dystonia: The spectrum of clinical manifestations in a large North American family. Neurology 1990; 40: 66–69

105. Nygaard T G, Takahashi H, Heiman G A et al. Long-term treatment response and fluorodopa positron emission tomographic scanning of parkinsonism in a family with dopa-responsive dystonia. Ann Neurol 1992; 32: 603–608

106. Fink J K, Barton N, Cohen W et al. Dystonia with marked diurnal variation associated with biopterin deficiency. Neurology 1988; 38: 707–711

107. Sawle G V, Leenders K L, Brooks D J et al. Dopa-responsive dystonia: [¹⁸F]Dopa positron emission tomography. Ann Neurol 1991; 30: 24–30

108. Sawle G V. Imaging the brain: Functional imaging. J Neurol Neurosurg Psychiat 1995; 58: 132–144

109. Rajput A H, Gibb W R G, Zhong X et al. Dopa-responsive dystonia — pathological and biochemical observations in a case. Ann Neurol 1994; 35: 396–402

110. Narbona J, Obeso J A, Tuñon T et al. Hemi-dystonia secondary to localised basal ganglia tumour. J Neurol Neurosurg Psychiat 1984; 47: 704–709

111. Schulze-Bonhage A, Ferbert A. Cervical dystonia as an isolated sign of a basal ganglia tumour. J Neurol Neurosurg Psychiat 1995; 58: 108–109

112. Lehéricy S, Vidailhet M, Dormont D et al. Striatopallidal and thalamic dystonia. Arch Neurol 1996; 53: 241–250

113. Molho E S, Factor S A. Basal ganglia infarction as a possible cause of cervical dystonia. Mov Dis 1993; 8: 213–216

114. Schwartz M, De Deyn P P, Van den Kerchove M, Pickut B A. Cervical dystonia as a probable consequence of focal cerebral lesion. Mov Dis 1995; 10: 797–798

115. Marsden C D, Obeso J A, Zarranz J J, Lang A E. The anatomical basis of the symptomatic hemidystonias. Brain 1985; 108: 463–483

116. Isaac K, Cohen J A. Post-traumatic torticollis. Neurology 1989; 39: 1642–1643

117. Abbruzzese G, Rizzo F, Dall'Agata D et al. Generalized dystonia with bilateral striatal computed-tomographic lucencies in a patient with human immunodeficiency virus infection. Eur Neurol 1990; 30: 271–273

118. Barton J J S, Cox T A, Calne D A. Involuntary ocular deviations and generalized dystonia in multiple sclerosis: A case report. J Neuro-Ophthalmol 1994; 14: 160–162

119. Krauss J K, Mohadjer M, Braus D F et al. Dystonia following head trauma: A report of nine patients and a review of the literature. Mov Dis 1992; 7: 263–272

120. Brett E M, Hoare R D, Sheehy M P, Marsden C D. Progressive hemi-dystonia due to focal basal ganglia lesion after mild head trauma. J Neurol Neurosurg Psychiat 1981; 44: 460

121. Gibb W R G, Lees A J, Marsden C D. Pathological reports of four patients presenting with cranial dystonias. Mov Dis 1988; 3: 211–221

122. Gille M, Jacquemin C, Kiame G et al. Myelinolyse centropontine avec ataxie cerebelleuse et dystonie. Revue Neurologique 1993; 149: 344–346

123. Salerno S M, Kurlan R, Joy S E, Shoulson I. Dystonia in central pontine myelinolysis without evidence of extrapontine myelinolysis. J Neurol Neurosurg Psychiat 1993; 56: 1221–1223

124. Uncini A, Di Muzio A, Thomas A et al. Hand dystonia secondary to demyelinating lesion. Acta Neurol Scand 1994; 90: 51–55

125. Cammarota A, Gershanik O S, García S, Lera G. Cervical dystonia due to spinal cord ependymoma: Involvement of cervical cord segments in the pathogenesis of dystonia. Mov Dis 1995; 10: 500–503

126. Gollomp S M, Fahn S. Transient dystonia as a complication of varicella. J Neurol Neurosurg Psychiat 1987; 50: 1228–1229

127. Lee M S, Rinne J O, Ceballos-Baumann A et al. Dystonia after head trauma. Neurology 1994; 44: 1374–1378

128. Mauro A J, Fahn S, Russman B. Hemidystonia following 'minor' head trauma. Ann Neurol 1980; 8: 108

129. Polk J L, Maragos V A, Nicholas J J. Cervical spondylotic myeloradiculopathy in dystonia. Arch Phys Med Rehab 1992; 73: 389–392

130. Drory V E, Neufeld M Y, Korczyn A D. Carpal tunnel syndrome: A complication of idiopathic torsion dystonia. Mov Dis 1991; 6: 82–84

chapter 7

Chorea

Guy Sawle

There are many causes of chorea. Broadly, there are a series of hereditary disorders of which the commonest is Huntington's disease, and there are also metabolic, infectious, and structural causes, the latter comprising both vascular and mass lesions. Chorea can also occur as a side-effect of certain drugs (see Chapter 11). Some of the conditions which commonly cause chorea also cause other abnormalities of movement, such as parkinsonism and dystonia.

Huntington's disease

History

George Huntington (1850–1916) was born on Long Island and grew up in a community where hereditary chorea was already known to his father and grandfather, who were both local family physicians. His only known written document 'On Chorea'[1] refers to a hereditary illness producing insanity and suicide, yet manifesting itself only in adult life. Huntington stated 'It begins as an ordinary chorea might begin, by the irregular and spasmodic action of certain muscles, as of the face, arms etc. These movements gradually increase, when muscles hitherto unaffected take on the spasmodic action until every muscle in the body becomes affected (except the involuntary ones), and the poor patient presents a spectacle which is anything but pleasing to witness'.

Epidemiology

Huntington's disease is found worldwide. The prevalence in the USA is around 5–7 per 100 000. Rates in Europe vary from around 0.5 (Finland) to 7.8 (Malta) per 100 000. The highest known prevalence is around Lake Maracaibo in Venezuela, where rates of around 700 per 100 000 have been estimated.[2]

Genetics

Huntington's disease is caused by an unstable expanded DNA trinucleotide (cytosine–adenosine–guanine, or CAG) repeat within the coding region for a protein

called huntingtin.[3] The gene (*IT15*) lies on the short arm of chromosome four (4p16.3). Most normal subjects have between 11 and 24 CAG repeats at this position in the huntingtin gene. Patients have a higher number of repeats (typically 37 or more). Most centres have found no overlap between the highest repeat number in normal controls and the lowest number in patients,[4] though some have reported a slight overlap (normal controls 9–34 repeats versus affected individuals 30–70;[5] normal controls 7–34 repeats versus affected individuals 27–102[6]). One possible explanation for patients with repeat lengths in the 'normal' range may be inaccuracies in diagnosis; in some cases, the pathology ultimately shows conditions other than Huntington's disease.[7] Exceptionally, careful studies have documented occasional subjects with long repeats who have remained healthy into extreme old age, such as a man aged 95 without classical signs of Huntington's disease despite a repeat length of 39.[8]

The repeat length varies from generation to generation. Whilst it may become shorter or longer in meiosis, the largest *increases* occur in paternal spermatogenesis.[4]

In a fully penetrant disease, how do we explain the appearance of apparently sporadic cases? Hitherto, such patients have been explained on the basis of misdiagnosis, non-paternity, or on the assumption that the affected parent must have died prior to clinical presentation (this argument being supported by the observation of occasional presentation in old age). The changes in CAG repeat length does, however, provide a potential genetic mechanism for new mutations. It appears that individuals who appear clinically as 'new mutations' have a parent with a repeat length at the upper limit of the normal range;[9] so mutation to Huntington's disease is associated with further expansion from an already large repeat length.

Since the gene was identified, many centres have explored the possibility of a relationship between the size of the triple repeat and various aspects of the disease. There is a clear relationship between the length of the repeat and the age of onset of the disease (Fig. 7.1).[10] It has been estimated that the repeat length accounts for approximately 50% of the variation in age at onset,[10] though this association becomes less clear-cut with later disease onset.[9] Measurement of the repeat length in presymptomatic subjects does not, therefore, provide a reliable estimate of the likely age of presentation. Whether the size of the repeat on the normal allele contributes to any of the clinical manifestations of the disease is presently unknown. Some authors have reported an inverse relationship between CAG repeat length and the rate of disease progression after presentation,[11,12] whilst others have found no such relationship.[13]

The mechanism whereby this apparently fully penetrant disorder usually causes no apparent harm until well into adult life is unknown.

Clinical features

The cardinal clinical features of Huntington's disease are the movement disorder, dementia and psychiatric features, usually in the context of a positive family history.

Because chorea is usually the first obvious clinical sign this led to the previous naming of the condition as Huntington's *chorea*. But patients with Huntington's disease also have other abnormal movements including myoclonus, parkinsonism and dystonia. Typically, chorea dominates the picture in the early stages, whilst parkinsonism and dystonia become more obvious later. All patients have abnormal eye movements, usually from very early on in the clinical phase of their illness.

Chorea

The chorea of Huntington's disease is typically more conspicuous in the face and upper limbs (CDs 7.1 and 7.2). A wide variety of movements are seen both between and within patients; though prolonged observation may show that some patients make particular movements more frequently than others. Early on, patients may be unaware of the movements; even those who know themselves to be at risk for the disease and are 'on the lookout' for involuntary movements may be unaware that they have begun. It is usually the secondary effects of the chorea, clumsiness and incoordination, which patients notice first.

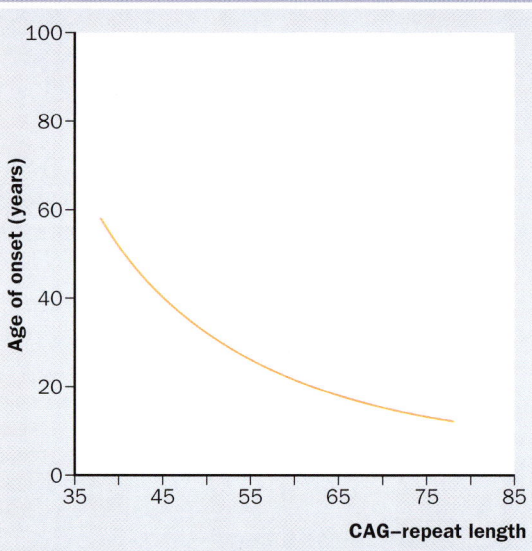

CAG REPEAT LENGTH VERSUS AGE OF ONSET

Figure 7.1. The relationship between CAG repeat length and age of onset in Huntington's disease. (Adapted from ref. 10.)

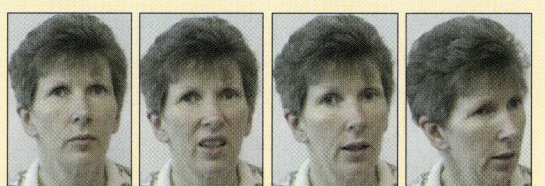

CD 7.1. Choreic facial movements.

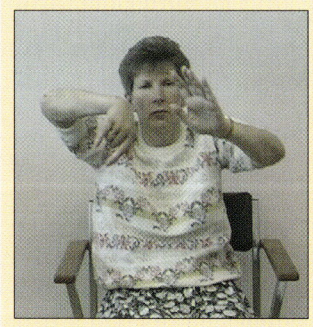

CD 7.2. Progression of chorea over three years in a patient with Huntington's disease.

Some patients incorporate their choreic movements into subsequent purposeful acts. Thus a jerk of the hand towards the face may be adopted and used as the first part of a movement to stroke the face or adjust spectacles (CD 7.7).

With more severe chorea, speech function becomes disturbed and intermittently halted. Feeding can be a problem, although usually less so than in patients with neuroacanthocytosis (see page 126). Chorea affecting the legs leads to a lurching appearance, with swaying, jerkiness, and falls.

Oculomotor disturbance

Patients with Huntington's disease are rarely aware that there is anything wrong with the way their eyes move. But clinical examination often shows slow and/or inaccurate saccades, and abnormal (quick phases of) optokinetic nystagmus. It is usual for the abnormalities to be more severe in the vertical than the horizontal plane.[14] They may have difficulty in initiating saccades without head movement. Patients with Huntington's disease are more distractible than normal, and they have difficulty in suppressing gaze towards a novel visual stimulus.[15,16] Pursuit movements may be slow and vergence limited. Horizontal saccadic latency and velocity have been shown to deteriorate over a 2-year period in untreated patients, leading to the suggestion that this measure might serve as a useful clinical marker of disease progression.[17]

Parkinsonism

Many patients with Huntington's disease show evidence of parkinsonism. In patients with the most usual choreic presentation, parkinsonism usually follows years later and in some cases it may be made more clinically obvious as a side-effect of drugs used to suppress the chorea (such as tetrabenazine).

In a minority, parkinsonism is the *presenting* motor symptom. This pattern of presentation is more common in patients with juvenile onset.

Myoclonus

Myoclonus is an uncommon feature of juvenile onset Huntington's disease.[18] Multifocal action myoclonus also rarely occurs in patients with adult-onset disease (see CD 9.1).[19,20] In some cases, treatment with valproic acid and/or clonazepam is beneficial.

Cognitive impairment

Patients with Huntington's disease have early problems with memory, arithmetic, and interpersonal relationships. They become slow, disorganized and inefficient in the performance of activities of daily living. By way of contrast, aphasia, agnosia and apraxia (all seen in Alzheimer's disease) are rare.

Part of the problem in communication in Huntington's disease is due to difficulty understanding prosody, with failure to follow changes in rhythm and tone in normal speech.

Psychiatric impairment

Folstein[21] surveyed 186 patients in Maryland, and using DSM-III criteria found 30% to have no definite psychiatric disorder, whilst 33% had affective disorder, 30% intermittent explosive disorder, 4.8% dysthymic disorder, 15.6% alcoholism, 5.9% antisocial personality and 5.9% schizophrenia.

Family members report irritability, which may amount to the 'intermittent explosive disorder' referred to above. There are often other personality changes too, including inappropriate behaviour such as standing too close to other people. Huntington's original description refers to abnormal sexual behaviour,[1] but this has not subsequently been a consistent finding.

Suicide is more common in Huntington's disease than in the general population. Various rates have been reported; in a recent Danish study similar rates were reported in affected patients (5.6%) and siblings (5.3%).[22] Whilst some of the siblings may have been asymptomatic carriers, it is likely that this high suicide rate also reflects the effect of this disease on genetically unaffected family members.

Gait

Patients with Huntington's disease have a gait abnormality which cannot all be explained on the basis of chorea. They are usually rather unsteady and adopt a broad base. Their chorea may be generally more severe when walking than when sitting quietly. Some have a chaotic gait pattern, with gross lurching and swaying movements (CD 7.3). Gait may be slowed, particularly in patients showing features of parkinsonism.

Imaging

Structural measurements using CT and MRI have been reported (Fig. 7.2). The bicaudate diameter is considered a sensitive measure of caudate atrophy in Huntington's disease. Patients who present in early life with an akinetic-rigid syndrome, and some who

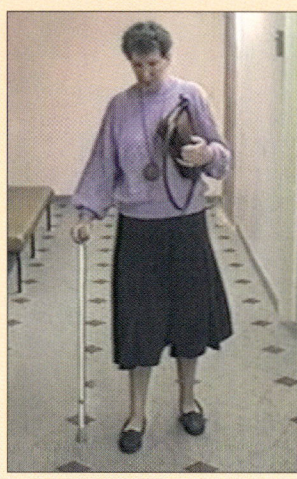

CD 7.3. Gait in Huntington's disease.

present later with chorea, have striatal hypointensity on T2-weighted MR images.[23]

Positron emission tomography (PET) scans using [^{11}C]flumazenil as tracer have shown reduced benzodiazepine receptor density in the caudate nucleus; using fluorodeoxyglucose as tracer, hypometabolism is seen not only in caudate but also in putamen and thalamus.[24]

PET striatal dopamine receptor studies using [^{11}C]SCH23390 (for D1 receptors) and [^{11}C]raclopride (for D2 receptors) show a severe and parallel reduction of the two types irrespective of whether patients present with chorea or an akinetic-rigid syndrome (Fig. 7.3).[25]

Some asymptomatic gene carriers also show parallel reductions in these two receptor types.[26]

Neuropathology

Atrophy is maximal in the caudate, putamen and globus pallidus, though the cerebral cortex is also atrophied with loss of frontal, temporal and parietal cross-sectional area (Fig. 7.4). There is an increase in the grey/white matter ratio. The amygdala and thalamus are also reduced in area.[27] Abnormal neurites and inclusion bodies are both visible in the cortex using immunostaining for ubiquitin (Figs. 7.5, 7.6). It has been suggested that the principal reason for pallidal atrophy is loss of striatopallidal fibres, rather than neurons.[28] Neuronal loss in the striatum is related to cell type. Of the three populations of striatal interneurons (one kind expressing somatostatin, neuropeptide Y and nitric oxide synthase (SS/NPY/NOS), another expressing acetylcholine, and the third expressing gamma-aminobutyric acid (GABA), the GABA neurons are affected first, though not in early disease. The cholinergic neurons become dysfunctional but do not degenerate severely, and the SS/NPY/NOS neurons are comparatively spared throughout. Of the striatal projection neurons, there is early loss of the projection to the external pallidum and substantia nigra pars reticulata; the projection to the substantia nigra pars compacta may occur even earlier, and the projection to the internal pallidum

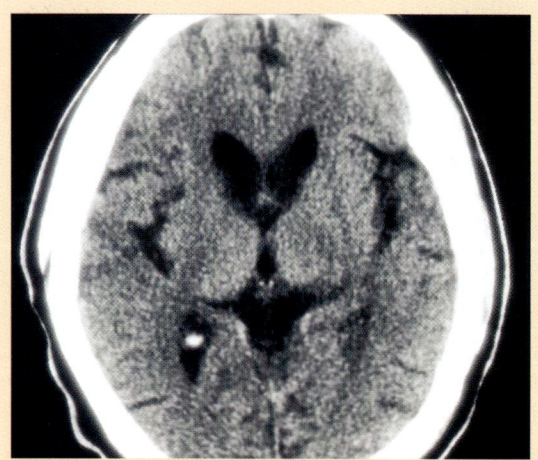

Figure 7.2. CT in advanced Huntington's disease showing ventricular dilation due to cortical and subcortical atrophy. (Courtesy of J. K. Niparko.)

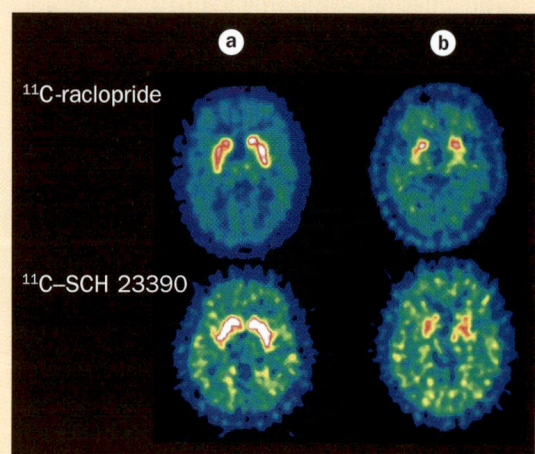

Figure 7.3. Raclopride (D2) and SCH23390 (D1) scans showing reduced binding of both tracers in stratum of (a) control and (b) a Huntington's disease patient. (Courtesy of N. Turjanski.)

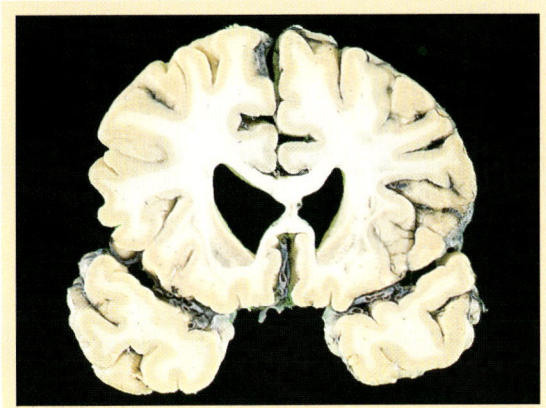

Figure 7.4. Cortical and subcortical atrophy in Huntington's disease. (Courtesy of J. Lowe.).

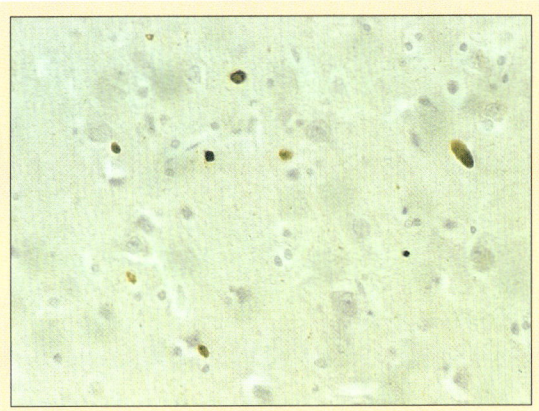

Figure 7.5. Huntington's disease. Anti-ubiquitin staining of cortical neurites. (Courtesy of J. Lowe.)

most likely occurs last.[29] Striatal afferent terminals, such as from the nigrostriatal projection, appear unimpaired. There is a significant positive correlation between the CAG repeat length and neuropathological severity in the striatum at postmortem.[30]

The function of huntingtin remains unclear at the time of writing, though the gene is expressed in a variety of tissues including brain, where in normal subjects the highest levels are seen in cerebellum, hippocampus, cerebral cortex, substantia nigra pars compacta, and pontine nuclei. Expression in the striatum is intermediate and in the globus pallidus low.[31] It is expressed predominantly in neurons. In patients, the distribution and levels of mRNA are comparable to controls in all areas except in the striatum where the intensity of labelling is much reduced.[31] The characteristic pattern of pathology found in Huntington's disease cannot therefore be accounted for by the expression of huntingtin.

Current speculation of the mechanism of the disease relates to a 'gain of function' effect, whereby the abnormal protein has acquired a new and lethal property;[32] so discovering what huntingtin *normally* does, may not help understand its role in the pathogenesis of Huntington's disease, since the abnormal polyglutamine could confer on the protein some entirely different property, such as altering protein transcription.

Animal models of Huntington's disease may be produced by injection of either 3-nitropropionic acid, or malonate, each of which inhibits succinate dehydrogenase, complex II of the mitochondrial respiratory

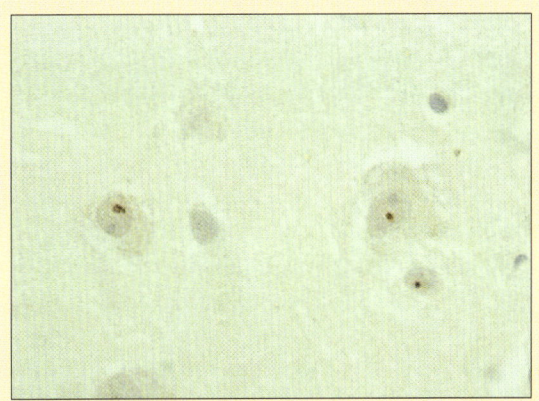

Figure 7.6. Huntington's disease. Anti-ubiquitin staining of cortical inclusion bodies. (Courtesy of J. Lowe.)

chain. Defects of complexes II, III and IV have been demonstrated in human caudate from patients with Huntington's disease. It has been argued that deficient energy metabolism may cause neuronal death through excitotoxic mechanisms, a suggestion supported by demonstration of increased glutamate levels in the caudate using magnetic resonance spectroscopy.[33] But for the moment there is no obvious connection between expanded CAG repeats and the excitotoxic mechanism speculated to be the ultimate cause of cell death in Huntington's disease.

Prognosis

The median duration of survival is independent of the age of onset, except in patients aged over 50 years at onset, where survival is slightly shorter, due to death from unrelated causes (Fig. 7.7).[34] Survival is slightly shorter for males, particularly if they inherit the disease from their father.

Drug treatment

No form of treatment has yet been shown to delay the onset or progression of Huntington's disease. Several agents are used for symptomatic control, however, and in some cases they have been subject to formal drug trials.

The suppression of chorea does not usually either improve or maintain functional ability,[35] so it is wrong to suppress the movements just because they are present. Sometimes, however, the chorea is severe enough to seriously hamper a patient's motor skills in which case a variety of agents may suppress the unwanted movements.

Several drugs act to suppress chorea via the reduction or interruption of dopaminergic transmission. These include dopamine receptor antagonists, and dopamine depleting agents such as tetrabenazine[36] and reserpine. The penalty of dopamine blockade or depletion is, of course, parkinsonism and sometimes akathisia, tardive dyskinesia or tardive dystonia.[37] Rarely, both neuroleptic agents and tetrabenazine can cause the so-called neuroleptic malignant syndrome.[38] Sedation is a common side-effect of some agents. Tetrabenazine often makes patients depressed. Since parkinsonism can develop as a consequence of the disease process itself, it is important to watch carefully to be sure that any antidopamine drugs being used are really still giving benefit in excess of impairment.

Sulpiride and risperidone have each been shown to improve functional activities as assessed by a functional disability scale.[39] Sulpiride has also been shown to have a modest effect on the eye movement abnormality.[40] In an open-label trial, clozapine was shown to improve chorea and to lead to an improvement in the activities of daily living.[41]

Very rarely, in patients who present with parkinsonism, a cautious trial of levodopa may produce some benefit.[42]

Depression in Huntington's disease is common and this aspect at least may be partially amenable to drug treatment. Rarely, patients with severe depression may be unresponsive to drug treatment, in which case electroconvulsive therapy (ECT) may have a role, particularly in patients with prominent delusions.[43]

SURVIVAL IN HUNTINGTON'S DISEASE

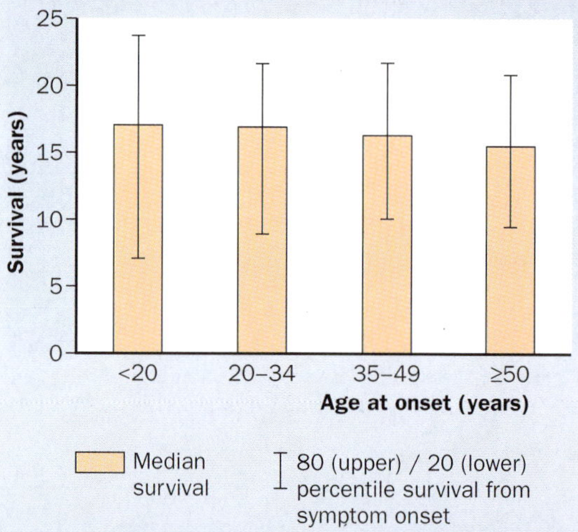

Figure 7.7. The relationship between survival and age at onset of symptoms in Huntington's disease. (Adapted from ref. 34.)

Leuprolide acetate (a gonadotrophin-releasing hormone agonist) has been used to ameliorate exhibitionism.[44]

Trials of agents with a putative neuroprotective effect have to date been disappointing. The first major controlled trial of an agent which it was hoped might have neuroprotective benefit used baclofen. The trial was based on the observation that baclofen retards corticostriatal release of glutamate and aspartate. Baclofen 60 mg per day had no better effect than placebo over a period of 30–42 months.[45]

In an effort to reduce oxidative stress, a prospective placebo-controlled double-blind study compared high dose d-alpha-tocopherol (which reduces oxyradical damage to cell membranes) with placebo. The study showed no overall benefit of the active drug, although *post hoc* analysis did show an effect on neurological symptoms in early disease.[46] A recent preliminary study showed tolerability of coenzyme Q10 in Huntington's disease, but no effect on rating scales over the short study period.[47] The results of longer-term studies are awaited. In a randomized double-blind placebo-controlled study, remacemide (an *N*-methyl-D-aspartate (NMDA) glutamate receptor ion channel blocker) was generally well tolerated. There were no significant differences between drug- and placebo-treated patients, though there was a trend to improvement in chorea in patients on remacemide.[48]

Neurotransplantation

Almost all of the patients who have undergone fetal cell implantation have had Parkinson's disease, even though there are a wide variety of effective alternative medical treatments for that condition. Why so? Almost certainly because of the apparent simplicity of nigral deafferentation leading to striatal dopamine deficiency. For several years interested scientists and clinicians have pondered and studied the applicability of a similar technique as treatment for Huntington's disease.

Whereas Parkinson's disease transplantation procedures utilize tissue from the fetal mesencephalon (a fraction of which would normally become the substantia nigra), harvesting tissue for a striatal graft in Huntington's disease would require donor tissue from that part of the fetal brain destined to become the adult striatum. The problem here is that at the stage of embryological development when the future striatal cells are at appropriate maturity to survive the harvesting and implantation procedure, they are intermingled with other cells which are destined to become adult cortex. And the difficulty with implanting such a cell mixture could be uncontrolled tissue growth.

Another difficulty is connected to the lack of successful treatments for Huntington's disease. In Parkinson's disease, the many drug trials have fuelled the need for reliable and agreed clinical rating scales. There are fewer such validated scales in Huntington's disease, although much work has been done to develop a Unified Huntington's Disease Rating Scale (UHDRS),[49] and a core assessment program for intracerebral transplantation in Huntington's disease (CAPIT-HD).[50]

Senile chorea

For many years, it has been recognized that elderly patients occasionally develop chorea without any obvious explanation and without a positive family history. The disorder was assumed to be separate from Huntington's disease, in which presentation is usually very much earlier. But then an influential study reexamined the issue of diagnosis in patients with 'senile chorea' and on the basis of the pathological findings it was concluded that the correct diagnosis was, in most cases, Huntington's disease. Various explanations for the lack of family history (including non-paternity and death of an affected parent prior to clinical presentation) were put forward.

With the advent of the gene test for Huntington's disease it has still more recently become possible to measure such patients' CAG repeat lengths. Some undoubtedly do have normal CAG repeats, confirming that they do *not* all have Huntington's disease.[51]

Sydenham's chorea

Despite the recognition of an association between rheumatic heart disease and chorea in the mid-nineteenth century, and the later realization of an association with group A streptococcal infection, we still do not know the exact aetiology of this disorder.

There has been a marked decline in the incidence of Sydenham's chorea in recent decades, although an increased incidence was reported in the late 1980s. In addition to the chorea, many patients have prominent behavioural change.[52] Psychiatric symptoms, including obsessive-compulsive symptoms, may be more common for decades after motor recovery.[53]

No single test can be used to make the diagnosis. EEG abnormalities are common (usually diffuse slowing), whilst CT brain scans are generally normal. Patients studied acutely with PET have increased putamen and caudate glucose metabolism, which may return to normal when the chorea settles.[54,55] CSF protein level and white cell count are normal, and oligoclonal immunoglobulin bands are not seen.[56] Upper and lower limb cortical somatosensory-evoked potentials are also normal.[56] Cardiolipin antibodies are absent in some patients,[57] but positive in others, particularly in patients with valvulitis.[58]

Sodium valproate has been reported an effective treatment.[59,60]

Systemic lupus erythematosus

With the decline in the incidence of rheumatic fever, systemic lupus erythematosus has become one of the more common causes of chorea, particularly in young women (CD 7.4). Many, but not all, cases are associated with circulating lupus anticoagulant, or antiphospholipid antibodies. Some patients have antiphospholipid antibodies, but without classical clinical features of lupus.

The neurological symptoms of lupus are legion and so patients may show other clinical signs, such as migraine, seizures, transient ischaemic attacks, stroke or neuropathy. Neuropsychiatric features are not unusual. When chorea occurs in lupus it may be the earliest sign of neurological involvement, and it may even antedate all other clinical signs by months or years. The movements may be focal or generalized. In some cases, chorea may appear for the first time during treatment with oestrogens (page 176),[61] during pregnancy (see below), or in the postpartum period.[62]

It is not clear whether the chorea is due to vascular damage to the basal ganglia, or due to immunological damage via circulating antibodies.

Imaging studies sometimes show basal ganglia lesions which are presumed to be vascular. Neuronal loss with widespread astroglial proliferation in the putamen has been reported at postmortem.[63]

The chorea may remit spontaneously within days, or continue for as long as years. In the first instance, treatment is usually directed to the underlying condition, and includes the use of corticosteroids, aspirin and anticoagulation. If persistent and troublesome, the involuntary movements can be treated with neuroleptic agents including haloperidol.

Chorea gravidarum

It has long been realized that women with a prior history of (usually Sydenham's) chorea may develop chorea again during pregnancy. With the decline in the incidence of Sydenham's chorea, however, most cases of chorea gravidarum nowadays are probably due to other conditions, such as systemic lupus erythematosus.[64] Rarely, chorea may develop in pregnancy without any relevant past medical history. In one patient who developed the disorder late in her first pregnancy and died of hyperthermia 2 weeks later, neuropathological examination showed striatal nerve cell loss and astrocytosis.[65] Rarely, chorea may recur in subsequent pregnancies.[66]

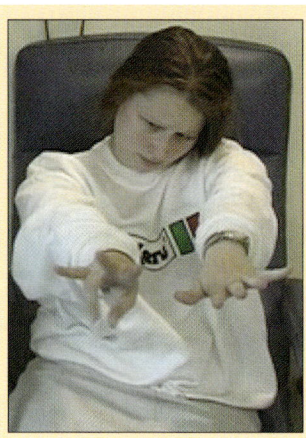

CD 7.4. Chorea in systemic lupus erythematosus.

Haloperidol has been recommended as a 'reasonably safe treatment' in the context of chorea in the second and third trimesters.[67]

Neuroacanthocytosis

Acanthocytes are spiky red blood cells (Fig. 7.8). Bassen and Kornzweig are credited with being the first (in 1950) to recognize an association between the presence of acanthocytes in peripheral blood and neurological disease.[68] In the late 1960s, reports of families with chorea and acanthocytosis were reported. Not all patients with neuroacanthocytosis have chorea; but it is the most common associated movement disorder. Acanthocytes are also seen in the McLeod syndrome.

Clinical features

Presentation is between middle childhood and the seventh decade of life (range 8–62, mean age of onset 32). The literature contains a small excess of male cases in comparison to female. The genetics remain uncertain. Most patients have a positive family history, but not all. Consanguinity has been a feature in some families. Both autosomal recessive and autosomal dominant inheritance have been proposed — the latter because of recorded cases of parent-to-child transmission.

Behavioural disturbance, personality change and cognitive impairment are all common clinical features. Of those showing general intellectual deterioration, some have memory impairment (including visuoperceptual deficits); many show a range of impairments in frontal lobe executive skills,[69] meaning a difficulty in

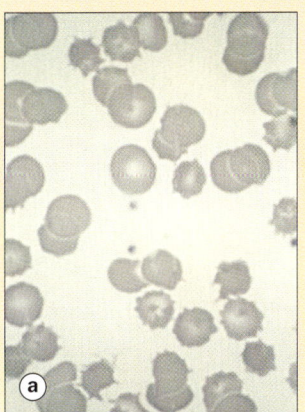

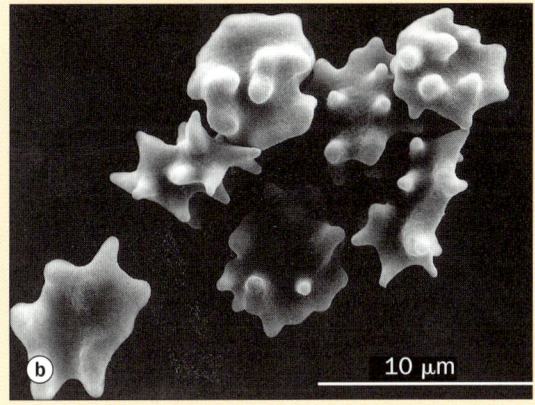

Figure 7.8. (a) Peripheral blood smear showing acanthocytes. (b) Scanning electron micrograph showing acanthocytes. (Courtesy of S. Bohlega

sustaining concentration over time, planning, monitoring and modifying behaviour appropriately in order to achieve a particular goal. Some patients show depression, anxiety, or obsessive compulsive behaviour.[70]

Many have chorea, which may affect the face as well as the limbs. Some patients present with dystonia rather than chorea and in such cases speech is often affected. Almost half may also suffer stereotyped tics. A minority develop a parkinsonian syndrome. Many patients have a mixture of these forms, though chorea when present is often dominant and it tends to involve the legs earlier and there are said to be fewer movements of the forehead and hands than are typically seen in patients with Huntington's chorea. A small minority of patients are detected by laboratory investigation, yet have no movement disorder.

This mixture of abnormal movements very often gives rise to dysarthria and patients may become virtually anarthric. A variety of involuntary vocalizations occur (but not usually the utterance of recognizable words) and many patients have orofacial dyskinesias. Involuntary biting of the lips, tongue, and the inside of the mouth can be a particular problem in these patients. Some develop dystonic tongue protrusion when attempting to eat.

Occasional patients have weakness or wasting; some are hypo- or areflexic and a few have extensor plantar responses. Almost half of affected patients have seizures which may be the first clinical manifestation.[71]

Haematology

Acanthocytes must be specifically looked for and fresh blood films are required; if blood is collected into ethylene-diamine-tetracetic acid (EDTA) blood tubes, then the film should be made within an hour of collection. Acanthocytes are dense, slightly contracted red cells bearing a number of irregularly spaced thorny surface projections, often with terminal bulbs. Occasional acanthocytes are seen in normal blood films. Patients with neuro-acanthocytosis usually have >3% acanthocytes. It may be necessary to send a series of blood films to the laboratory in order to identify acanthocytes, because even in patients subsequently shown to have neuroacathocytosis, up to several initial blood films may appear normal.

Non-haematological investigations

Creatine kinase is commonly raised; in exceptional patients the level may be >1000 IU/l. Serum lipoprotein electrophoresis is normal (in contrast to the abnormal pattern seen in patients with abetalipoproteinaemia, Bassen Kornzweig syndrome). CT brain scans may show cerebral and/or caudate atrophy and MRI scan may show abnormal signal return from the putamen also. Sensory action potentials are often abnormal whereas motor nerve conduction is usually unimpaired. PET scans of patients with neuroacanthocytosis using fluorodopa as tracer have shown normal caudate and anterior putamen uptake, but a loss of posterior putamen signal, much as seen in the early stages of Parkinson's disease. PET studies using raclopride as tracer have shown markedly reduced D2 receptor density in the striatum, compatible with a loss of the D2 receptor bearing striatal neurones.[72]

Pathology

In nerve biopsy specimens there may be a reduction in the large myelinated fibre populations together with histological features suggestive of regeneration following axonal degeneration.

At postmortem, lateral ventricular enlargement is usual (Fig. 7.9). Both caudate and putamen are atrophic with neuronal loss and gliosis. Small and medium sized striatal neurons are particularly depleted. The globus pallidus is almost as severely affected, whilst the thalamus, substantia nigra[73] and anterior horns of the spinal cord show neuronal loss with gliosis in some cases only. Brain areas which are consistently spared include the subthalamic nucleus, cerebral cortex, cerebellum, pons and medulla.[74]

Treatment and prognosis

There is no specific treatment for this condition. Seizures are treated with anticonvulsants. Tics, chorea and dystonia are treated in the usual way. There have not been any controlled trials with any of these medications.

Of those patients who have been reported at postmortem, the mean interval from diagnosis to death has been 14 (range 7–24) years. At the time of reporting, surviving patients have been alive from diagnosis for a mean of 9 (range 3–33) years; this latter rather low average figure may reflect the recent recognition of this disorder, rather than a genuine short survival.

McLeod syndrome

This is an X-linked condition with abnormal expression of the Kell blood group. Kell is a complex blood group system with more than 20 serologically

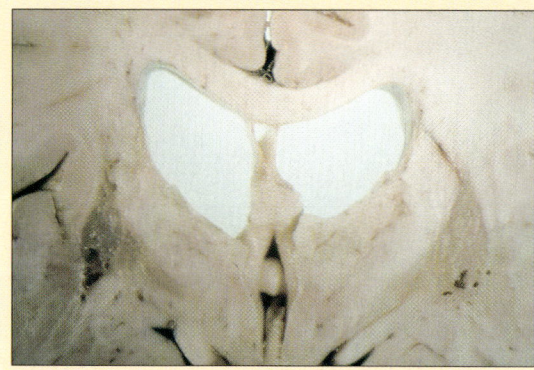

Figure 7.9. Severe atrophy of the caudate nuclei with dilatation of anterior horns of lateral ventricles in neuroacanthocytosis. (Courtesy of R. Hardie.)

recognized erythrocyte antigens. It is the next most important blood group system after ABO and Rhesus in determining transfusion compatibility. All patients with the McLeod syndrome are male. They all have elevated creatine kinase. A benign myopathy has been described and some patients were historically said to have chorea.

Hemiballismus

The movements of hemiballismus are big. They are mostly proximal, irregular and vigorous (CD 7.5). There are often other associated movements, typically chorea.[75,76] The movements generally stop during sleep.

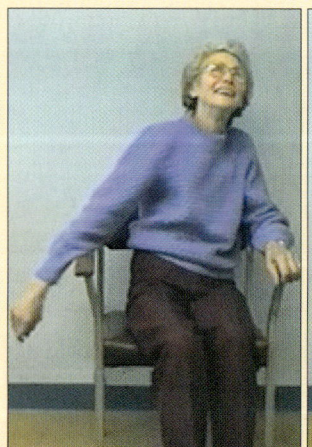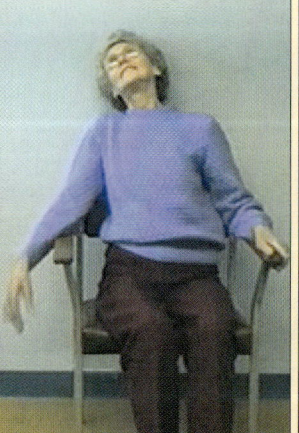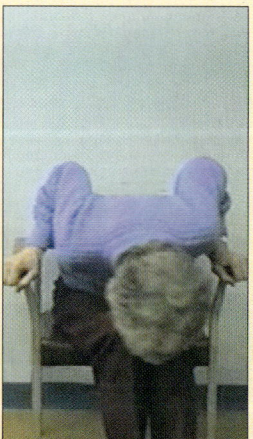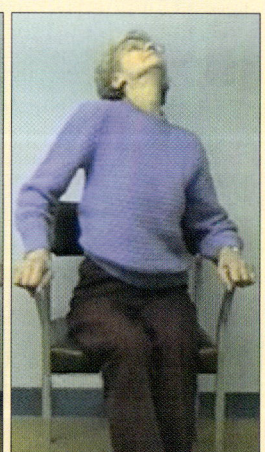

CD 7.5. Hemiballismus before treatment.

Patients cannot suppress the movements, at least not for more than a moment or two. Thankfully the disorder is usually unilateral, although when (as is often the case) the trunk is involved, this still leads to massive whole-body movements. Very rarely the disorder is bilateral (biballism) when drug induced or due to a system disease.

Hemiballismus is much less common than chorea, with an incidence of around 1 in 500 000, and comprising less than 1% of patients referred to a movement disorder clinic.[76]

When a lesion is found on imaging or at postmortem, it is classically sited in the subthalamic nucleus. With the increasing sophistication of imaging methods, not only are appropriate lesions seen more frequently, but many patients also have lesions in other sites too. There have been a small number of reports of patients who appear only to have *ipsilateral* striatal lesions on imaging studies.[77]

Most lesions causing hemiballismus are vascular, including both ischaemia and haemorrhage; nevertheless, many other causes have been recognized, including tumours, multiple sclerosis, head trauma, tuberculosis, systemic lupus erythematosus, scleroderma, thalamotomy, syphilis, hyperglycaemia, and a variety of drugs (including the oral contraceptive, phenytoin, levodopa and neuroleptics).[78] In recent years there have been a number of reports of hemiballismus associated with toxoplasmosis and AIDS.[79,80]

Where the underlying cause is a sudden event, such as a stroke, the onset of the abnormal movements may be immediate, or delayed for at least a period of several weeks.

In patients with a vascular aetiology, the age at onset is usually around 65–75. Patients with a more exotic aetiology may present at a much earlier age.

Treatment and prognosis

Even though spontaneous improvement is usual in patients with a vascular aetiology, short-term drug treatment is appropriate because of the severity and danger of the involuntary movements (CD 7.6). In many cases it is possible to reduce and stop all drugs after 2 or 3 months. Neuroleptic agents including haloperidol, pimozide and sulpiride are effective. Tetrabenazine, reserpine, clonazepam, clozapine[81]

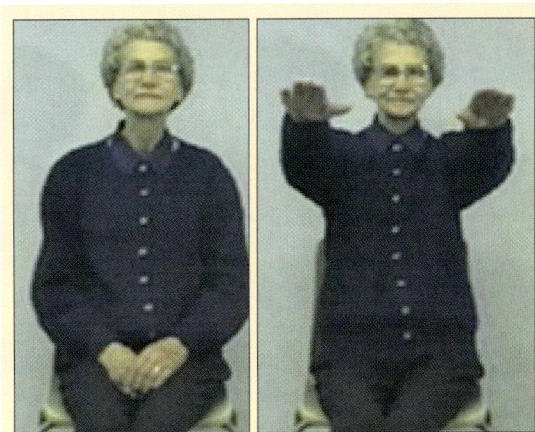

CD 7.6. Hemiballismus during treatment.

and sodium valproate[82,83] have also been tried with some success. Rarely, in drug resistant cases, a stereotactic ventral intermediate thalamotomy has been effective,[84] as has chronic thalamic stimulation.[85]

Vascular chorea

Less commonly, vascular disease may cause chorea rather than hemiballismus. The responsible lesions may be found in the caudate, putamen, thalamus or corona radiata. The onset of symptoms is usually sudden, and gradual improvement occurs with time (CD 7.7). The symptoms are typically unilateral and may involve a single limb. Perhaps more surprising is the frequency with which broadly similar vascular lesions are noted in the basal ganglia as incidental findings, without history of any kind of movement disorder at all.

Miscellaneous causes of chorea

Although as a disease of white matter, multiple sclerosis rarely gives rise to any kind of movement disorder other than tremor, chorea and hemiballismus have been described in a few patients in whom MRI lesions have been demonstrated in the basal ganglia, including the subthalamic nucleus.[86] In some cases, the signs have subsequently improved or disappeared, consistent with an attack of multiple sclerosis.

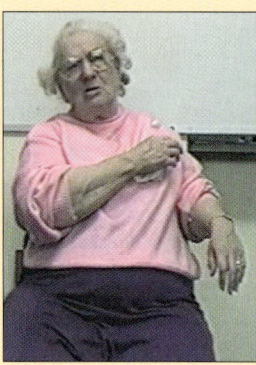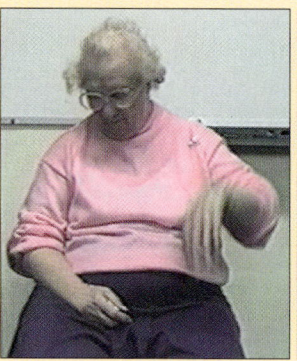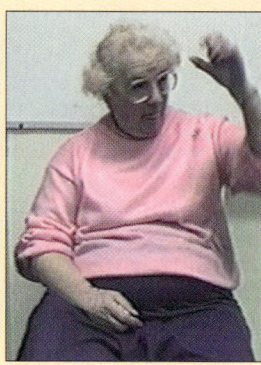

CD 7.7. Vascular chorea in the arm and face.

Patients with polycythaemia vera may develop generalized chorea, which may even be the presenting symptom of the disorder. It is presumed that the increased viscosity impairs cerebral blood flow; certainly the movement disorder usually improves when the condition is treated and the viscosity lowered.

Rarely, metastatic or other tumours (including CNS lymphoma) may present with chorea.[76]

Abscesses causing chorea have been described, and chorea due to toxoplasma infection associated with AIDS has recently been recognized.

A variety of perturbations of electrolyte or hormonal balance have been associated with chorea, including hypo- and hypernatraemia, hypocalcaemia, hypomagnesaemia, hypoglycaemia, hypoparathyroidism and hyperthyroidism. Of these, the commonest is probably hyperthyroidism.[87]

References

1. Huntington G. On chorea. Med Surg Rep 1872; 26: 320–321

2. Avila-Giron R. Medical and social aspects of Huntington's chorea in the state of Zulia, Venezuela. Adv Neurol 1973; 1: 261–266

3. The Huntington's disease collaborative research group. A novel gene containing a trinucleotide repeat that is expanded and unstable in Huntington's disease chromosomes. Cell 1993; 72: 971–983

4. Duyao M, Ambrose C, Myers R et al. Trinucleotide repeat length instability and age of onset in Huntington's disease. Nature Gen 1993; 4: 387–392

5. Snell R G, MacMillan J C, Cheadle J P et al. Relationship between trinucleotide repeat expansion and phenotypic variation in Huntington's disease. Nature Gen 1993; 4: 393–397

6. Craufurd D, Dodge A. Mutation size and age at onset in Huntington's disease. J Med Gen 1993; 30: 1008–1011

7. Xuereb J H, MacMillan J C, Snell R et al. Neuropathological diagnosis and CAG repeat expansion in Huntington's disease. J Neurol Neurosurg Psychiat 1996; 60: 78–81

8. Rubinsztein D C, Leggo J, Coles et al. Phenotypic characterization of individuals with 30–40 CAG repeats in the Huntington disease (HD) gene reveals HD cases with 36 repeats and apparently normal elderly individuals with 36–39 repeats. Am J Hum Gen 1996; 59: 16–22

9. Myers R H, MacDonald M E, Koroshetz W J et al. De novo expression of a (CAG)(n) repeat in sporadic Huntington's disease. Nature Gen 1993; 5: 168–173

10. Andrew S E, Goldberg Y P, Kremer B et al. The relationship between trinucleotide (CAG) repeat length and clinical features of Huntington's disease. Nature Gen 1993; 4: 398–403

11. Illarioshkin SN, Igarashi S, Onodera O et al. Trinucleotide repeat length and rate of progression of Huntington's disease. Ann Neurol 1994; 36: 630–635

12. Brandt J, Bylsma F W, Gross R et al. Trinucleotide repeat length and clinical presentation in Huntington's disease. Neurology 1996; 46: 527–531

13. Kieburtz K, MacDonald M, Shih C et al. Trinucleotide repeat length and progression of illness in Huntington's disease. J Med Gen 1994; 31: 872–874

14. Avanzini G, Girotti F, Caraceni T, Spreafico R. Oculomotor disorders in Huntington's chorea. J Neurol Neurosurg Psychiat 1979; 42: 581–589

15. Leigh R J, Newman S A, Folstein S E et al. Abnormal ocular motor control in Huntington's disease. Neurology 1983; 33: 1268–1275

16. Lasker A G, Zee D S, Hain T C et al. Saccades in Huntington's disease: Initiation defects and distractibility. Neurology 1987; 37: 364–370

17. Rubin A J, King W M, Reinbold K A, Shoulson I. Quantitative longitudinal assessment of saccades in Huntington's disease. J Clin Neuro-Ophthalmol 1993; 13: 59–66

18. Jervis G A. Huntington's chorea in childhood. Arch Neurol 1963; 9: 244–257

19. Carella F, Scaioli V, Ciano C et al. Adult onset myoclonic Huntington's disease. Mov Dis 1993; 8: 201–205

20. Vogel C M, Drury I, Terry L C, Young A B. Myoclonus in adult Huntington's disease. Ann Neurol 1991; 29: 213–215

21. Folstein S E. Huntington's disease: A disorder of families. Baltimore: John Hopkins University Press, 1989

22. Sorensen S A, Fenger K. Causes of death in patients with Huntington's disease and in unaffected first degree relatives. J Med Gen 1992; 29: 911–914

23. Oliva D, Carella F, Savoiardo M et al. Clinical and magnetic resonance features of the classic and akinetic-rigid variants of Huntington's disease. Arch Neurol 1993; 50: 17–19

24. Holthoff V A, Koeppe R A, Frey K A et al. Positron emission tomography measures of benzodiazepine receptors in Huntington's disease. Ann Neurol 1993; 34: 76–81

25. Turjanski N, Weeks R, Dolan R et al. Striatal D1 and D2 receptor binding in patients with Huntington's disease and other choreas. A PET study. Brain 1995; 118: 689–696

26. Weeks R A, Piccini P, Harding A E, Brooks D J. Striatal D1 and D2 dopamine receptor loss in asymptomatic mutation carriers of Huntington's disease. Ann Neurol 1996; 40: 49–54

27. Mann D M A, Oliver R, Snowden J S. The topographic distribution of brain atrophy in Huntington's disease and progressive supranuclear palsy. Acta Neuropathol 1993; 85: 553–559

28. Wakai M, Takahashi A, Hashizume Y. A histometrical study on the globus pallidus in Huntington's disease. J Neurol Sci 1993; 119: 18 27

29. Albin R L. Selective neurodegeneration in Huntington's disease. Ann Neurol 1995; 38: 835–836

30. Furtado S, Suchowersky O, Rewcastle B et al. Relationship between trinucleotide repeats and neuropathological changes in Huntington's disease. Ann Neurol 1996; 39: 132–136

31. Landwehrmeyer G B, McNeil S M, Dure L S I V et al. Huntington's disease gene: Regional and cellular expression in brain of normal and affected individuals. Ann Neurol 1995; 37: 218–230

32. Albin R L, Tagle D A. Genetics and molecular biology of Huntington's disease. Trends Neurosci 1995; 18: 11–14

33. Taylor-Robinson S D, Weeks R A, Sargentoni J et al. Evidence for glutamate excitotoxicity in Huntington's disease with proton magnetic resonance spectroscopy. Lancet 1994; 343: 1170

34. Roos R A C, Hermans J, Vegtervan der Vlis M et al. Duration of illness in Huntington's disease is not related to age at onset. J Neurol Neurosurg Psychiat 1993; 56: 98–100

35. Shoulson I. Huntington's disease: Functional capacities in patients treated with neuroleptic and antidepressant drugs. Neurology 1981; 31: 1333–1335

36. Jankovic J, Orman J. Tetrabenazine therapy of dystonia, chorea, tics, and other dyskinesias. Neurology 1988; 38: 391–394

37. Schott K, Ried S, Stevens S, Dichgans J. Neuroleptically induced dystonia in Huntington's disease: A case report. Eur Neurol 1989; 29: 39–40

38. Burke R E, Fahn S, Mayeux R et al. Neuroleptic malignant syndrome caused by dopamine-depleting drugs in a patient with Huntington disease. Neurology 1981; 31: 1022–1026

39. Reveley M A, Dursun S M, Andrews H. A comparative trial use of sulpiride and risperidone in Huntington's disease: A pilot study. J Psychopharmacol 1996; 10: 162–165

40. Reveley M A, Dursun S M, Andrews H. Improvement of abnorma saccadic eye movements in Huntington's disease by sulpiride: A case study. J Psychopharmacol 1994; 8: 262–265

41. Bonuccelli U, Ceravolo R, Maremmani C et al. Clozapine in Huntington's chorea. Neurology 1994; 44: 821–823

42. Jongen P J, Renier W O, Gabreels F J. Seven cases of Huntington's chorea in childhood and levodopa-induced improvement in the hypokinetic-rigid form. Clin Neurol Neurosurg 1980; 82: 251

43. Ranen N G, Peyser C E, Folstein S E. ECT as a treatment for depression in Huntington's disease. J Neuropsychiatr Clin Neurosci 1994; 6: 154–159

44. Rich S S, Ovsiew F. Leuprolide for exhibitionism in Huntington's disease. Mov Dis 1994; 9: 353–357

45. Shoulson I, Odoroff C, Oakes D et al. A controlled clinical trial of baclofen as protective therapy in early Huntington's disease. Ann Neurol 1989; 25: 252–259

46. Peyser C E, Folstein M, Chase G A et al. Trial of d-alpha-tocopherol in Huntington's disease. Am J Psych 1995; 152: 1771–1775

47. Feigin A, Kieburtz K, Como P et al. Assessment of coenzyme Q10 tolerability in Huntington's disease. Mov Dis 1996; 11: 321–323

48. Kieburtz K, Feigin A, McDermott M et al. A controlled trial of remacemide hydrochloride in Huntington's disease. Mov Dis 1996; 11: 273–277

49. Kieburtz K, Penney J B, Como P et al. Unified Huntington's disease rating scale: Reliability and consistency. Mov Dis 1996; 11: 136–142

50. Quinn N, Brown R, Craufurd D et al. Core assessment program for intracerebral transplantation in Huntington's disease (CAPIT-HD). Mov Dis 1996; 11: 143–150

51. Shinotoh H, Calne D B, Snow B et al. Normal CAG repeat length in the Huntington's disease gene in senile chorea. Neurology 1994; 39: 192–195

52. Swedo S E, Leonard H L, Schapiro M B et al. Sydenham's chorea: Physical and psychological symptoms of St Vitus dance. Pediatrics 1993; 91: 706–713

53. Swedo S E, Rapoport J L, Cheslow D L et al. High prevalence of obsessive-compulsive symptoms in patients with Sydenham's chorea. Am J Psychiat 1989; 146: 246–249

54. Goldman S, Amron D, Szliwowski H B et al. Reversible striatal hypermetabolism in a case of Sydenham's chorea. Mov Dis 1993; 8: 355–358

55. Weindl A, Kuwert T, Leenders K L et al. Increased striatal glucose consumption in Sydenham's chorea. Mov Dis 1993; 8: 437–444

56. Gledhill R F, Thompson P D. Standard neurodiagnostic tests in Sydenham's chorea. J Neurol Neurosurg Psychiat 1990; 53: 534–535

57. Asherson R A, Hughes G R V, Gledhill R, Quinn N P. Absence of antibodies to cardiolipin in patients with Huntington's chorea, Sydenham's chorea and acute rheumatic fever. J Neurol Neurosurg Psychiat 1988; 51: 1458–1488

58. Figueroa F, Berrios X, Gutierrez M et al. Anticardiolipin antibodies in acute rheumatic fever. J Rheumatol 1992; 19: 1175–1180

59. Dhanaraj M, Radhakrishnan A R, Srinivas K, Sayeed Z A. Sodium valproate in Sydenham's chorea. Neurology 1985; 35: 114–115

60. Daoud A S, Zaki M, Shakir R, AlSaleh Q. Effectiveness of sodium valproate in the treatment of Sydenham's chorea. Neurology 1990; 40: 1140–1141

61. Omdal R, Roalso S. Chorea gravidarum and chorea associated with oral contraceptives — diseases due to antiphospholipid antibodies? Acta Neurol Scand 1992; 86: 219–220

62. Thomas D, Byrne P D, Travers R L. Systemic lupus erythematosus presenting as post-partum chorea. Aus N Z J Med 1979; 9: 568–570

63. Kuroe K, Kurahaski K, Nakano I, et al. A neuropathological study of a case of lupus erythematosus with chorea. J Neurol Sci 1994; 123: 59–63

64. Agrawal B L, Foa R P. Collagen vascular disease appearing as chorea gravidarum. Arch Neurol 1982; 39: 192–193

65. Ichikawa K, Kim R C, Collins G H, Givelber H. Chorea gravidarum. Report of a fatal case with neuropathological examination. Arch Neurol 1980; 37: 429–432

66. Ghanem Q. Recurrent chorea gravidarum in four pregnancies. Can J Neurol Sci 1985; 12: 136–138

67. Donaldson J O. Control of chorea gravidarum with haloperidol. Obstet Gynaecol 1982; 59: 381–382

68. Bassen F A, Kornzweig A L. Malformations of the erythrocytes in a case of atypical retinitis pigmentosa. Blood 1950; 5: 381–387

69. Kartsounis L D, Hardie R J. The pattern of cognitive impairments in neuroacanthocytosis. Arch Neurol 1996; 53: 77–80

70. Hardie R J, Pullon H W H, Harding A E et al. Neuroacanthocytosis. A clinical, haematological and pathological study of 19 cases. Brain 1991; 114: 13–49

71. Schwartz M S, Monro P S, Leigh P N. Epilepsy as the presenting feature of neuroacanthocytosis in siblings. J Neurol 1992; 239: 261–262

72. Brooks D J, Ibanez V, Playford E D et al. Presynaptic and postsynaptic striatal dopaminergic function in neuroacanthocytosis: A positron emission tomographic study. Ann Neurol 1991; 30: 166–171

73. Rinne J O, Daniel S E, Scaravilli F et al. Nigral degeneration in neuroacanthocytosis. Neurology 1994; 44: 1629–1632

74. Rinne J O, Daniel S E, Scaravilli F et al. The neuropathological features of neuroacanthocytosis. Mov Dis 1994; 9: 297–304

75. Klawans H L, Moses H, Nausieda P A et al. Treatment and prognosis of hemiballismus. N Engl J Med 1976; 295: 1348–1350

76. Dewey R B, Jankovic J. Hemiballism–hemichorea: Clinical and pharmacologic findings in 21 patients. Arch Neurol 1989; 46: 862–867

77. Borgohain R, Singh A K, Thadani R et al. Hemiballismus due to an ipsilateral striatal haemorrhage: An unusual localization. J Neurol Sci 1995; 130: 22–24

78. Vidakovic A, Dragasevic N, Kostic V S. Hemiballism: Report of 25 cases. J Neurol Neurosurg Psychiat 1994; 57: 945–949

79. Sanchez Ramos J R, Factor S A, Weiner W J, Marquez J. Hemichorea–hemiballismus associated with acquired immune deficiency syndrome and cerebral toxoplasmosis. Mov Dis 1989; 3: 266–273

80. Awada A. Hemiballisme revelateur d'une toxoplasmose cerebrale et d'un syndrome d'immunodeficience acquise. Revue Neurologique 1993; 149: 421–423

81. Bashir K, Manyam B V. Clozapine for the control of hemiballismus. Clin Neuropharmacol 1994; 17: 477–480

82. Lenton R J, Copti M, Smith R G. Hemiballismus treated with sodium valproate. Br Med J 1981; 283: 17–18

83. Chandra V, Wharton S, Spunt A L. Amelioration of hemiballismus with sodium valproate. Ann Neurol 1982; 12: 407

84. Levesque M F, Markham C H. Ventral intermediate thalamotomy for posttraumatic hemiballismus. Stereotactic Funct Neurosurg 1992; 58: 26–29

85. Tsubokawa T, Katayama Y, Yamamoto T. Control of persistent hemiballismus by chronic thalamic stimulation. Report of two cases. J Neurosurg 1995; 82: 501–505

86. Tranchant C, Bhatia K P, Marsden C D. Movement disorders in multiple sclerosis. Mov Dis 1995; 10: 418–423

87. Delwaide P J, Schoenen J. Hyperthyroidism as a cause of persistent choreic movements. Acta Neurol Scand 1987; 58: 309

chapter 8

Tics and related disorders

Graham Lennox

Phenomenology

Tics are the most variable and pleomorphic of the movement disorders. The movements range from simple brief rapid movements of a single body part to complex sequences of coordinated movements. Complex tics may look like normal movements, including meaningful gestures, but are irresistible, repetitive, purposeless and unwanted. Unlike many other movement disorders, they are usually easy to imitate. These *motor tics* are mirrored in a similarly diverse range of *vocal tics*, from brief elementary noises to words and phrases. Both motor and vocal tics may be preceded by a sensation — and an urge to make the movement — which is transiently relieved by the tic itself; these premonitory feelings are sometimes referred to as *sensory tics*. Most patients can temporarily suppress the tics but this is usually accompanied by mounting inner tension and followed by a flurry of noises or movements as soon as the effort is relaxed. For many patients the tics therefore have a compulsive quality and are not entirely involuntary; some may deliberately make the movement or noise to ease the inner tension. Tics are sometimes relieved by intense distraction (including sexual arousal), alcohol or fever.

They are often aggravated by anxiety, irritation or self-consciousness as well as, paradoxically, by relaxation.

Examples of the various forms of tics are given in Table 8.1. The distinction between simple and complex tics is arbitrary (CD 8.1). Complex tics shade off towards more prolonged motor activities such as the rituals associated with obsessive compulsive disorder and the stereotypies associated with learning disability, both of which may coexist with tics. Simple motor tics can usually be distinguished from myoclonic jerks by their suppressibility. At any given time they usually

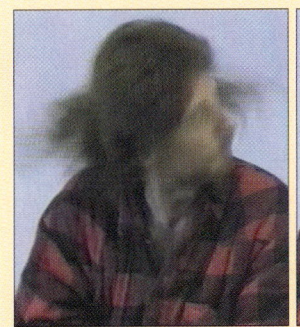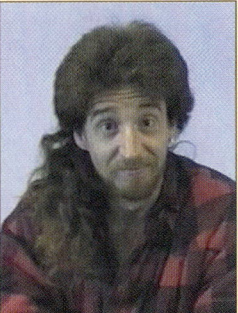

CD 8.1. Complex motor tic involving neck and face.

● **Table 8.1.** Classification of tics

Type of tic	Examples
Simple motor tics	Blinking; grimacing; shrugging; tongue protruding; contracting platysma, rectus abdominis or glutei
Complex motor tics	Head shaking; shoulder rolling; touching; jumping; squatting; spitting; imitating the movements of others (echopraxia); making obscene gestures (copropraxia)
Simple vocal tics	Sniffing; grunting; throat clearing; coughing; humming; yelping; barking
Complex vocal tics	Saying or shouting obscene words or phrases (coprolalia); repeating the same word spontaneously (palilalia) or in response to the speech of other people (echolalia)
Associated phenomena	
'Sensory tics'	A sensation usually within a body part but occasionally perceived as external, which may be relieved by movement
'Mental tics'	Repetitive thoughts which resemble echolalia, palilalia and coprolalia but are not verbalized; occasionally these may be described as mental images of the word or phrase

have a more restricted distribution than chorea. People with complex motor tics often have some slower and more prolonged movements within their tic repertoire which resemble dystonia, such as head movements which look rather like torticollis. Again it is the subjective qualities of these so-called *dystonic tics* which distinguish them from the involuntary movements and postures of dystonia.

Motor tics typically wax and wane in severity over weeks and months, and change in their form and distribution over years. Mildly affected patients may experience periods of complete remission.

The most common forms of vocal tics are simple sounds like sniffs or grunts. More complex vocal tics such as coprolalia (i.e. the unwanted and inappropriate utterance of obscenities) are actually rare, even in the syndrome of Gilles de la Tourette with which they are particularly associated. Patients with complex vocal tics often go to great lengths to disguise or conceal the noises.

Public awareness of tic disorders is slowly increasing, but most patients still present to neurologists late, after unhappy attempts by family and friends to suppress the movements by scolding or teasing, and unhelpful consultations in ear, nose and throat, allergy, ophthalmology, or psychiatry clinics depending on the form of the tics. Ironically, the tics themselves may be least noticeable during the neurological examination. If this is the case then you can either ask the patient to mimic the movements or noises, which will sometimes precipitate the tics themselves, or give the patient the impression that your attention is directed elsewhere (by writing your case notes or talking to their family) and covertly observe the release of the tics that this often brings. The best place to see tics is often the waiting room of a movement disorders clinic.

Aetiology

The causes of tics are summarized in Table 8.2. The transient tic disorder of childhood is very common, affecting up to 15% of children, especially boys. The tics are usually mild and often involve only a single movement such as winking or grimacing. Chronic tic disorder is defined on the basis of its persistence, and more commonly involves more than one tic. Gilles de la Tourette's syndrome is described in more detail below.

● **Table 8.2.** Causes of tics

Idiopathic

Transient tic disorder
Motor or vocal tic(s) but not both
Lasts more than 1 but less than 12 months
Onset before the age of 21 years
Not due to any secondary cause

Chronic motor or vocal tic disorder
Definition is the same as transient tic disorder except duration more than 12 months without a sustained remission
Adult-onset variants of this condition occur

Gilles de la Tourette's syndrome
Multiple motor tics and at least one vocal tic
Onset before the age of 21 years (although similar late-onset cases are described)

Secondary

Tics as components of specific neurodegenerative diseases
Huntington's disease
Neuroacanthocytosis

Tics in association with neurodevelopmental disorders
Learning disability (including cases with identifiable genetic causes such as chromosome translocations), autism and schizophrenia

Tics following acute brain injury
Stroke (where the tics may be unilateral), encephalitis (especially encephalitis lethargica), Sydenham's chorea, head injury, carbon monoxide poisoning, hypoglycaemia, etc.

Tics related to drug exposure
CNS stimulants (including amphetamines and cocaine), levodopa, neuroleptics ('tardive Tourettism'), carbamazepine, phenytoin, barbiturates, quinolone antibiotics etc.

Many identifiable brain disorders can give rise to tics.[1–3] Only a tiny minority of patients with Huntington's disease present with tics rather than the usual initial manifestations of chorea or cognitive impairment. So-called secondary Tourettism (Fig. 8.1) (i.e. where features of Gilles de la Tourette's syndrome occur in an established case of another disease) is, however, relatively common in established Huntington's disease; patients often have periods with simple vocal tics, involuntary echolalia, palilalia and coprolalia, and suppressible movements including complex compulsions amongst the

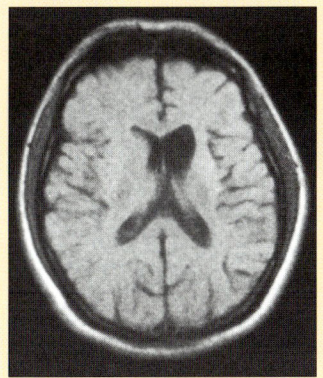

Figure 8.1. Secondary Tourettism.

A previously healthy 32-year-old man abruptly developed abnormal movements of his right arm and leg. He described an irresistible urge to shrug his shoulder or extend his leg, which was worse in public places like buses and at times of stress like job interviews. He could suppress the movements for several minutes but reported that this made him feel unbearably tense. After a month he started sniffing and grunting uncontrollably, and would shout 'Fuck' and 'Shit' on the bus. Examination confirmed the presence of motor and vocal tics; he was slightly aggressive and had hypometric saccades but had no other abnormalities. An MR brain scan showed a mature infarct of the head of the left caudate nucleus. Routine investigations were unremarkable and he declined cerebral angiography. His tics subsided with sulpiride 200 mg twice daily.

chorea. The motor and vocal tics that accompanied encephalitis lethargica were termed klazomania and were of particular historical importance, convincing many neurologists for the first time that tic disorders might have a neurological rather than a behavioural basis. Vocal tics and involuntary orofacial movements are common in neuroacanthocytosis, but can occur in a range of other degenerative, metabolic and postinfectious disorders including Wilson's disease and Sydenham's chorea. Tics are an unusual complication of a range of acute brain injuries, but rarely occur in isolation.

The observation that tics may occur at the same time as parkinsonism in some of these conditions has important implications when it comes to developing pathophysiological models of tic disorders.[4]

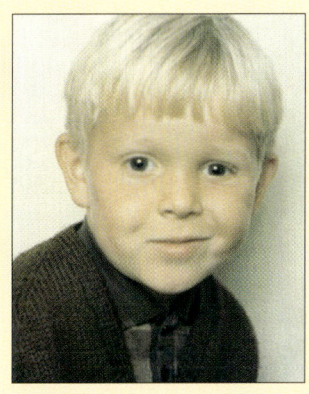

Figure 8.2. Left-sided facial tic in boy aged 8 years.

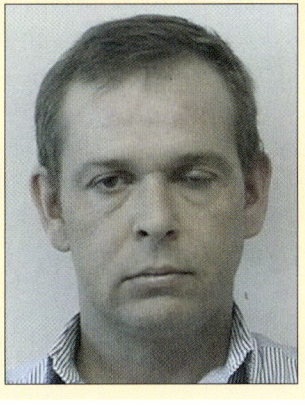

CD 8.2. Chronic facial tic. (Same patient as in Fig. 8.2.)

The diagnostic approach to a child with a single tic

A single tic, whether motor or vocal, is best managed with masterly inactivity, especially in young boys where they are so very common (Fig. 8.2). In the majority of cases the tic remits spontaneously, and requires no investigation or treatment.

Even where it persists as a chronic tic disorder (CD 8.2), further investigation is unlikely to be rewarding unless there are features in the history or on examination to suggest a secondary cause. It is sensible, as always, to have a low threshold for screening for Wilson's disease but even this will usually declare itself in the form of evolving neurological problems over the course of a few months. The prognosis of chronic tic disorders is less favourable, and many of these children keep their tic throughout adult life to some degree: it becomes part of their behavioural repertoire (and, in the case of public figures, a great help to impressionists). Treatment is rarely requested but a few patients with a complex and embarrassing tic may be relieved by intermittent treatment with the drugs described below.

Where both motor and vocal tics develop, Gilles de la Tourette's syndrome should be considered.

Gilles de la Tourette's syndrome

Georges Gilles de la Tourette (Fig. 8.3) came across the syndrome that bears his name (or, in a regrettable if understandable recent trend, merely the final part of his surname) through serendipity, after he translated Beard's description of the 'jumping Frenchmen of Maine'.[5] On joining Charcot as the *chef de clinique* at the Salpetriere he was given the task of bringing order to 'the chaos of the choreas'. He set out to find more jumping Frenchmen, in the belief that they should be thicker on the ground in Paris than in New England. He did not discover any, but in his search he came across six people with a similar pattern of involuntary jerks and vocalizations. In 1885 he reported these and three other cases in a paper entitled '*Etude sur an affection nerveuse characterisee par l'incoordination motrice accompangnee d'echolalie et coprolalie*'.[6] He described a syndrome which began in childhood and waxed and waned throughout life, and that affected men more than women. He identified cases of above-average intelligence as well as cases with learning disability. He also recognized an association with psychiatric illness in other family members.

It is now realized that Gilles de la Tourette's syndrome is common. Epidemiological studies are beset with problems of definition and ascertainment (especially in relation to mild cases), but recent large-scale studies suggest a prevalence of at least 5 per 10 000[7,8] (i.e. about 25 000 patients in the UK and 110 000 in the USA) with three- or fourfold higher prevalence rates amongst boys than girls. A recent survey of children in mainstream schools found a much higher prevalence of 2.9%;[9] most of these children had not come to medical attention and had mild forms of the disorder which did not require treatment. Gilles de la Tourette's syndrome is found at similar rates and with similar clinical features across a wide range of different cultures.[10]

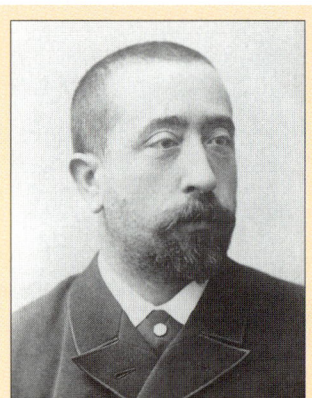

Figure 8.3. Georges Gilles de la Tourette.

Georges Albert Edouard Brutus Gilles de la Tourette was born in 1857. He became one of Charcot's favourite pupils at the Salpetriere in Paris, making a particular study of hysteria and hypnosis. He described his syndrome in 1885. In 1893 he was shot in the back of the neck by a deluded former patient but recovered completely, only to go on and develop neurosyphilis from which he died in Switzerland in 1904.

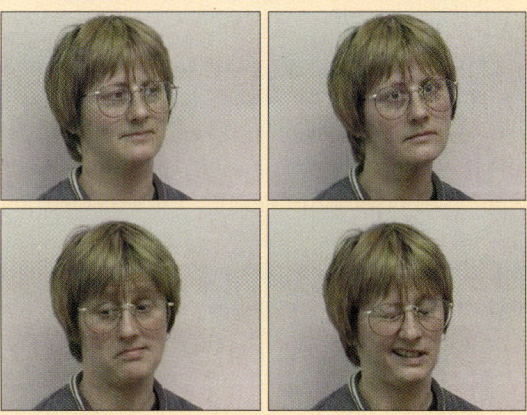

CD 8.3. Facial tics in Gilles de la Tourette syndrome.

Clinical features

The core features are multiple motor and vocal tics, occurring many times each day in bouts (CD 8.3).[3] The motor tics usually begin first, at a mean age of 7 years but with a range between 2 and 15 years. Boys tend to have an earlier age of onset than girls. They are often initially simple tics like blinking, but usually gradually evolve to more complex facial and limb movements and gait abnormalities. They are often accompanied by premonitory sensory phenomena which are relieved by the movements themselves;[11] articulate patients say this is like the feeling before a sneeze or like an itch that they have to scratch. The motor tics typically vary in severity, and change in form and distribution over the years, tending to become more complex with increasing age. They are often especially troublesome during adolescence and early adult life, settling down a little thereafter.

Vocal tics usually begin later, at a mean age of 11 years but with a range of 5 to 21 years. Again these are usually simple sniffs, coughs or grunts to begin with. Later a wide range of more bizarre noises may occur, including yelping and barking, as may repetitive retching or vomiting. Vocal tics involving utterances are less common. Coprolalia is frankly rare in affected children. Although Gilles de la Tourette regarded it as a core feature of the syndrome, it tends to be seen mainly in severely affected adults attending specialist clinics; it probably occurs in only a few percent of unselected patients. The obscenities themselves vary somewhat from culture to culture, but tend to be the most offensive available words. Many patients learn to abbreviate them ('Fuh, fuh, fuh ...') to lessen their embarrassment. Palilalia (where the patient repeats the last phrase, word or syllable of their own speech) is rather more common, affecting 6–15% of patients.[3] Many more patients 'internalize' their coprolalia and palilalia, tending to rehearse the words over and over again in their minds without actually speaking them, in a vivid and intrusive way. Echolalia (repeating the words or sounds of others) is probably more common again, affecting 11–44% of patients.

All of these speech phenomena have counterparts in non-verbal communication. Patients with Gilles de la Tourette's syndrome may find it impossible to resist making obscene gestures (copropraxia) or copying the gestures of others (echopraxia). They may also develop complex movements with a more definitely compulsive basis. A compulsion is a repetitive and seemingly purposeful behaviour performed in a stereotyped way and accompanied by a subjective sense that it must be carried out. Many patients with Gilles de la Tourette's syndrome have simple compulsions, like forced touching where for example the patient taps all the door knobs or radiators as he walks along a corridor. Others perform more complex and ritualized acts.

Indeed patients with Gilles de la Tourette's syndrome can develop any or all of the features of obsessive-compulsive disorder, like repetitive checking of locks and switches, and rituals which often involve mathematical rules (like turning on the spot seven times before crossing a doorway). They may also develop obsessional (i.e. recurrent and unwanted) thoughts and impulses; for example, a patient may experience intrusive and upsetting thoughts of harm-

ing her baby every time she sees a sharp knife in her kitchen. A few patients develop obsessional thoughts and compulsions relating to self-injury (like eye-poking), and these can lead to permanent physical damage. There is some evidence that these sorts of obsessive-compulsive phenomena, involving forced touching or violent thoughts, may be more common in Gilles de la Tourette's syndrome than they are in patients with obsessive-compulsive disorder without tics, who in turn are more likely to have repetitive hand washing and other classical phenomena relating to fear of contamination.[12,13]

Mild symptoms of obsessive-compulsive disorder are helpful in supporting a diagnosis of Gilles de la Tourette's syndrome; where severe symptoms occur they are often more disabling than the tics, and become the main focus of treatment. One can often obtain a family history of obsessive-compulsive disorder (without tics) in Gilles de la Tourette's syndrome, but must be careful about putting diagnostic weight on this sort of second-hand information. A recent study of the first-degree relatives of 87 probands with Gilles de la Tourette's syndrome found only background rates of obsessive-compulsive disorder,[14] casting doubt on the previous assumption that the two conditions might share common genetic risk factors or even be allelic variants.

Patients with Gilles de la Tourette's syndrome also experience a range of other psychiatric symptoms.[15] They have a higher prevalence of anxiety and depression than control groups. These are particularly common in patients with longstanding disabling disease[16] and may relate more to the social stigma of Gilles de la Tourette's syndrome than any biological factors. In children with Gilles de la Tourette's syndrome there appears to be a strong association with attention deficit hyperactivity disorder, although the magnitude and basis of the association remain a matter of debate.[17] In severe cases of Gilles de la Tourette's syndrome of the kind that are concentrated in specialized clinics, there is an apparent association with eating disorders, substance abuse and personality disorder, but it is not clear that there is any such association in the condition as a whole.

Most patients with Gilles de la Tourette's syndrome have no other abnormalities on routine neurological examination, although an excess of left-handedness and minor neurological signs such as slight reflex asymmetry or clumsiness have been described.[18] Careful neurophthalmological studies have shown subtle impairments of eye movement, including increased latency of antisaccades, but these are not apparent at the bedside.[19] Patients often appear impulsive and may find it difficult to sustain attention during cognitive tests. Most patients have normal intelligence (and the condition has been described in at least one genius: see Fig. 8.4), but there is a definite subgroup with learning disability of varying degree. Indeed surveys of people in special schools for the learning disabled have found a very high prevalence of Gilles de la Tourette's syndrome, and the condition may be underdiagnosed in this setting.[20] Gilles de la Tourette's syndrome does not cause progressive cognitive impairment.

The severity of Gilles de la Tourette's syndrome varies hugely. Milder cases — which are very common — may present incidentally; movement disorder specialists often pass the time in airport departure lounges by diagnosing the condition amongst the other travellers. Such cases usually have little or no disability as a result of their tics and compulsions and may naturally resent having the condition drawn to their attention. Mild cases may improve or even remit as the patient enters the third and fourth decades. Moderately and severely affected cases tend to seek medical advice, and are less likely to remit completely.

The diagnostic approach to a patient with both motor and vocal tics

The first clinical issue is to be sure that the movements and noises are indeed tics, and therefore suppressible with a subjective component, rather than manifestations of chorea or myoclonus. The second consideration is the possibility of secondary Tourettism. It is important to make sure that there has been no history of neuroleptic drug exposure, which can lead to so-called tardive Tourettism. Likewise a history of acute brain insults such as trauma or carbon monoxide poisoning must be

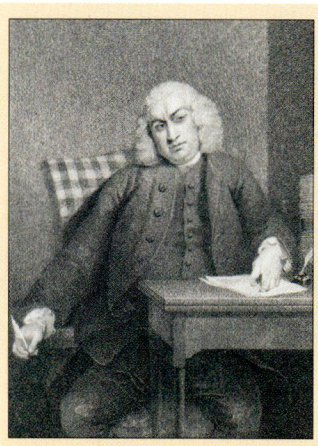

Figure 8.4. Dr. Samuel Johnson and his Gilles de la Tourette's syndrome.[62] (Courtesy of George Bernard Science Photo Library.)

Dr. Johnson wrote his renowned dictionary, essays and literary biographies and became one of the foremost figures of eighteenth century London despite having Gilles de la Tourette's syndrome. The features were recorded by famous contemporaries:

Motor tics 'He has an infirmity of the convulsive kind, that attacks him sometimes, so as to make him a sad spectacle.' (Alexander Pope, the poet)
'His mouth is almost constantly opening and shutting as if he were chewing. He has a strange method of frequently twisting his fingers and twisting his hands. His body is in continual agitation seesawing up and down; his feet are never a moment quiet; and in short his whole person is in perpetual motion.' (Fanny Burney, diarist)

Vocal tics 'In the intervals of articulating he made various sounds with his mouth, sometimes as if ruminating, or what is called chewing the cud, sometimes giving a half whistle, sometimes making his tongue play backwards from the roof of his mouth as if clucking like a hen, and sometimes protruding it against his upper gums in front as if pronouncing quickly under his breath *too, too, too*.' (James Boswell, biographer)

Suppressibility 'He could sit motionless, when he was told to do so, as well as any other man.' (Sir Joshua Reynolds, artist — who painted Johnson's portrait)

Compulsions 'As he lurched along, his head rolling from side to side, he would be at particular pains to avoid treading on any pavement crack and insist on touching every post in his path.' (James Boswell, biographer)

excluded. Further investigation may be needed where there is a family history of a neurological disorder (other than Gilles de la Tourette's syndrome or obsessive-compulsive disorder) and where there are neurological signs that cannot be explained by a diagnosis of Gilles de la Tourette's syndrome. In severe tic syndromes the movements may be so florid that one cannot be certain that there is not an element of chorea or dystonia, and eye movements may appear distractible. It is, therefore, occasionally necessary to exclude Huntington's disease by genetic testing, neuroacanthocytosis by repeated blood films, Wilson's disease by copper studies and so on. Any other definite neurological deficits require an alternative explanation and must be investigated on their own merits. In the very rare situation of an acute onset severe tic syndrome then investigations for encephalitis including MR brain scanning, EEG and lumbar puncture, together with a screen for recent streptococcal infection are justified. In tic syndromes presenting well into adult life the diagnosis of Gilles de la Tourette's syndrome must be made with care: late-onset cases have been described but are very unusual, and investigations should include brain imaging to rule out vascular disease.

There are, however, no established ancillary tests for Gilles de la Tourette's syndrome itself, and in most cases the diagnosis can be confidently made on clinical grounds. Routine blood tests and brain imaging are normal. Research-based forms of brain imaging are of some interest because of the faint light they shed on the biology of the disorder, but as yet have no place in diagnosis.

Brain imaging

The literature on brain imaging in Gilles de la Tourette's syndrome is characterized mainly by conflicting reports. It would be fair to summarize these by saying that no clear consensus about the biological basis of the disorder has yet emerged. Routine scanning reveals no relevant abnormalities of the structure of the brain (although there have been many case reports describing a wide range of incidental findings).[3] More detailed structural imaging studies using volumetric MRI have suggested that there may be a loss of the normal slight asymmetry of the caudate nuclei,[21] but studies measuring the cross-sectional area of the corpus callosum have suggested either an increase or a decrease (albeit in different age groups).[22,23]

Similar confusion occurs in single photon emission computed tomography (SPECT) studies,[24] which have been reported as showing reduction in blood flow through either right[25] or left[26,27] basal ganglia. Other studies have shown no such asymmetry of blood flow, but have shown changes in dopaminergic markers. For example, Wolf and colleagues[28] used the radioligand iodobenzamide (IBZM) to study D2-receptor binding in five pairs of monozygotic twins who were discordant for their severity of Gilles de la Tourette's syndrome. They found greater IBZM binding in the caudate nuclei of the more severely affected twin.

Positron emission tomography (PET) ligand studies have not, however, shown any consistent changes in dopaminergic systems. In metabolic studies, there have been anecdotal reports of caudate hypermetabolism, whereas covariance analysis of group $[^{18}F]$ fluoro-deoxyglucose suggests that there may be a relative increase in glucose metabolism in lateral premotor cortex, supplementary motor cortex and midbrain, reflecting a non-specific increase in cortical motor activity, yet a reduction in metabolism in caudate, lentiform, thalamic, and hypothalamic nuclei which perhaps reflects underactivity of an inhibitory network.[29] The involvement of the midbrain in these circuits is supported by a case report in which tics remitted after the dorsal midbrain was damaged by Wernicke's encephalopathy due to hyperemesis.[30]

Functional MRI techniques have only just started to examine Gilles de la Tourette's syndrome, but have the theoretical ability to assess the fluctuating motor and vocal tics more or less as they happen. One study has already shown widespread changes in activation (both positive and negative) during the act of tic suppression.[31]

Histopathology and postmortem neurochemistry

Relatively few brains from patients with Gilles de la Tourette's syndrome have been examined using modern pathological methods. Routine histopathology is normal. A small-scale immunohistochemical study revealed a reduction in dynorphin-positive woolly fibres in parts of the globus pallidus in some but not all cases.[32]

Again postmortem neurochemistry has produced conflicting findings, at least in part because of their small sample sizes and the confounding effects of drug treatment. There does not appear to be any abnormality of dopamine receptor binding, but an increase in dopamine reuptake site binding has been reported.[33] As previously mentioned, tics can emerge in the presence of parkinsonism (or vice versa) making it unlikely that Gilles de la Tourette's syndrome could be explained by any simple dopaminergic mechanism.[4] No major abnormality of cholinergic, noradrenergic, serotoninergic, glutamatergic or GABAergic systems has been consistently identified.

Genetics

Although environmental factors probably influence the expression of the disease,[34] both twin studies and family studies suggest that the aetiology of Gilles de la Tourette's syndrome has a major genetic component. The mechanism of this remains elusive,[35] and traditional genetic linkage studies have been hampered by difficulties in defining the phenotype; should one count as affected just those members of a kindred who have motor and vocal tics, or should one include relatives with obsessive-compulsive disorder or other psychiatric problems that are associated with Gilles de la Tourette's syndrome? A second problem is a lack of a definite genetic model. Family studies with a broad definition of the phenotype suggest that the condition may have an autosomal dominant pattern of inheritance with low penetrance, but a huge range of other possibilities have been proposed including an intermediate pattern in which a single copy of a susceptibility allele confers some risk of developing the condition but two copies increase this risk, bilineal transmission, and complex models with one or two major susceptibility genes operating against a multifactorial background.[36,37] Further complexity comes from the suggestion that Gilles de la Tourette's syndrome may be influenced by the phenomenon of genomic imprinting, with an earlier age of onset,[38] and perhaps also differences in phenotype,[39,40] in patients who have inherited the condition from their mothers. Further genetic studies using the robust sib-pair technique may get around these problems within the next few years.

In the meantime, candidate gene studies have met with no success, with no consistent linkage for example to the genes for dopamine receptors, synthetic enzymes or transporters etc, and conventional linkage studies have been unsuccessful despite screening almost all the human genome.[37]

Immunology

Against the background of these genetic disappointments, there has been considerable interest in recent observations suggesting a possible role for autoimmunity in Gilles de la Tourette's syndrome. In particular, studies in children have suggested that a form of obsessive-compulsive disorder, with hyperactivity and sometimes tics, may come on abruptly after a beta-haemolytic streptococcal infection.[41] This condition, which has been given the acronym PANDAS (paediatric autoimmune neuropsychiatric disorder associated with streptococcal infection), appears to be associated with a specific B-cell antigen which is known to confer susceptibility to rheumatic fever,[42,43] and with an antineuronal antibody.[44] The relationship between PANDAS and the classical self-limiting Sydenham's chorea on the one hand, and with Gilles de la Tourette's syndrome on the other, is not yet clear.

Management

Many patients are relieved to be given an accurate diagnosis. They usually welcome a careful explanation of the organic basis of their apparently wilful and bizarre behaviour. Detailed written information, for example from self-help groups, is immensely valuable. The diagnosis may come as more of a shock to family members, who may feel guilty if they have previously tried to control the tics through admonishment and also because of the potential genetic aetiology of the disease. In younger patients it is important to make sure that their teachers have an understanding of the diagnosis and its educational implications.

Once the diagnosis has been explained, the next step is to ask the patient whether they want any specific form of treatment. Many patients are happy simply to have a diagnosis, and regard their Gilles de la Tourette's syndrome as part and parcel of their personality (which in a way it is). The clinician should encourage the patient to consider that treatment is not mandatory. If the tics are not particularly disabling, then clearly the prospect of drug therapy (with its attendant risk of adverse effects) will be unattractive.

In the US, many clinicians begin treatment with the alpha-2-adrenergic agonist clonidine either orally or as a transdermal patch.[45] The main problems are sedation and lack of efficacy, but this approach avoids the risk of tardive dyskinesia that is associated with neuroleptic drugs. In the UK clonidine is generally reserved for cases with additional problems due to attention deficit hyperactivity disorder. A recent alternative in this situation is another alpha-2-adrenergic agonist, guanfacine, which appears to be well-tolerated.[46,47]

Clonazepam is another low-potency drug that is sometimes helpful in patients with mild tics and few other symptoms. Again sedation is the main adverse effect but occasionally it releases an unwanted tendency to impulsive behaviour. Many other drugs have been tried in this setting, including various opioids (including naltrexone and tramadol) and marijuana but there are insufficient data to recommend them in routine practice.

The most powerful treatments for both motor and vocal tics are the dopamine receptor antagonists. Although controlled trials are few, they have shown little difference in efficacy between the different neuroleptic drugs.[48] Haloperidol is the traditional drug (which is alone in being licensed for Gilles de la Tourette's syndrome) against which newer drugs like sulpiride and pimozide are compared. These newer drugs certainly cause fewer side-effects, especially sedation, and should generally be tried first. As always, it is a good idea to titrate slowly from the smallest possible starting dose towards the lowest maintenance dose that provides acceptable symptom control. Pimozide can prolong the QT interval, so an ECG before and after initiating treatment is advised.

The great majority of patients will obtain satisfactory benefit from this sort of treatment, but some find all these neuroleptic drugs sedating to an unacceptable degree. They may comment that they miss the impulsive flashes of inspiration or wit which Oliver Sacks has suggested may be the mental equivalent of their tics. Such patients may wish to try alternative neuroleptics like olanzapine[49] which may be less sedating but where there is only anecdotal evidence of efficacy.

One of the main concerns about using neuroleptic drugs is the risk of inducing tardive dyskinesia,[50] which is probably small but has been described even with some of the newer neuroleptic drugs.[51] One way around this may be to use the dopamine depleting drug tetrabenazine instead. Tetrabenazine has been shown to be an effective therapy[52] although side-effects such as depression and sedation are common. Somewhat surprisingly, recent studies have suggested that dopamine agonists such as pergolide may also be effective in relieving tics, especially in patients who also report symptoms similar to restless legs syndrome.[53]

Complex tics and compulsive phenomena are harder to treat. Milder cases may be helped by behavioural psychotherapy, although the effectiveness of this in Gilles de la Tourette's syndrome has never been fully evaluated. Selective serotonin reuptake inhibitors (such as fluoxetine, paroxetine, fluvoxamine and sertraline) have been shown to have beneficial effects in more severe cases,[54] as has the tricyclic antidepressant clomipramine. In clinical practice one often finds that a patient initially responds well to one of these drugs, only for the symptoms to gradually return after a few months. Such cases can be managed by rotating through three or four drugs in turn. An alternative strategy is to try the neuroleptic risperidone, either alone or in addition to a selective serotonin reuptake inhibitor.[55,56] In very severe cases, psychosurgery has been tried with limited success (Fig. 8.5).[57,58]

It is particularly difficult to manage attention deficit hyperactivity disorder where it occurs in children with Gilles de la Tourette's syndrome. The central stimulants like methylphenidate and dexamphetamine which are used in attention deficit hyperactivity disorder can exacerbate tics. It may be necessary to take this risk in order to allow the child to engage in a normal education and recent studies suggest that the risk is small so long as the doses are titrated carefully.[59,60]

Stereotypies and mannerisms

There is an arbitrary distinction between the more complex forms of motor tics and sterotypies. Lees[61] defines stereotypies as purposeless voluntary movements carried out in a uniform repetitive fashion often for long periods of time and at the expense of all other activities (CD 8.4). The movements tend to be more prolonged than tics, and to involve larger areas of the body. Stereotypies are particularly common in people with learning disability, autism or schizophrenia, where communication difficulties can make it hard to be sure that the movements are truly voluntary rather than compulsive. In this setting, the traditional approach to management is behavioural, with distraction and

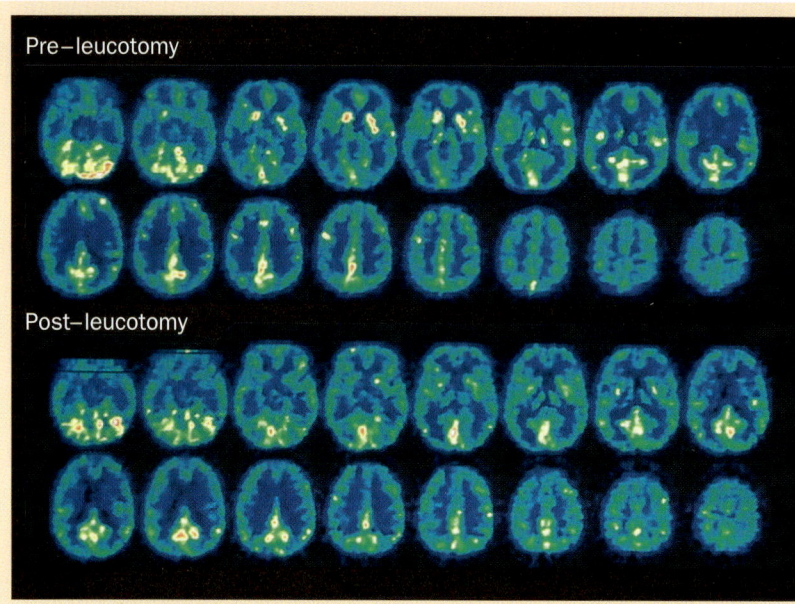

Pre–leucotomy

Post–leucotomy

Figure 8.5. PET scan of oxygen metabolism in a patient with Tourette's syndrome before and after limbic leucotomy. (Note the reduction in basal ganglia metabolism following surgery.)

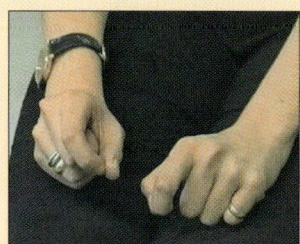

CD 8.4. Stereotypy following anoxia.

Lees[61] defines a mannerism as a bizarre mode of carrying out a purposeful act which usually occurs as a result of the incorporation of a stereotyped action into goal-directed behaviour. It is the useful outcome which distinguishes mannerisms from stereotypies; for example, a patient rocks back and forth for hours on end whilst running his fingers through his hair would be said to have a stereotypy but a patient who rocked back and forth whenever he combed his hair for normal social purposes would be said to have a mannerism. Mannerisms are not necessarily indicative of any underlying neurological dysfunction, but are more common in patients who are institutionalized for any reason.

encouragement. Stereotypies are sometimes suppressed by neuroleptic therapy, but this is a risky long-term approach because the movements may re-emerge with greater severity whilst the patient is still on treatment (rather like tardive dyskinesia).

Further reading

Kurlan K (ed) Handbook of Tourette's syndrome and related tic and behavioural disorders. New York: Marcel Dekker, 1993

Lees A J. Tics and related disorders. Edinburgh: Churchill Livingstone, 1985

Robertson M M, Stern J S. Tic disorders: new developments in Tourette syndrome and related disorders. Curr Opin Neurol 1998; 11: 373–380

References

1. Bruun R D, Shapiro A K. Differential diagnosis of Gilles de la Tourette's syndrome. J Nerv Ment Dis 1972; 155: 328–332

2. Sacks O W. Acquired Tourettism in adult life. In: Friedhoff A J, Chase T N (eds) Gilles de la Tourette syndrome (Advances in Neurology volume 35). New York: Raven Press, 1992

3. Robertson M M. The Gilles de la Tourette syndrome: the current status. Br J Psychiat 1989; 154: 147–169

4. Kumar R, Lang A E. Coexistence of tics and parkinsonism: evidence for non-dopaminergic mechanisms in tic pathogenesis. Neurology 1997; 49: 1699–1701

5. Lees A J. George Gilles de la Tourette: the man and his times. Revue Neurologique (Paris) 1986; 142: 808–816

6. Gilles de la Tourette G. Etude sur une affection nerveuse characterisee par de l'incoordination motrice accompagnee d'echolalie et de copralalie. Arch Neurol 1885; 9: 19–42, 158–200

7. Bruun R D. Gilles de la Tourette's syndrome: an overview of clinical experience. J Am Acad Child Psychiat 1984; 23, 126–133

8. Apter A, Pauls D L, Bleich A et al. A population based epidemiological study of Tourette syndrome among adolescents in Israel. In: Chase T N, Friedhoff A J, Cohen D J (eds) Tourette syndrome: genetics, neurobiology and treatment (Advances in Neurology volume 58). New York: Raven Press, 1992, 61–65

9. Mason A, Banerjee S, Eapen V et al. The prevalence of Gilles de la Tourette's syndrome in a mainstream school population. Dev Med Child Neurol 1998; 4: 292–296

10. Staley D, Wand R, Shady G. Tourette disorder: a cross cultural review. Compr Psychiat 1997; 38: 6–16

11. Chee K-Y, Sachdev P. A controlled study of sensory tics in Gilles de la Tourette syndrome and obsessive-compulsive disorder using a structured interview. J Neurol Neurosurg Psychiat 1997; 62: 188–192

12. Eaten V, Robertson M M, Alsobrook J P, Pauls D L. Obsessive compulsive symptoms in Gilles de la Tourette syndrome and obsessive compulsive disorder: differences by diagnosis and family history. Am J Med Gen 1997; 74: 432–438

13. Zohar A H, Pauls D L, Ratzoni G et al. Obsessive–compulsive disorder with and without tics in an epidemiological sample of adolescents. Am J Psychiat 1997; 154: 274–276

14. Hebebrand J, Klug B, Fimmers R et al. Rates for tic disorders and obsessive–compulsive symptomatology in families of children and adolescents with Gilles de la Tourette syndrome. J Psychiat Res 1997; 31: 519–530

15. Robertson M M, Banerjee S, Fox Hiley P J, Tannock C. Personality disorder and psychopathology in Tourette's syndrome: a controlled study. Br J Psychiat 1997; 171: 283–286

16. Robertson M M, Trimble M R, Lees A J. The psychopathology of the Gilles de la Tourette syndrome: a phenomenological analysis. Br J Psychiat 1988; 152: 383–390

17. Wodrick D L, Benjamin E, Lachar D. Tourette's syndrome and psychopathology in a child psychiatry setting. J Am Acad Child Adolesc Psychiat 1997; 36: 1618–1624

18. Lees A J, Robertson M, Trimble M R et al. A clinical study of Gilles de la Tourette syndrome in the United Kingdom. J Neurol Neurosurg Psychiat 1984; 47: 1–8

19. Straube A, Mennicken J-B, Riedel M et al. Saccades in Gilles de la Tourette syndrome. Mov Dis 1997; 12: 536–546

20. Eapen V, Robertson M M, Zeitlin H, Kurlan R. Gilles de la Tourette's syndrome in special education schools: a United Kingdom study. J Neurol 1997; 244: 378–382

21. Moriaty J, Varma A R, Stevens J et al. A volumetric MRI study of Gilles de la Tourette's syndrome. Neurology 1997; 49: 419–425

22. Baumgardner T L, Singer H S, Denckla M B et al. Corpus callosum morphology in children with Tourette syndrome and attention deficit hyperactivity disorder. Neurology 1996; 47: 477–482

23. Peterson B S, Leckman J, Duncan J. Corpus callosum morphology from magnetic resonance images in Tourette's syndrome. Psychiat Res 1994; 55: 85–99

24. Robertson M M. D2 be or not to be?: Neuroimaging of monozygotic twins with Tourette syndrome suggests that increased binding by dopamine D2 receptors contributes to the disease phenotype. Nature Med 1996; 2: 1076–1077

25. Klieger P S, Fett K A, Dimitsopulos T, Kurlan R. Asymmetry of basal ganglia perfusion in Tourette's syndrome shown by Technetium-99m-HMPAO SPECT. J Nucl Med 1997; 38: 188–191

26. Riddle M, Rasmussen A, Woods S, Hoffer P B. SPECT imaging of cerebral blood flow in Tourette's syndrome. In: Chase T N, Friedhoff A J, Cohen D J (eds) Tourette syndrome: genetics, neurobiology and treatment (Advances in Neurology volume 58). New York: Raven Press, 1992, 207–211

27. Sieg K, Buckingham D, Gaffney G et al. Technetium-99m-HMPAO SPECT imaging of Gilles de la Tourette's syndrome. Clin Nucl Med 1993; 18: 255

28. Wolf S S, Jines D W, Knable M B et al. Tourette syndrome: prediction of phenotypic variation in monozygotic twins by caudate nucleus D2 receptor binding. Science 1996; 273: 1225–1227

29. Eidelberg D, Moeller J R, Antonini A et al. The metabolic anatomy of Tourette's syndrome. Neurology 1997; 48: 927–934

30. Pantoni L, Poggesi L, Repice A, Inzitari D. Disappearance of motor tics after Wernicke's encephalopathy in a patient with Tourette's syndrome. Neurology 1997; 48: 381–383

31. Peterson B S, Skudlarski P, Anderson A W et al. A functional magnetic resonance imaging study of tic suppression in Tourette syndrome. Arch Gen Psychiat 1998; 54: 326–333

32. Haber S N, Wolfer D. Basal ganglia peptidergic staining in Tourette syndrome. In: Chase T N, Friedhoff A J, Cohen D J (eds) Tourette syndrome: genetics, neurobiology and treatment (Advances in Neurology, volume 58). New York: Raven, 1992, 145–150

33. Singer H S. Neurobiology of Tourette syndrome. Neurol Clin 1997; 15: 357–379

34. Leckman J F, Dolansky E S, Hardin M T. Perinatal factors in the expression of Tourette's syndrome: an exploratory study. J Am Acad Child Adolesc Psychiat 1990; 29: 220–226

35. Patel P I. Quest for the elusive genetic basis of Tourette syndrome. Am J Hum Gen 1996; 59: 980–982

36. Walkup J T, LaBuda M C, Singer H S et al. Family study and segregation analysis of Tourette syndrome: evidence for a mixed model of inheritance. Am J Hum Gen 1997; 59: 684–693

37. Alsobrook J P, Pauls D L. The genetics of Tourette syndrome. Neurol Clin 1997; 15: 381–392

38. Eapen V, O'Neil J, Gurling H M D, Robertson M M. Sex of parent transmission effect in Tourette's syndrome: evidence for an earlier age of onset in maternally transmitted cases suggests a genomic imprinting effect. Neurology 1997; 48: 934–937

39. Lichter D G, Jackson L A, Schachter M. Clinical evidence of genomic imprinting in Tourette's syndrome. Neurology 1995; 45: 924–928

40. Caron C, Brassard A, Merette C. Genomic imprinting in Tourette's syndrome (letter). Neurology 1997; 49: 636–638

41. Swedo S E, Leonard H L, Garvey M et al. Pediatric autoimmune neuropsychiatric disorders associated with streptococcal infections: clinical description of the first 50 cases. Am J Psychiat 1998; 155: 264–271

42. Swedo S E, Leonard H L, Mittleman B B et al. Identification of children with pediatric autoimmune neuropsychiatric disorders associated with streptococcal infections by a marker associated with rheumatic fever. Am J Psychiat 1997; 154: 110–112

43. Murphy T K, Goodman W K, Fudge M W et al. B lymphocyte antigen D8/17: a peripheral marker for childhood-onset obsessive-compulsive disorder and Tourette's syndrome. Am J Psychiat 1997; 154: 402–407

44. Laurino J P, Hallet J, Kiessling L S et al. An immunoassay for anti-neuronal antibodies associated with involuntary repetitive movement disorders. Ann Clin Lab Sci 1997; 27: 230–235

45. Leckman J M, Detlor J, Harcherick D F et al. Short and long-term treatment of Tourette's syndrome with clonidine: a clinical perspective. Neurology 1985; 35: 343–351

46. Chappell P B, Riddle M A, Scahill L et al. Guanfacine treatment of comorbid attention-deficit hyperactivity disorder and Tourette's syndrome: preliminary clinical experience. J Am Acad Child Psychiat 1995; 34: 1140–1146

47. Cohn L M, Caliendo G C. Guanfacine use in children with attention deficit hyperactivity disorder (letter). Ann Pharmacol 1997; 31: 918–919

48. Sallee F R, Nesbitt L, Jackson C et al. Relative efficacy of haloperidol and pimozide in children and adolescents with Tourette's disorder. Am J Psychiat 1997; 154: 1057–1062

49. Bhadrinah B R. Olanzepine in Tourette syndrome (letter). Br J Psychiat 1998; 172: 366

50. Silverstein F S, Johnston M V. Risks of neuroleptic drugs in children. J Child Neurol 1987; 2: 41–43

51. Roan A B, Malone R P. Tics with risperidone withdrawal (letter). J Am Acad Child Psychiat 1997; 36: 162–163

52. Jankovic J, Beach J. Long-term effects of tetrabenazine in hyperkinetic movement disorders. Neurology 1997; 48: 358–362

53. Lipinski J F, Sallee F R, Jackson C, Sethuraman G. Dopamine agonist treatment of Tourette disorder in children: results of an open-label trial of pergolide. Mov Dis 1997; 12: 402–407

54. Riddle M A, Hardin M T, King R A et al. Fluoxetine treatment of children and adolescents with Tourette's and obsessive-compulsive disorders: preliminary clinical experience. J Am Acad Adolesc Child Psychiat 1990; 29: 45–48

55. Robertson M M, Scull D A, Eapen V, Trimble M R. Risperidone in the treatment of Tourette syndrome: a retrospective case note study. J Psychopharmacol 1996; 10: 317–320

56. Stein D J, Bouwer C, Hawkridge S, Emsley R A. Risperidone augmentation of serotonin reuptake inhibitors in obsessive-compulsive and related disorders. J Clin Psychiat 1997; 58: 119–122

57. Rausch S, Baer L, Cosgrove G R, Jenike M A. Neurosurgical treatment of Tourette's syndrome: a critical review. Compr Psychiat 1995; 36: 141–156

58. Sawle G V, Lees A J, Hymas N F et al. The metabolic effect of limbic leucotomy in Gilles de la Tourette syndrome. J Neurol Neurosurg Psychiat 1993; 56: 1016–1019

59. Nolan E E, Gadow K D. Children with ADHD and tic disorder and their classmates: behavioural normalisation with methylphenidate. J Am Acad Adolesc Child Psychiat 1997; 36: 597–604

60. Castellanos F X, Giedd J N, Elia J et al. Controlled stimulant treatment of ADHD and comorbid Tourette's syndrome: effects of stimulant and dose. J Am Acad Adolesc Child Psychiat 1997; 36: 589–596

61. Lees A J. Tics and related disorders. Edinburgh: Churchill Livingstone, 1985

62. Murray T J. Dr Samuel Johnson's movement disorder. Br Med J 1979; 1: 1610–1614

chapter 9

Myoclonus

Peter Brown

Introduction

Myoclonus is defined as shock-like involuntary movements arising from the central nervous system. Most often these are due to brief bursts of muscle activity, resulting in positive myoclonus. Jerks, however, may also result from sudden short inhibitions of ongoing tonic muscle activity, termed negative myoclonus. Myoclonus may be physiological, such as hiccups, or due to a variety of hereditary or acquired conditions (Table 9.1).

● **Table 9.1.** Aetiological classification of myoclonus

Symptomatic myoclonus (progressive or static encephalopathy dominates)	Toxic encephalopathies:
	    Heavy metal poisons
	    Drugs

Storage disease:
    Lafora's disease
    Lipidosis
    Ceroid-lipofuscinosis
    Sialidosis
	Paraneoplastic encephalopathies

	Physical encephalopathies:
	    Posthypoxia (Lance Adams syndrome)
	    Post-traumatic

Spinocerebellar degenerations:
    Baltic myoclonus (Unverricht–Lundborg disease)
    Ataxia telangiectasia
	Focal CNS damage:
	    Vascular
	    Tumour
	    Trauma
	    Syringomyelia

Basal ganglia degenerations:
    Wilson's disease
    Torsion dystonia
    Hallervorden–Spatz disease
    Progressive supranuclear palsy
    Huntington's disease
    Multiple system atrophy
    Corticobasal degeneration
    Dentato-rubro-pallido-luysian atrophy
	Epileptic myoclonus (seizures dominate; no encephalopathy, at least initially)

	Fragments of epilepsy:
	    Isolated epileptic myoclonic jerks
	    Epileptic myoclonic jerks
	    Photosensitive myoclonus
	    Myoclonic absences in petit mal

Mitochondrial encephalopathies	Childhood myoclonic epilepsies:
	    Benign myoclonus of infancy
	    Infantile spasms

Dementias:
    Creutzfeldt–Jakob disease
    Alzheimer's disease
	Myoclonic astatic epilepsy (Lennox–Gastaut)

Malabsorption syndromes:
    Whipple's disease
    Coeliac disease
	Cryptogenic myoclonic epilepsy (Aicardi)

	Benign familial myoclonic epilepsy (Rabot)
Biotin-responsive encephalopathy	**Essential myoclonus (no other neurological deficit)**

Viral encephalopathies:
    Subacute sclerosing panencephalitis
    Encephalitis lethargica
    Postinfectious encephalitis
    Infantile polymyoclonus
	Hereditary essential myoclonus

	Sporadic essential myoclonus
	Periodic movements of sleep

Metabolic encephalopathies:
    Hepatic failure
    Renal failure
    Hyponatraemia
    Hypoglycaemia
	Physiological myoclonus

	Sleep jerks Hiccups

The underlying cause of pathological myoclonus is only correctable infrequently, and in most cases symptomatic treatment is all that is possible. Although aetiological classifications have not proven very useful in predicting the response to drugs, electrophysiological investigations have been able to distinguish several different pathophysiological mechanisms with therapeutic implications.

Cortical myoclonus

Cortical myoclonus is the result of an abnormal discharge in the sensorimotor cortex, and rapidly conducting corticospinal pathways. It may consist of reflex myoclonus, spontaneous jerks or myoclonus elicited by voluntary action, and may be focal or multifocal. It is characterized by brief bursts of electromyographic activity (EMG), usually less than 70 ms in duration. EMG bursts are preceded by pathological enlargement of the cortical components of the sensory-evoked potential in reflex jerks, or a time-locked cortical correlate in the electroencephalographic activity (EEG) in action or spontaneous myoclonus (Fig. 9.1). In each case the relevant EEG wave precedes the EMG burst by an interval more or less appropriate for conduction in the fastest corticospinal pathways. For the intrinsic muscles of the hand this interval is about 20 ms. Although the EEG waves prior to the jerks are often several tens of microvolts in amplitude, averaging techniques, such as back-averaging, are usually necessary to identify their morphology and distribution.

This is the classical view of cortical myoclonus. However, over the last few years two further physiological abnormalities have been identified, which, when present, contribute to disability. The first of these is the presence of both positive and negative myoclonus in some patients. In the latter, a brief silencing of muscle activity of cortical origin occurs. Sudden lapses in posture result, particularly noticeable during gait, and tend to be more resistant to drug treatment than positive reflex or action myoclonus. The second abnormality consists of the spread of myoclonic activity within and between the sensorimotor cortices in some patients with multifocal myoclonus, so that bilateral or generalized jerks also occur.[1] Spread is somatotopic, and cranial nerve innervated muscles are activated rostrocaudally, unlike the caudorostral activation seen

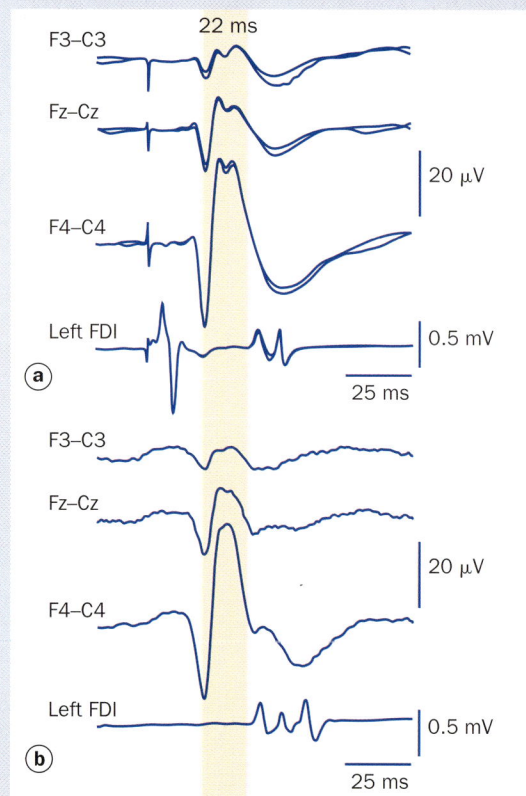

CORTICAL SENSORY- EVOKED POTENTIALS

Figure 9.1. (a) Cortical sensory-evoked potentials to electrical stimulation of the left ulnar nerve at the wrist; (b) back-averaged EEG activity preceding voluntary action jerks in a patient with coeliac disease and cortical myoclonus. A giant EEG wave is recorded, largest contralateral to the stimulated or moved hand. The positive (downgoing) component of the wave precedes the reflex response (a) or action jerk (b) by 22 ms, an interval appropriate for conduction from motor cortex to hand via the fastest pyramidal pathways. (From ref. 6 with permission.)

in hyperekplexia. The cortical inhibitory processes, which would normally keep spread in check, are deficient in cortical myoclonus. This can be shown *in vivo* using the technique of transcutaneous stimulation of the motor cortex. A conditioning magnetic shock to either the ipsilateral or contralateral motor cortex normally inhibits the response to a succeeding test shock, demonstrating the presence of both corticocortical and transcallosal inhibition in healthy subjects. Both types of inhibition are severely impaired in patients with cortical myoclonus and evidence of cortical spread of myoclonic activity.[2]

Aetiology and clinical features

Cortical myoclonus is most marked in the distal limb, and in focal forms is usually confined to this site. If widespread, myoclonus is multifocal, and, in many cases, punctuated by additional bilateral or generalized jerks. The latter are associated with more marked disability (CD 9.1).[2] Reflex jerks may be elicited by touch and tap, or visual stimuli. Sensitivity to auditory stimuli suggests a startle syndrome, although some patients may have a combination of cortical myoclonus and pathological startle. Multifocal jerks occurring with voluntary action are very suggestive of a cortical origin for the myoclonus. As well as involving arm function, jerks may affect speech and gait. Extra-ocular muscles are spared.

Focal cortical myoclonus is usually due to vascular or neoplastic lesions of the sensorimotor cortex. When spontaneous jerks are frequent, focal cortical myoclonus is often called epilepsia partialis continua. Multifocal myoclonus may occur in posthypoxic encephalopathy, or as part of a progressive illness, as in the syndromes of progressive myoclonic ataxia and progressive myoclonic epilepsy. The former describes those patients with prominent myoclonus and ataxia, but little in the way of epilepsy or progressive dementia. The term encompasses the Ramsay Hunt syndrome. Progressive myoclonic ataxia is most commonly due to a spinocerebellar degeneration such as Unverricht–Lundborg disease, mitochondrial encephalopathy or coeliac-related encephalopathy. Progressive myoclonic epilepsy describes those patients with myoclonus, severe epilepsy and relentless cognitive decline. The commonest causes are sialidosis, Lafora's disease, lipidosis, ceroid-lipofuscinosis, dentato-rubro-pallido-luysian atrophy and Huntington's disease, although mitochondrial encephalopathy can also be responsible. Cortical myoclonus may also be a relatively minor aspect of several degenerative diseases, where the clinical picture is dominated by other features. Examples are multiple system atrophy and Alzheimer's disease. Multifocal myoclonus, particularly of the hands, may be present in corticobasal degeneration (page 42–43) (CD 3.5), but it seems likely that the myoclonus in this condition is subserved by different pathways to classical cortical myoclonus.[3] In particular, cortical sensory-evoked potentials are not giant, and the latency of reflex responses is very short, raising the possibility of a direct relay of somatosensory afferent input to the motor cortex without involvement of the sensory cortex.

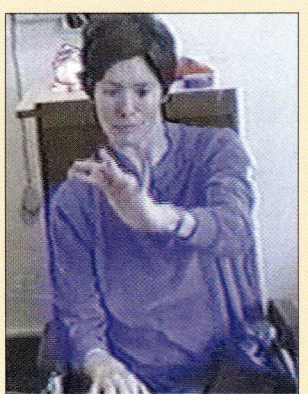

CD 9.1. Cortical myoclonus in Huntington's disease.

Myoclonus due to a static posthypoxic encephalopathy, as first described by Lance and Adams,[4] is a particularly common and difficult problem. These patients have multifocal action myoclonus, often in combination with some bilateral or generalized jerks, and a variable degree of stimulus sensitivity. Disability following the hypoxic event is often severe, but it has been realized recently that late improvement in the myoclonic syndrome and the level of disability can occur years after onset.[5] Some patients are eventually able to discontinue antimyoclonic medication and to walk unaided. Cognitive deficits are found in about half of cases, but are usually mild. Epilepsy may be a problem in the first year, particularly during the initial period of posthypoxic coma, but thereafter only persists in the minority of cases. Other neurological deficits are rare.

Treatment

Drug treatment is aimed primarily at bolstering deficient inhibitory processes. In particular, a reduction of 25–50% of gamma-aminobutyric acid (GABA) levels has been reported in the cerebrospinal fluid of patients with posthypoxic myoclonus and progressive myoclonic epilepsy, and GABAergic drugs form the cornerstone of treatment.[7] Of these sodium valproate is the most effective, and increases cortical GABA levels as well as potentiating GABA postsynaptic inhibitory activity. The drug is introduced slowly, with most patients needing doses of 1200 to 2000 mg/day. Transient gastro-intestinal upset may occur during initial treatment, usually with nausea and vomiting, but sometimes with abdominal pain and diarrhoea. Hair loss, tremor, hepatotoxicity and drowsiness may also occur.

Benzodiazepines and barbiturates facilitate GABAergic transmission by effects on the GABA receptor–ionophore complex. Clonazepam is the most useful antimyoclonic agent. Large doses of clonazepam are often necessary (as much as 15 mg/day). Undue drowsiness and ataxia are the only major side-effects and can be largely overcome by gradually increasing the dosage. Abrupt reductions and withdrawals can result in a marked deterioration in myoclonus and withdrawal fits. Tolerance may develop over a period of several months in some patients. Primidone and phenobarbitone are occasionally useful.

Piracetam is a relatively recent addition to the therapeutic armoury in myoclonus.[8] Although structurally similar to GABA, it does not elicit specific GABAergic effects nor modify GABA levels in the brain, and its mechanism of action remains unknown. The drug's effectiveness is largely limited to cortical myoclonus, regardless of aetiology. This suggests that, where possible, electrophysiological assessment of the physiological type of myoclonus should be undertaken before considering treatment with the drug. Piracetam is well tolerated and does not alter blood levels of other anticonvulsants. In particular, it is non-sedating. It is usually prescribed as add-on therapy, but can be effective when given alone. Therapeutic dosages range from 2.4 to 21.6 g. Abrupt withdrawal of piracetam has been associated with a severe worsening of myoclonus and seizures in a minority of patients.

Disturbances of serotoninergic function have also been incriminated in cortical myoclonus. Lhermitte *et al.* first reported the dramatic effect of the serotonin precursor 5-hydroxytryptophan (5-HTP) in a patient with posthypoxic action myoclonus.[9] Cerebrospinal fluid (CSF) concentrations of the principal metabolite of serotonin, 5-hydroxyindoleacetic acid, are reduced in these patients.[7] However, treatment with serotonin precursors is poorly tolerated and, nowadays, only used as a last resort.

Phenytoin and carbamazepine are helpful in only a minority of patients. In others, particularly those with Unverricht–Lundborg disease, phenytoin may exacerbate myoclonus. Carbamazepine may rarely worsen myoclonic seizures. Vigabatrin, an irreversible inhibitor of GABA transaminase, surprisingly does not seem very useful. It may lead to a paradoxical increase in myoclonus in some patients, or, occasionally, myoclonus in its own right.[10]

In summary, the treatments of first choice in cortical myoclonus are sodium valproate and clonazepam. However, most patients only gain adequate relief from their myoclonus when drugs are used in combination. Gait disturbance tends to be the most resistant feature and a bouncy unsteady gait with frequent falls may persist despite control of action and reflex myoclonus in the upper limbs. Obeso *et al.* found that the combination of clonazepam, primidone and either sodium valproate, piracetam or both was necessary to provide substantial relief from myoclonus and that the latter was not possible with monotherapy.[11] Polytherapy is generally well tolerated, but doses may be limited by ataxia and drowsiness. Piracetam has particular advantages in these circumstances, as its addition to existing treatments is rarely accompanied by sedation.

Brainstem myoclonus and the startle syndrome

Brainstem myoclonus usually leads to generalized myoclonic jerks, as in brainstem reticular reflex myoclonus and hyperekplexia. Focal forms are rare, although diaphragmatic myoclonus may arise in the rostral medulla.[12] Palatal myoclonus is best considered as a form of tremor. The most striking clinical characteristic of the generalized forms of brainstem myoclonus is the exaggerated motor response to unexpected auditory and, sometimes, somaesthetic and visual stimuli. Hyperekplexia is the commonest cause of the startle syndrome (Table 9.2).

Hyperekplexia

Hyperekplexia may be idiopathic, inherited as an autosomal dominant condition, or symptomatic. The pathophysiology of the abnormal startle response in hyperekplexia was, until recently, unclear. Theories relating the abnormal startle reflex to brainstem reticular reflex or cortical myoclonus have not been substantiated. Although pathologically enlarged cortical somatosensory-evoked potentials (SEPs) and

● **Table 9.2.** Aetiology of the startle syndrome

Pathological exaggeration of the normal startle reflex

Hereditary hyperekplexia

Symptomatic hyperekplexia

    Static encephalopathies
        posthypoxic encephalopathy
        post-traumatic encephalopathy

    Brainstem encephalitis
        sarcoidosis
        viral encephalomyelitis
        jerking stiff person syndrome
        demyelination
        paraneoplastic

    Structural
        brainstem haemorrhage/infarct

Idiopathic

Brainstem reticular reflex myoclonus

    posthypoxic encephalopathy
    brainstem encephalitis
    uraemia

Unknown physiology

    hexosaminidase A deficiency
    startle epilepsy
    Gilles de la Tourette syndrome
    Jumping, Latah and Myriachit

Psychogenic startle

EMG ACTIVITY

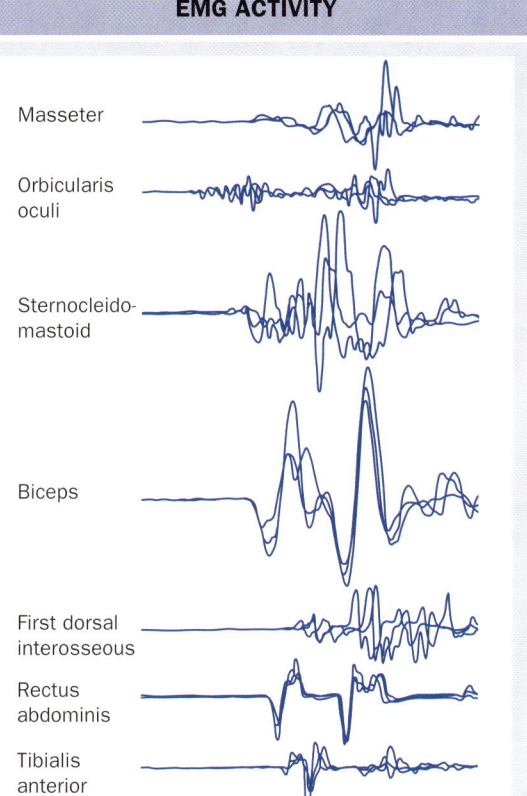

Figure 9.2. The EMG activity in the abnormal startle response elicited by auditory stimulation in a patient with symptomatic hyperekplexia. The unrectified EMG activity in three single trials is superimposed. Each trial was started at the point of presentation of a 124 dB tone. Following the normal auditory blink reflex, EMG activity was recorded first in sternocleidomastoid, and then later in masseter and trunk and limb muscles. The latencies to the intrinsic hand muscles of the hand and foot were disproportionately long. (From ref. 14 with permission.)

enhanced C responses have been reported in hyperekplexia, this is not a uniform finding and no cortical correlate has been found on back-averaging the EEG activity prior to the startle responses. There is now general agreement that the response in hereditary and symptomatic hyperekplexia is a pathological exaggeration of the normal startle reflex.[13–15] Both types of response are the result of activity in a common reflex centre in the lower brainstem. Thus (when allowance is made for the blink reflex which is usually elicited concurrently) the first EMG activity in the startle is recorded in sternocleidomastoid, with other cranial, trunk and limb muscles following in an orderly fashion, as myoclonic activity spreads up the brainstem and down the spinal cord (Fig. 9.2). Caudal muscles are recruited relatively slowly, and involvement of the intrinsic hand and foot muscles is disproportionately delayed. Thus hyperekplexia is defined as a pathological exaggeration of the startle response.

The reflex jerks to auditory, somaesthetic or visual stimuli involve many muscles, both proximal and distal, bilaterally and synchronously to produce a sudden shock-like movement usually involving a grimace, abduction of the arms, and flexion of the neck, trunk, elbows, hips and knees. Thus the reflex jerks resemble the normal startle reaction in general character, although, clinically, they are greatly exaggerated in amplitude, more extensive in distribution and habituate poorly. Somaesthetic stimuli are most effective when applied to the mantle area; that is the head, face and upper chest. Kurczynski reported two cases from the same family where, in addition to unexpected noises, only touch to the tip of the nose would elicit a startle response.[16]

Many patients also exhibit generalized tonic spasms with unexpected stimuli, and it is these that lead to frequent injury and which are the most disabling feature of the condition.[14,17] The pathophysiology of these tonic spasms is not known. They may be brainstem phenomena or the result of activity in the motor and supplementary motor cortex, as in startle epilepsy. Tonic spasms consist of a generalized stiffening, lasting a few seconds, usually in response to unexpected somaesthetic or acoustic stimuli (Fig. 9.3a). During these tonic spasms patients are unable to take any protective action and, if erect, fall stiffly to the ground, without losing consciousness. When present, tonic spasms tend to dominate the clinical picture. The tonic episodes are quite different to the brief, generalized startle reflexes seen in these patients and occur less frequently than the latter. They begin a few seconds after an unexpected sound, separated in time from the earlier startle response (Fig. 9.3b). These tonic responses are distinct from the tonic spasms of multiple sclerosis, which are usually painful, unilateral and rarely stimulus sensitive.

Patients may also experience excessive jerking, particularly during or when going off to sleep.[14,17] These paroxysms of jerking involve repetitive flexion of all four limbs, especially the legs. They are usually spontaneous. Consciousness is preserved in diurnal attacks, although jerking may be severe enough to cause incontinence of urine. The pathophysiology of the episodes of jerking, like that of the tonic spasms, is unclear.

Carbamazepine, phenytoin and the benzodiazepines, particularly clonazepam, form the mainstay of treatment, which is directed at the disabling tonic spasms rather than the exaggerated startle responses.

Hereditary hyperekplexia

Hereditary hyperekplexia is due to a mutation in the alpha-1 subunit of the glycine receptor, which may lead to altered ligand binding or disturbance of the chloride ion channel part of the receptor.[18] Glycine receptors are widely distributed within the central nervous system, and this change in the alpha-1 subunit may account for the range of abnormalities which can be present in this

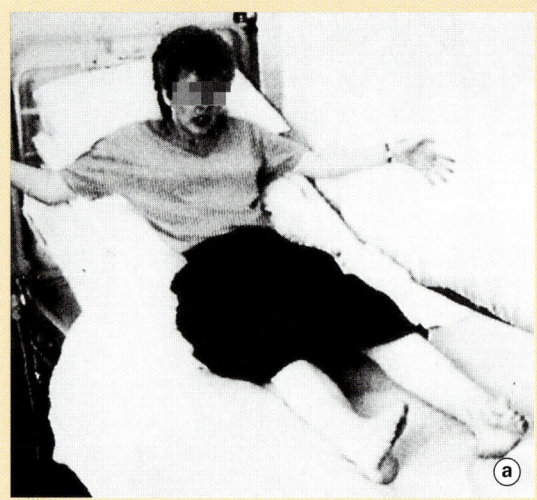

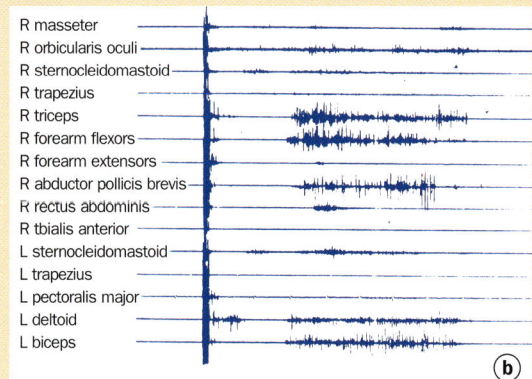

Figure 9.3. (a) A tonic spasm elicited by an unexpected noise in a patient with hereditary hyperekplexia. The shoulders are abducted, the elbows and knees extended, and the feet plantar flexed. The tonic spasm lasted 15 seconds, during which consciousness was retained; (b) EMG record of the tonic spasm occurring after an unexpected sound (delivered 1.9s after the start of the trace) in a patient with symptomatic hyperekplexia. The tonic spasm starts about 2 seconds after the stimulus and is clearly separate from the very rapid and brief startle response. (From ref. 14 with permission.)

condition. Stiffness and apnoeic attacks as a baby, hyper-reflexia, a hesitant wide-based gait, epilepsy, and low intelligence may occur in addition to an exaggerated startle, tonic spasms and paroxysms of jerking.[17]

The clinical and electrophysiological findings vary between members of the same family, and many relatives may only have an excessive startle reaction, without other neurological abnormalities. The mutation in the glycine receptor has not, as yet, been demonstrated in these minor forms.

Idiopathic and symptomatic hyperekplexia

Clinically, idiopathic and symptomatic hyperekplexia are usually only distinguished from hereditary hyperekplexia by the absence of a family history and the presence of any signs attributable to the underlying disease in symptomatic forms. Patients have an exaggerated startle reflex, with or without tonic spasms and paroxysms of jerking. Tonic spasms are occasionally complicated by laryngeal spasm, with the risk of respiratory arrest.[19] So far sporadic cases have not been found to have mutations in the glycine receptor. Symptomatic hyperekplexia is usually due to brainstem disease (Table 9.2).

Startle epilepsy

Startle epilepsy, as described by Alajouanine and Gastaut,[20] can readily be distinguished from hyperekplexia, although similar pathophysiological mechanisms may operate in the tonic episodes of each condition. Startle epilepsy is seen in the setting of early brain damage, usually perinatal anoxia. Virtually all patients have a hemiparesis and mental retardation is common. Seizures begin in childhood or adolescence and tend to be frequent. They consist of tonic spasms, lasting up to 30 seconds, with preservation of consciousness. The spasms are typically asymmetrical and predominately involve the paretic limbs. They may be elicited by unexpected auditory, visual or somaesthetic stimulation, or occur spontaneously. Other seizure types occur in about a quarter of patients.

Cranial imaging is abnormal in the majority of cases, usually showing unilateral atrophy involving the lateral central and pericentral cortex. The interictal EEG is generally abnormal with localized or diffuse slow waves and spikes. Ictal scalp-recorded EEG shows a fast low amplitude discharge often preceded by a high voltage spike at the vertex. Using depth electrodes the tonic seizures have been shown to originate in the motor or supplementary motor cortex.[21]

Brainstem reticular reflex myoclonus

This rare form of generalized myoclonus may occur in posthypoxic encephalopathy, brainstem encephalitis and uraemia. It responds to anticonvulsant drugs, particularly clonazepam and sodium valproate.

Clinically, it is usually readily distinguished from hyperekplexia by the frequent occurrence of spontaneous, as well as reflex, jerks to auditory and somaesthetic stimulation. The latter are most effective over the distal limbs, rather than the mantle area typical of hyperekplexia. The basic pattern of muscle recruitment in the jerks is similar to that recorded in hyperekplexia in so far as activity seems to spread from the caudal brainstem. EMG activity is recorded first in trapezius and sternocleidomastoid, and later in other cranial, trunk and limb muscles. The relative latencies to onset of reflex EMG activity in these muscles increases with the distance of their respective segmental innervations from the lower brainstem.[22]

These generalized jerks are believed, therefore, to arise in the reticular formation of the caudal brainstem. Despite this, several important electrophysiological distinctions exist between brainstem reticular reflex myoclonus and hyperekplexia, making it likely that their origins within the bulbopontine reticular formation are different. The difference between the relative latencies of trunk and limb muscles is small in the jerks of brainstem reticular reflex myoclonus, indicating that the spinal motor pathways are rapidly conducting, with velocities comparable to those of rapidly conducting pyramidal pathways. This is in contrast to the findings in hyperekplexia. Also, in reticular reflex myoclonus the relative latencies of the intrinsic hand and foot muscles are not disproportionately prolonged.[23]

Startle responses with unknown physiology

There remain several other conditions in which an exaggerated startle is a prominent feature, but the physiology of the motor response is unclear (Table 9.2). Infantile GM2 gangliosidosis (Tay–Sachs and Sandhoff's diseases) is characterized by hypotonia, irritability and abnormal startle responses in infancy. Developmental regression, progressive blindness with a cherry red macular spot, deafness, seizures and spasticity ensue. Death usually occurs before the third year. The physiology of the abnormal startle is unknown in this condition, but a relationship to the normal startle or Moro response seems unlikely as the motor response consists of a sudden extension of the arms, head and trunk.

Tics in Gilles de la Tourette's syndrome usually are spontaneous, but sometimes may be triggered by external stimuli and have the appearance of an exaggerated startle response. They rarely represent a diagnostic problem as the other clinical features of Gilles de la Tourette's syndrome are distinctive. In Jumping, Latah and Myriachit unexpected sensory stimulation leads to an initial violent start followed by automatic speech or behaviour, such as echolalia, echopraxia or the assumption of a defensive posture.

Essential myoclonus

Essential myoclonus is commonly inherited as an autosomal dominant trait with variable penetrance and expression, when it is termed hereditary essential myoclonus (the terms essential familial myoclonus, familial myoclonia, ballistic overflow myoclonus and benign essential myoclonus have also been used). The diagnostic criteria for this condition have been set out by Mahloudji and Pikielny[24] and are shown in Table 9.3. The jerks are present at rest, but become more marked with action. They are worst around the neck and proximal arms, and dramatically improve with alcohol. In many cases there is also evidence of dystonic posturing or a family history of dystonia (CD 9.2). Sporadic cases are very similar and may be examples of hereditary essential myoclonus with incomplete penetrance, new mutations or truly sporadic phenocopies. Some families with idiopathic dystonia may have family members with jerks (termed myoclonic dystonia), but myoclonus is not found in the absence of dystonia and does not show a dramatic response to alcohol, distinguishing these families from those with hereditary essential myoclonus.[25]

Myoclonic jerks arise from a distortion of the normal reciprocal activation pattern of ballistic movements, so that muscle activity is no longer restricted to appropriate muscles. EMG activity may also be prolonged, with conspicuous cocontraction. Stimulus sensitivity is not a prominent feature, although jerks can sometimes be provoked by unexpected loud noises. Cortical somatosensory-evoked potentials are normal. Back-averaging of the EEG activity preceding jerks reveals no cortical correlate or an unusual generalized wave preceding the jerks by a longer interval than seen in cortical myoclonus.

The available but limited pharmacological evidence suggests a cholinergic–serotoninergic imbalance. Therapeutic trials have shown moderate benefit from benztropine mesylate and 5-HTP, although the latter is poorly tolerated. The deterioration of the myoclonus following parenteral physostigmine also supports a relative cholinergic overactivity. Antiepileptic treatments are not helpful, with the possible exception of clonazepam. Drug treatments generally fail to match the amelioration seen with alcohol, and as a result there is a real danger of alcoholism in this condition.

Spinal myoclonus

The spinal cord possesses both local segmental organization and long propriospinal pathways linking activity across many segments. Pathological activity in either system can lead to myoclonus.

	Table 9.3. Diagnostic criteria for hereditary essential myoclonus
1	Onset under 20 years old
2	Males and females equally affected
3	Myoclonus with a benign course, compatible with an active life of normal span
4	Dominant mode of inheritance, but with variable severity
5	Absence of seizures, dementia, gross ataxia and other neurological deficits
6	Normal EEG

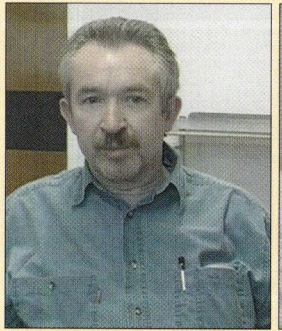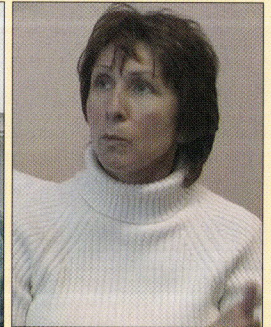

CD 9.2. Two siblings with essential myoclonus.

Propriospinal myoclonus

In this form of myoclonus a spinal myoclonic generator recruits axial muscles up and down the spinal cord via long propriospinal pathways (CD 9.3).[26,27] The disorder generally develops in middle age, and follows cervical trauma, albeit mild, in about half of cases (Table 9.4). Its course is relatively benign, with a history of involuntary jerking stretching back as far as 25 years. Myoclonus usually takes the form of axial flexion jerks involving the neck, trunk, and hips, although a minority of patients may have truncal extension jerks (Fig. 9.4). It may occur spontaneously, particularly on lying flat, or be precipitated by somaesthetic stimuli. Myoclonic EMG activity usually consists of repetitive bursts with a frequency of 1–7 Hz. EMG bursts can be quite long, lasting several hundred milliseconds. The jerks may be stimulus sensitive, particularly to taps to the abdomen, biceps or patella tendons. The orderly recruitment of rostral and caudal segments from a given spinal focus often confirms a spinal origin for the myoclonus, although it is not always possible to distinguish such a pattern of activation. Clonazepam has proven the most effective treatment for propriospinal myoclonus, and leads to partial improvement in over half of patients. Other anticonvulsants have been largely unhelpful.

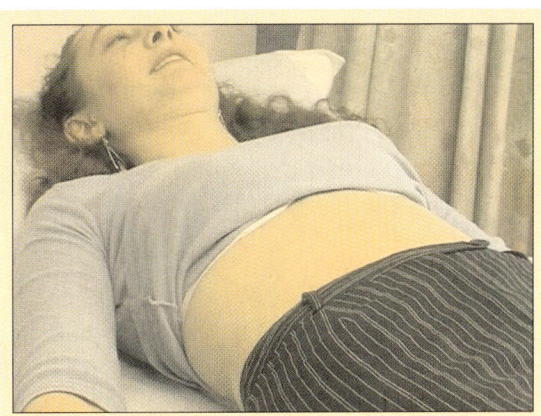

CD 9.3. Propriospinal myoclonus.

● **Table 9.4.** Aetiology of propriospinal myoclonus

Idiopathic

Trauma
Intrinsic cord tumour
Demyelination
Herpes zoster myelitis
HTLV III
Inflammatory

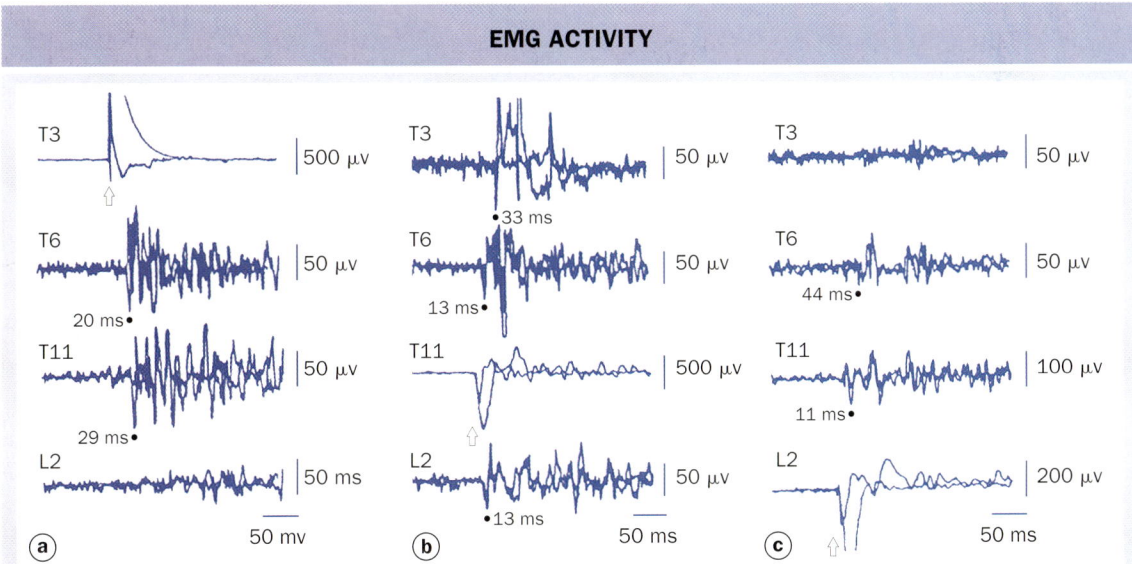

EMG ACTIVITY

Figure 9.4. EMG recordings from erector spinae at various vertebral levels from the third thoracic vertebra (T3) to the second lumbar vertebra (L2) in a patient with stimulus-sensitive propriospinal myoclonus. Two recordings are superimposed. Jerks were elicited by tapping one of the electrodes (arrowed). Latencies are given with respect to the stimulus artefact. Propagation occurs in both rostrocaudal (a,b) and caudorostral (b,c) directions. (From ref. 29 with permission.)

Segmental spinal myoclonus

Segmental spinal myoclonus is often symptomatic of an underlying lesion, such as an intrinsic or extrinsic malignancy, syringomyelia (CD 9.4) or viral myelitis (Table 9.5). It is confined to one or a few contiguous myotomes, and is most often rhythmic, the frequency of jerks varying between 1–2 per minute to 240 per minute (Fig. 9.5). EMG bursts may be up to 1000 ms in duration. Clues to a spinal origin are the independence from supraspinal influences and persistence of myoclonus in sleep. The condition may or may not be stimulus sensitive.

This form of spinal myoclonus is believed to result from the isolation of spinal motorneurones from inhibitory influences or from direct cellular injury.[28] Treatment is that of the underlying cause, where this is possible. Symptomatic treatment is only moderately effective. Clonazepam is the drug of first choice and, in dosages of up to 6 mg daily, may diminish or abolish myoclonus. Diazepam, carbamazepine and tetrabenazine have been useful in occasional cases.

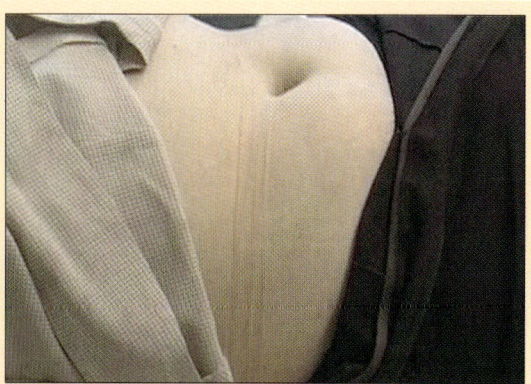

CD 9.4. Segmental myoclonus due to syringomyelia.

● **Table 9.5.** Aetiology of segmental spinal myoclonus

Developmental Arteriovenous malformations Syringomyelia
Intradural and extradural malignancy Paraneoplastic
Cervical spondylosis Ischaemic myelopathy Trauma Radiotherapy Spinal anaesthesia
Herpes zoster HTLV III Encephalitis lethargica

RHYTHMIC SPINAL SEGMENTAL MYOCLONUS

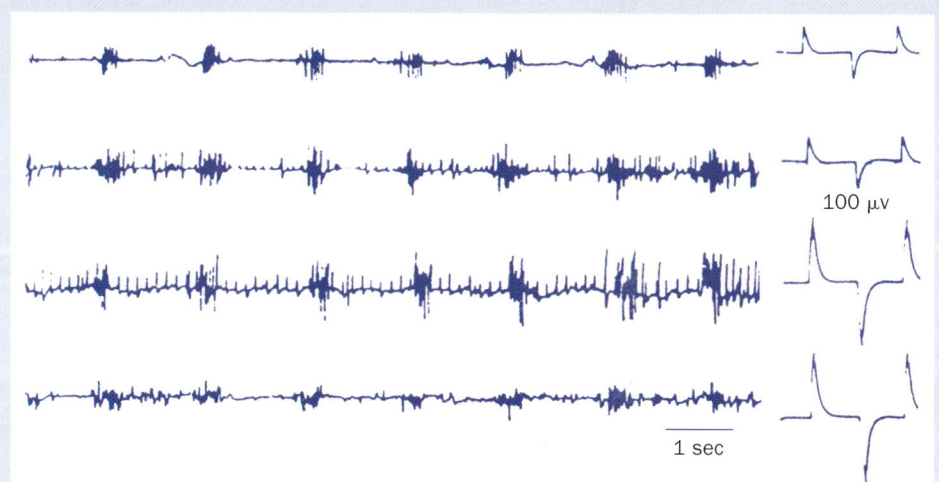

100 µv

1 sec

Figure 9.5. Rhythmic spinal segmental myoclonus in a patient with an astrocytoma of the cervical cord. (From ref. 30 with permission.)

References

1. Brown P, Day B L, Rothwell J C et al. Intrahemispheric and interhemispheric spread of cerebral cortical myoclonic activity and its relevance to epilepsy. Brain 1991; 114: 2333–2351

2. Brown P, Ridding M C, Werhahn K J, Rothwell J C, Marsden C D. Abnormalities of the balance between inhibition and excitation in the motor cortex of patients with cortical myoclonus. Brain 1996; 119: 309–318

3. Thompson P D, Day B L, Rothwell J C, Brown P, Britton T C, Marsden C D. The myoclonus in corticobasal degeneration. Evidence for two forms of cortical reflex myoclonus. Brain 1994; 117: 1197–1207

4. Lance J W, Adams R D. The syndrome of intention or action myoclonus as a sequel to hypoxic encephalopathy. Brain 1963; 86: 111–136

5. Werhahn K J, Brown P, Thompson P D, Marsden C D. The clinical features and prognosis of chronic post-hypoxic myoclonus. Mov Dis 1997; 12: 216–220

6. Bhatia K P, Brown P, Gregory R, Lennox G G, Manji H, Thompson P D, Ellison D W, Marsden C D. Progressive myoclonic ataxia associated with coeliac disease: the myoclonus is of cortical origin, but the pathology is in the cerebellum. Brain 1995; 118: 1087–1093

7. Van Woert M H, Rosenbaum D, Chung E. Biochemistry and therapeutics of posthypoxic myoclonus. Adv Neurol 1986; 43: 171–182

8. Brown P, Steiger M J, Thompson P D et al. Effectiveness of piracetam in cortical myoclonus. Mov Dis 1993; 8: 63–68

9. Lhermitte F, Peterfalvi M, Marteau R et al. Analyse pharmacologique d'un cas de myoclonus d'intention et d'action postanoxique. Rev Neurol 1971; 124: 21–31

10. Marciani M G, Maschio M, Spanedda F, Iani C, Gigli G L, Bernardi G. Development of myoclonus in patients with partial epilepsy during treatment with vigabatrin: an electroencephalographic study. Acta Neurol Scand 1995; 91: 1–5

11. Obeso J A, Artieda J, Rothwell J C et al. The treatment of severe action myoclonus. Brain 1988; 112: 765–777

12. Chen R, Remtulla H, Bolton C F. Electrophysiological study of diaphragmatic myoclonus. J Neurol Neurosurg Psychiat 1995; 58: 480–483

13. Brown P, Rothwell J C, Thompson P D, Britton T C, Day B L, Marsden C D. New observations on the normal auditory startle reflex in man. Brain 1991; 114: 1891–1902

14. Brown P, Rothwell J C, Thompson P D et al. The hyperekplexias and their relationship to the normal startle reflex. Brain 1991; 114: 1903–1928

15. Matsumoto J, Fuhr P, Nigro M, Hallet M. Physiological abnormalities in hereditary hyperekplexia. Ann Neurol 1992; 32: 41–50

16. Kurczynski T W. Hyperekplexia. Arch Neurol 1983; 40: 246–248

17. Suhren O, Bruyn G W, Tuynman J A. Hyperekplexia: a hereditary startle syndrome. J Neurol Sci 1966; 3: 577–605

18. Shiang R, Ryan S G, Zhu Y, Hahn A F, O'Connell P, Wasmuth J J. Mutations in the alpha1 subunit of the inhibitory glycine receptor cause the dominant neurologic disorder, hyperekplexia. Nature Genet 1993; 5: 351–357

19. Kullmann D M, Howard R S, Miller D H, Hirsch N P, Brown P, Marsden C D. Brainstem encephalopathy with stimulus-sensitive myoclonus leading to respiratory arrest: a description of two cases and review of the literature. Mov Dis 1996; 11: 715–718

20. Alajouanine T, Gastaut H. La syncinesie-sursaut et l'epilepsie-sursaut a declanchement sensoriel ou sensitif inopine. I. Les fais anatomo-cliniques (15 observations). Rev Neurol 1955; 93: 29–41

21. Chauvel P, Trottier S, Vignal J P, Bancaud J. Somatomotor seizures of frontal lobe origin. Adv Neurol 1992; 57: 185–232

22. Hallet M, Chadwick D, Adam J et al. Reticular reflex myoclonus: a physiological type of human post-hypoxic myoclonus. J Neurol Neurosurg Psychiat 1977; 40: 253–264

23. Brown P, Thompson P D, Rothwell J C, Day B L, Marsden C D. A case of post-anoxic encephalopathy with cortical action and brainstem reticular reflex myoclonus. Mov Dis 1991; 6: 139–144

24. Mahloudjii M, Pikeilny R T. Hereditary essential myoclonus. Brain 1967; 90: 669–674

25. Quinn N P. Essential myoclonus and myoclonic dystonia. Mov Dis 1996; 11: 119–124

26. Brown P, Thompson P D, Rothwell J C et al. Axial myoclonus of propriospinal origin. Brain 1991; 114: 197–214

27. Brown P, Rothwell J C, Thompson P D, et al. Propriospinal myoclonus: evidence for spinal 'pattern' generators in man. Mov Dis 1994; 9: 571–576

28. Swanson P D, Luttrell C N, Magladery J W. Myoclonus: a report of 67 cases and review of the literature. Medicine 1962; 41: 339–356

29. Schulz-Bonhage A, Knott H, Ferbert A. Pure stimulus-sensitive truncal myoclonus of propriospinal origin. Mov Dis 1996; 11: 87–90

30. Garcin R, Rondot P, Guiot G. Rhythmic myoclonus of the right arm as the presenting symptom of the cervical cord tumour. Brain 1968; 91: 75–84

chapter 10

Movement disorders during sleep

Guy Sawle

Few of us are personally aware of movement disorders during sleep. Some of the following conditions are therefore of more concern to patients' sleeping partners or family than to the patients themselves.

Of the conditions which cause troublesome movements in sleep, epilepsy is perhaps most important. Patients who have generalized tonic clonic seizure are usually easily recognized on the basis of clinical history including a witness description of the attack(s). Some other paroxysmal nocturnal attacks fall into the grey area between epilepsy and movement disorder neurology.

Restless legs syndrome and periodic limb movements during sleep

The close association of these two conditions justifies the inclusion of the former in this chapter. It would otherwise be a technical misfit because the symptoms of the restless legs syndrome do not occur during sleep; rather they *stop* patients from sleeping.

Ekbom is credited as having been the first to describe this syndrome as a clinical entity.[1] It comprises irresistible leg movements, usually accompanied by creeping sensations deep in the limbs. The symptoms are worse when patients try to rest, particularly when they lie down in an effort to go to sleep. Patients describe their sensory symptoms variously as pins and needles, prickling, feelings of tension, aching and so on. These symptoms are briefly and partially eased by either moving the legs in 'fidgeting' or walking around, or else rubbing them.

Many patients with the restless legs syndrome also have stereotyped repetitive movements during sleep. These movements are called periodic limb movements during sleep. The movements comprise extension of the big toe and dorsiflexion of the ankle, sometimes also flexion of the knee and hip. The individual movements last from half a second to 5 seconds and they occur every 20–40 seconds in clusters spanning minutes or hours. They are most common in stage 2 sleep, occur less commonly in stage 3 and 4 sleep and are not seen during rapid eye movement (REM) sleep. Many patients sleep through the movements, which are therefore more disturbing to their sleeping partners than to themselves. But the movements can be severe enough to wake patients from sleep if they are not otherwise woken by a complaining partner (Figs. 10.1, 10.2).

Periodic limb movements during sleep are common in the otherwise healthy population. Although rarely reported below 30 years, they occur in 5% of those aged 30–50 years and almost 30% of those aged over 50 years. Periodic limb movements during sleep also occur in patients with a variety of other sleep disorders, including narcolepsy (9%), sleep apnoea (14%), insomnia (18%), and other hypersomnias (10%).[2]

Factors known to worsen the symptoms of restless legs syndrome include pregnancy, caffeine, fatigue and heat. Both the restless legs and the periodic movements have been reported in connection with other medical conditions, including uraemia, anaemia, leukaemia, neuropathies (including, but not limited to, those caused by diabetes and amyloid), myelopathies, rheumatoid arthritis, fibromyositis, chronic lung disease, Isaac's syndrome, stiff-man syndrome, Huntington's disease, and amyotrophic lateral sclerosis. Some drugs including tricyclic antidepressants and lithium carbonate can precipitate this syndrome, as may withdrawal from several agents including anticonvulsants, benzodiazepines, barbiturates and other hypnotics.[3] Around 15% of patients report occasional spontaneous remissions lasting for a month or more.[4]

Some authors have used the term nocturnal myoclonus to include periodic movements of sleep, and these terms have even been used interchangeably. This term is best avoided as periodic movements of sleep are not a form of myoclonus. There are other conditions in which myoclonus does occur in sleep, and these are discussed below.

It is important to differentiate the restless legs syndrome from akathisia in which sensory symptoms

POLYSOMNOGRAPHY: PERIODIC LIMB MOVEMENTS DURING SLEEP

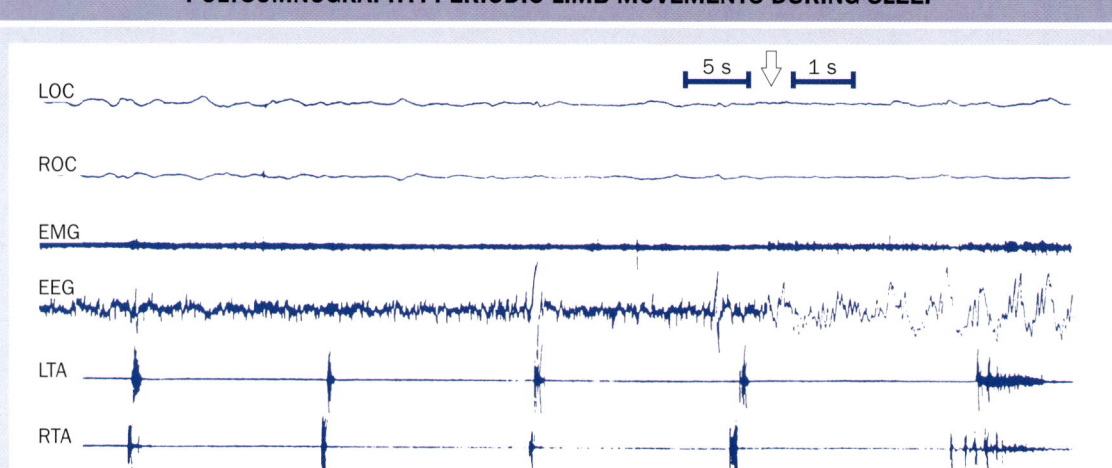

Figure 10.1. Polysomnogram showing periodic movements of sleep. Bilateral leg movements are seen to occur approximately every 20 seconds. LOC, left electro-oculogram; ROC, right electro-oculogram; EMG, chin electromyogram; EEG, left central electroencephalogram; LTA, left tibialis anterior EMG; RTA, right tibialis anterior EMG. Arrow points to a change of chart speed from 3 mm/sec to 15 mm/sec. (Adapted from ref. 3.)

HYPNOGRAMS IN PLMS

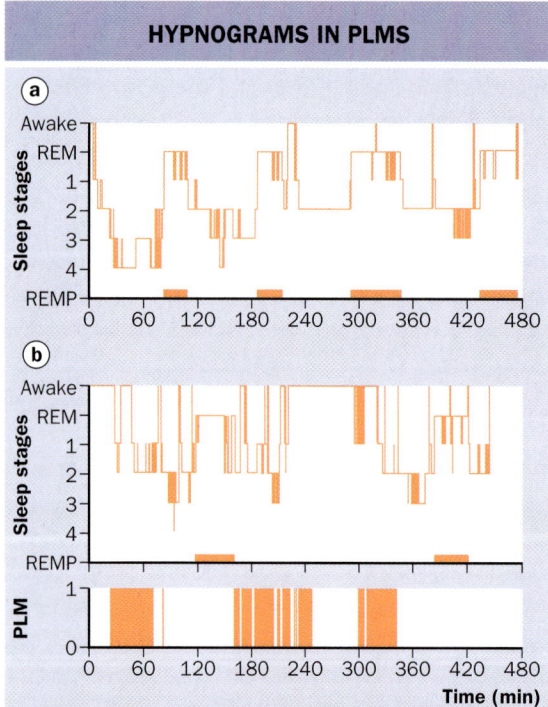

Figure 10.2. Hypnograms of a normal subject (a) and a patient with periodic movements during sleep (b). The leg movements occur in stage 1 and stage 2 of sleep. The patient takes longer to get to sleep, has more awakenings, and less stage 3 and stage 4 sleep than the control. REMP, REM period; PLM, period limb movements.

are less prominent and the relationship between the movements and sensory disturbance is less apparent. Patients with akathisia usually give a history of prior neuroleptic exposure (page 168) (CD 11.1).

The cause of the movements is uncertain. Electrophysiological examination of affected patients has shown a variety of abnormalities, including changes in the blink response, long-latency limb responses, somatosensory-evoked potentials and H reflexes. Such a broad range of abnormal findings (none of which are found consistently in all patients) has been put forward as evidence of a central neurological mechanism which may be responsible both for the restless legs syndrome and the periodic limb movements during sleep.[5,6]

Treatment

The three most effective groups of drugs which help the restless legs syndrome and periodic limb movements during sleep are dopaminergic drugs, benzodiazepines and opiates. All have merits and disadvantages.

Dopaminergic drugs

Levodopa taken as a single dose before bedtime (typically 200 mg with a decarboxylase inhibitor) improves patients' ability to get off to sleep and reduces the involuntary limb movements during the night.[7] There may, however, be a rebound effect with more severe movements in the latter part of the night and a rebound of worse symptoms on waking in the morning. Slow-release levodopa may be a better option.

Benzodiazepines

A variety of benzodiazepines are prescribed principally for their hypnotic effect and it is perhaps unsurprising that several have been shown to enable patients with the restless legs syndrome to get off to sleep more easily. Clonazepam (0.5–2.0 mg) has been studied most, and is generally regarded as an effective treatment,[8,9] as is temazepam (the latter causing less daytime sedation).

Opiates

Although effective in reducing both the restless legs symptoms and the periodic movements,[10] opiates (such as codeine, methadone and oxycodone) are best avoided when possible because of the risk of dependency. Nevertheless, a low dose of a weak opiate at bedtime is sometimes appropriate. Naloxone blocks the effect of opiates on these disorders.

Other treatments

Baclofen has been reported to increase total sleep time. This may be through a sedative effect, since sleep monitoring shows that it actually *increases* the number of leg movements during sleep.[11] Cognitive behavioural therapy has been compared with clonazepam and shown to be similarly effective in improving sleep time. The behavioural therapy reduced daytime napping (which increased in the clonazepam group), though clonazepam was more effective in reducing night-time arousals.[12]

Sleep-related myoclonus

Several kinds of myoclonus are associated with sleep.

Hypnic jerks

Many people have experienced a sudden jerk of the body, just at the point of falling asleep. These movements are called hypnic jerks, or 'sleep starts', and they are considered to be normal. They are brief and occur during light sleep. In some cases patients report an accompanying falling sensation or even a vivid hallucination. These movements may involve any part or the whole of the body. They are noticed more often after sleep deprivation, or under stress. Reassurance is usually the only action necessary.

Benign sleep myoclonus

This disorder is most common in neonates, when the term 'benign neonatal sleep myoclonus' is generally used. Affected infants develop myoclonic jerks within the first few weeks of life. The jerks occur only during sleep. They are not epileptic (though they may be misdiagnosed as such). Investigations, including EEG during the jerks, are normal. The movements usually stop within a few months, and subsequent neurological development is normal.[13-15] Similar nocturnal jerks can be seen in adults, by which age the condition is more common in men than women and the jerks affect mainly the face and hands. The movements can occur repeatedly over hours, spanning both REM and non-REM sleep.

Nocturnal head-banging

Nocturnal head-banging (also referred to as jactatio capitis nocturnis) comprises a stereotyped rhythmic movement which occurs principally in children, beginning prior to sleep onset and sustained into light sleep. Most patients stop by the age of 10, but rarely it persists, usually in the context of mental retardation. Exceptionally, the disorder continues into adult life in otherwise healthy individuals, in which case treatment with clonazepam has been reported (anecdotally) to be effective.[16]

Nocturnal paroxysmal dystonia

Under the heading 'hypnogenic paroxysmal dystonia', Lugaresi and colleagues described several patients with nocturnal attacks during non-REM sleep comprising often violent movements with a tonic phase of variable duration.[16] Although the heart and respiratory rate changed during the attacks, the EEG did not and the attacks were thought *not* to be epileptic, despite several of the patients having daytime fits and the nocturnal attacks responding to carbamazepine and sodium valproate.[17] The attacks may be sufficiently frequent to cause sleep fragmentation, as a consequence of which patients may present with complaints of excessive daytime somnolence.[17]

Much of the literature on this condition relates to the vexed question of whether or not it is a kind of epilepsy. Some patients with nocturnal 'dystonia' have occasional attacks which lead on to a convulsive seizure with changes on surface EEG, suggesting that these attacks at least are due to epilepsy, presumably from a focus in the orbital/medial frontal lobe.[18] Clinical examination of the attacks does not allow any definite distinction to be drawn between the clinical features of nocturnal paroxysmal dystonia, daytime frontal lobe seizures, or nocturnal attacks of known epileptic origin.[19] Positron emission tomography (PET) scans using fluorodeoxyglucose as tracer may show frontal or frontotemporal hypometabolic foci.[20]

So at least some of the patients with nocturnal paroxysmal dystonia probably have epilepsy. Whether epilepsy accounts for *all* such attacks remains unknown. No evidence of epilepsy was found in three members of a single family with dystonic attacks occurring in non-REM sleep,[21] though frontal lobe epilepsy can occur as a familial condition with autosomal dominant inheritance and it is often misdiagnosed — as night terrors, nightmares, hysteria, or paroxysmal nocturnal dystonia![22]

Attacks of nocturnal dystonia (unresponsive to carbamazepine, but responsive to acetazolamide) have also been reported after severe head trauma.[23]

Other movement disorders during sleep

It is said that most movement disorders stop in sleep. Whilst this is generally true, quite a number of dyskinetic movements (including those characteristic of Parkinson's disease, Gilles de la Tourette syndrome, Huntington's disease and both primary and secondary dystonia) can be seen occasionally during unequivocal sleep. Such movements generally occur either in stage 1 sleep, or after awakenings or lightenings of sleep.[24]

Other conditions which have been reported to sometimes continue at least into light sleep include palatal myoclonus,[25] and the syndrome of painful legs and moving toes.[26] Hemifacial spasm continues 'deeper' into sleep than most of these disorders with some movements occurring in REM sleep also.[27]

Fatal familial insomnia

One of the most striking sleep-related neurological disorders is fatal familial insomnia, a dominantly inherited prion protein disease (a D178N mutation encoding methionine at position 129)[28] in which the anterior and dorsomedial nuclei of the thalamus bear the brunt of the pathological changes (Fig. 10.3).[29] Clinical onset is usually between 35 and 60 years of age, with rapid progression to death over 6 months to 3 years. Affected members of successive generations may die at widely differing ages.[30]

The initial symptoms are usually progressive insomnia with autonomic features including hyperhidrosis, hyperthermia, tachycardia, irregular respirations and hypertension, and motor symptoms including ataxia, myoclonus, and pyramidal signs.[26]

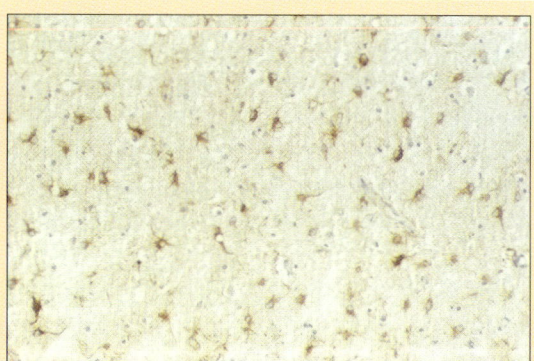

Figure 10.3. The dorsomedial nucleus of the thalamus in fatal familial insomnia exhibits severe astrocytosis, with numerous reactive astrocytes staining brown using an antibody technique for glial fibrillary acidic protein. (Courtesy of J. W. Ironside.)

References

1. Ekbom K A. Restless legs syndrome. Acta Med Scand 1945; (158 Suppl.): 1–123

2. Coleman R M, Pollak C P, Weitzman E D. Periodic movements in sleep (nocturnal myoclonus): Relation to sleep disorders. Ann Neurol 1979; 8: 416–421

3. Montplaisir J, Godbout R, Pelletier G, Warnes H. Restless legs syndrome and periodic limb movements during sleep. In: Kryger M H, Roth T, Dement W C (eds), Principles and practice of sleep medicine. Philadelphia: WB Saunders, 1994: 589–597

4. Walters A S, Hickey K, Maltzman J et al. A questionnaire study of 138 patients with restless legs syndrome: The 'night-walkers' survey. Neurology 1996; 46: 92–95

5. Wechsler L R, Stakes J W, Shahani B T, Busis N A. Periodic leg movements of sleep (nocturnal myoclonus): An electrophysiological study. Ann Neurol 1986; 19: 168–173

6. Martinelli P, Coccagna G, Lugaresi E. Nocturnal myoclonus, restless legs syndrome, and abnormal electrophysiological findings. Ann Neurol 1987; 21: 515

7. Maccario M, Lustman L I. Paroxysmal nocturnal dystonia presenting as excessive daytime somnolence. Arch Neurol 1990; 47: 291–294

8. Boghen D. Successful treatment of restless legs with clonazepam. Ann Neurol 1980; 8: 341

9. Matthews W B. Treatment of the restless legs syndrome with clonazepam. Br Med J 1979; 281: 751

10. Trzepacz P T, Violette J, Sateia M J. Response to opioids in three patients with the restless legs syndrome. Am J Psychiat 1984; 141: 993–995

11. Guilleminault C, Flagg W. Effect of baclofen on sleep-related periodic leg movements. Ann Neurol 1984; 15: 234–239

12. Edinger J D, Fins A I, Sullivan R J et al. Comparison of cognitive-behavioral therapy and clonazepam for treating periodic limb movement disorder. Sleep 1996; 19: 442–444

13. Di Capua M, Fusco L, Ricci S, Vigevano F. Benign neonatal sleep myoclonus: Clinical features and video-polygraphic recordings. Mov Dis 1993; 8: 191–194

14. Coulter D L, Allen R J. Benign neonatal sleep myoclonus. Arch Neurol 1982; 39: 191–192

15. Resnick T J, Moshé S L, Perotta L, Chambers H J. Benign neonatal sleep myoclonus. Relationship to sleep states. Arch Neurol 1986; 43: 266–268

16. Chisholm T, Morehouse R L. Adult headbanging: Sleep studies and treatment. Sleep 1996; 19: 343–346

17. Lugaresi E, Cirignotta F. Hypnogenic paroxysmal dystonia: Epileptic seizure or a new syndrome? Sleep 1981; 4: 129–138

18. Tinuper P, Cerullo A, Cirignotta F et al. Nocturnal paroxysmal dystonia with short-lasting attacks: Three cases with evidence for an epileptic frontal lobe origin of seizures. Epilepsia 1990; 31: 549–556

19. Meierkord H, Fish D R, Smith S J M et al. Is nocturnal paroxysmal dystonia a form of frontal lobe epilepsy? Mov Dis 1992; 7: 38–42

20. Sellal F, Hirsch E, Maquet P et al. Abnormal paroxysmal movements during sleep: Hypnogenic paroxysmal dystonia or focal epilepsy? Revue Neurologique 1991; 147: 121–128

21. Lee B I, Lesser R P, Pippenger C E et al. Familial paroxysmal hypnogenic dystonia. Neurology 1985; 35: 1357–1360

22. Scheffer I E, Bhatia K P, Lopes-Cendes I et al. Autosomal dominant frontal epilepsy misdiagnosed as sleep disorder. Lancet 1994; 343: 515–517

23. Biary N, Singh B, Bahou Y et al. Posttraumatic paroxysmal nocturnal hemidystonia. Mov Dis 1994; 9: 98–99

24. Fish D R, Sawyers D, Allen P J et al. The effect of sleep on the dyskinetic movements in Parkinson's disease, Gilles de la Tourette syndrome, Huntington's disease, and torsion dystonia. Arch Neurol 1991; 48: 210–214

25. Kayed K, Sjaastad O, Magnussen I, Marvik R. Palatal myoclonus during sleep. Sleep 1983; 6: 130–136

26. Spillane J D, Nathan P W, Kelly R E, Marsden C D. Painful legs and moving toes. Brain 1971; 94: 541–556

27. Montagna P, Imbriaco A, Zucconi M et al. Hemifacial spasm in sleep. Neurology 1986; 36: 270–273

28. Manetto V, Medori R, Cortelli P et al. Fatal familial insomnia: Clinical and pathologic study of five new cases. Neurology 1992; 42: 312–319

29. Lugaresi E, Medori R, Montagna P et al. Fatal familial insomnia and dysautonomia with selective degeneration of thalamic nuclei. N Engl J Med 1986; 315: 997–1003

30. Silburn P, Cervenáková L, Varghese et al. Fatal familial insomnia: A seventh family. Neurology 1996; 47: 1326–1328

chapter 11

Drug-induced movement disorders

Cynthia Comella

Drug-induced movement disorders arise secondary to the administration of pharmacological agents. Drugs may either create a new movement disorder in a normal brain, or activate an underlying susceptibility arising from previous but quiescent brain injury or subclinical degenerative processes. In almost all instances, drug-induced movement disorders are reversible, resolving after discontinuation of the offending drug. Tardive dyskinesia is the important exception to the general rule, with a potentially permanent movement disorder occurring where none existed before. Drug-induced movement disorders may manifest as any of the general categories of spontaneously occurring movement disorders.[1]

This chapter will focus on the spectrum of commonly occurring movement disorders associated with a variety of pharmacological agents including dopamine receptor antagonists (acute, subacute and chronic), dopamine receptor agonists, stimulant agents, and other frequently used drugs (hormone, anticonvulsants, antidepressant medications).

Dopamine receptor antagonists: acute and subacute effects

Acute dystonic reactions
Clinical manifestations and epidemiology
Acute dystonic reactions typically occur within days to weeks of initiating neuroleptic therapy[2] and affect approximately 10–30% of neuroleptic treated patients.[2–5] Although the classic neuroleptics are most often the cause of acute dystonia, tetrabenazine, a compound with combined dopamine receptor blocking and dopamine depleting properties, may also cause 'acute' dystonia whilst the dose is being increased.[6] Risk factors for neuroleptic-induced dystonia include younger age, male gender, more potent class and higher dose of neuroleptic administered. Children and young adults with a previous history of neuroleptic-induced dystonic reactions, and adults who later receive large

doses of high-potency neuroleptic, are at the highest risk for acute neuroleptic-induced dystonia.[7,8] Subjects who lack the cytochrome p450 enzyme CYP2D6 and are poor metabolizers of a range of antipsychotic drugs are no more susceptible to acute dystonic reactions than others.[9]

Acute dystonic reactions typically occur early in the course of neuroleptic treatment, in contrast to drug-induced parkinsonism and tardive dyskinesia which most commonly occur after chronic neuroleptic therapy. The onset of neuroleptic-induced dystonic reactions is usually within 1–2 days of the first dose of neuroleptic, although patients receiving long-term neuroleptics may also experience this side-effect after an increase in dose.[3] The symptoms may be intermittent at first, with periods of relative normality alternating with recurrence of dystonia.

The most dramatic of the acute dystonic reactions is oculogyric crisis, the hallmark of which is a forceful involuntary upward deviation and convergence of the eyes. This may present as no more than a mild intermittent upward eye movement, or it may be evident as a pronounced and sustained spasm of eye deviation. Frequently associated with these remarkable eye spasms is cervical dystonia with backward (retrocollic) or horizontal (torticollic) head postures; also involuntary jaw opening with tongue thrusting. The epidemic of von Economo's encephalitis in the early 1900s was frequently associated with recurrent oculogyric crisis. Many early descriptions of the patients with this disorder describe oculogyric crises in vivid detail. With the disappearance of von Economo's encephalitis, oculogyric crises were rarely reported until the introduction of neuroleptics in the 1950s. Neuroleptic treatment is now the most common cause of acute oculogyric crisis.

Other types of acute dystonic reactions include generalized dystonia, torticollis, trismus, and opisthotonus.[3,10] In addition to the involuntary movements, some patients experience mild or even extreme pain during the dystonic episodes. Although acute neuroleptic-induced dystonia may be dramatic in its appearance, subtle forms also occur, manifesting as jaw tightening, difficulty in speaking or upward eye deviation without other associated findings. These symptoms may be misdiagnosed as a worsening of the underlying psychiatric condition. Even when severe, the bizarre appearance of the movements and the intermittent nature of the symptoms have led physicians to mistakenly treat these patients for an exacerbation of psychosis or as hysteria.

Pathophysiology

The pathophysiology of neuroleptic-induced dystonia has been attributed to the blockade of dopamine receptors. Both D1 and D2 receptors appear to be involved, but the precise mechanism is unknown.[11] Excessive cholinergic activity has also been suggested as the underlying mechanism, largely based on clinical experience showing improvement of neuroleptic-induced dystonia with anticholinergic agents and the reduced occurrence of dystonia with neuroleptic agents having high anticholinergic activity.[12–14]

The delay in onset of symptoms from a few hours to a few days following the administration of a single dose of neuroleptic, at a stage when plasma levels of neuroleptic are declining, suggests that acute blockade of dopamine receptors is not the initiating factor.[11] An imbalance between dopaminergic and cholinergic activities has been proposed.

Treatment

A general approach for the treatment of acute neuroleptic-induced movement disorders is outlined in Table 11.1.

Effective treatment of an acute neuroleptic-induced dystonia is primarily with anticholinergic agents. Benztropine (Cogentin), trihexphenidyl (Artane), biperidine (Akineton) and the antihistaminic agents such as diphenhydramine (Benedryl) are the mainstays of therapy. The acute onset of symptoms and the abnormal head posture with associated buccolingual and laryngeal involvement may prevent oral administration, making parenteral administration necessary. Benztropine and diphenhydramine are each available for parenteral administration and are given in an initial dose of 0.5 and 25 mg respectively. The major side-effects of anticholinergic therapy are

Table 11.1. General approach for treatment of acute neuroleptic-induced movement disorders

Neuroleptic-induced disorder	Treatment
Any acute neuroleptic-induced disorder	Reduce or discontinue neuroleptic
	Replace neuroleptic with an atypical neuroleptic
Parkinsonism	Anticholinergic agent
	Amantadine
Dystonia	Anticholinergic agent
Oculogyric crisis	Benzodiazepine
Akathisia	Beta-blocking agent
	Anticholinergic agent
	Benzodiazepine
	Clonidine
	?Codeine
	?Tetrabenazine

dry mouth, urinary retention, and memory loss or delirium. Uncommonly, these agents may also exacerbate narrow angle glaucoma and can even lead to blindness in susceptible patients.[15] If an anticholinergic agent fails to provide relief, parenteral benzodiazepines may be useful. When the acute symptoms subside, oral may be substituted for parenteral therapy and given for at least 2 or 3 days and sometimes for as long as 1–4 weeks. A gradual reduction in anticholinergic or benzodiazepine dose is recommended before discontinuation to prevent withdrawal effects and to discern whether recovery from neuroleptic-induced dystonia is complete.[16]

Drug-induced parkinsonism
Clinical manifestations and epidemiology

In the 1950s, the development of chlorpromazine provided the first effective treatment for severe psychiatric disorders. Dopamine receptor antagonists have subsequently been used to treat a variety of medical and psychiatric disorders. Soon after the introduction of chlorpromazine into clinical practice, reports of a secondary parkinsonian syndrome started to appear.[17] Initially, it was believed that drug-induced parkinsonism was a necessary side-effect in achieving efficacy for psychosis.[18,19] Drug-induced parkinsonism was considered a 'necessary evil' if psychosis was to be improved. This belief was subsequently refuted with wider clinical experience.

Drug-induced parkinsonism has been estimated to occur in 10–15% of psychotic patients treated with neuroleptic agents. In some centres, drug-induced parkinsonism is the most frequent neuroleptic-induced movement disorder.[20] Bollini and colleagues conducted a meta-analysis of 22 studies comparing a variety of neuroleptic-induced side-effects and found that drug-induced parkinsonism was the most frequent, and was most severe in those receiving the highest doses of neuroleptics.[21] Other drugs with dopamine receptor antagonizing effects may also cause drug-induced parkinsonism, such as metoclopramide and prochlor-perazine (which are used to treat dizziness, vertigo, nausea and vomiting). Details of the common neuroleptic agents are given in Table 11.2.

The symptoms of drug-induced parkinsonism typically begin within days of initiating or increasing neuroleptic dose, with 75% of cases occurring in the first month and 90% by 3 months of neuroleptic initiation or increase.[10] The clinical symptoms and signs mimic those of idiopathic Parkinson's disease and can include tremor, rigidity, bradykinesia, akinesia, and postural reflex impairment. Although symmetry of parkinsonian symptoms was once considered to distinguish drug-induced parkinsonism from idiopathic Parkinson's disease, it was later recognized that the only reliable indicator is a history of dopamine receptor blocking drug use and a resolution of these symptoms with discontinuation of the offending agent.[22] The symptoms of drug-induced parkinsonism usually resolve within 3 months of discontinuation of the offending neuroleptic. In some patients, however, symptoms may persist much longer or indefinitely.[23] There have been reports of parkinsonism which began while on neuroleptic but continued to progress despite discontinuation of the agent. Whether this represents tardive parkinsonism or the coincidental occurrence of Parkinson's disease while on neuroleptic is not known.[24]

In contrast to the neuroleptic-induced acute dystonic reactions, the risk of drug-induced parkinsonism is greater in women. The potency of the neuroleptic also appears to increase the risk for drug-induced parkinsonism. Other factors have been inconsistently identified as potential risk factors for drug-induced parkinsonism. These include older age, recent use of neuroleptic, and severity of tardive dyskinesia.[25] Some clinicians have suggested that the greatest risk of drug-induced parkinsonism is in patients with presymptomatic Parkinson's disease, who have a reduced reserve of dopamine and also may be more susceptible to further reductions in dopamine activity.

Pathophysiology

The motor symptoms of idiopathic Parkinson's disease arise secondary to the loss of the pigmented

● **Table 11.2.** Common neuroleptic agents: relative equivalences and tendency to cause adverse effects.[16]

Class	Drug	Relative equivalence	Drug-induced parkinsonism	Sedation	Anticholinergic properties
Phenothiazines					
Aliphatic	Chlorpromazine	100	Moderate	Marked	Marked
Piperidine	Thioridazine	100	Mild	Marked	Marked
Piperazine	Perphenazine	10	Marked	Mild	Moderate
	Trifluoperazine	5	Marked	Mild	Mild
	Fluphenazine	2	Marked	Mild	Mild
Non-phenothiazines					
Thioxanthene	Thiothixene	4	Marked	Mild	Mild
Butyrophenone	Haloperidol	2	Marked	Mild	Mild
Dibenzoxazepine	Loxapine	10	Moderate	Moderate	Moderate
Dibenzazepine	Clozapine	50	Minimal	Marked	Marked
Diphenylbutylpiperidone	Pimozide	1	Marked	Mild	Mild
Benzisoxazole	Risperidone	6	Mild	Minimal	None
Dihydroindolone	Molindone	10	Moderate	Moderate	Moderate

dopamine-producing cells in the substantia nigra, a presynaptic cause of parkinsonism. Neuroleptic agents block the dopamine receptors in the nigrostriatal system and therefore give rise to postsynaptic parkinsonism. Blockade of dopamine receptors is thought to lead to excess release of dopamine and development of dopamine receptor denervation supersensitivity, a process considered to underlie the development of tardive dyskinesia.

Reserpine and tetrabenazine are both catecholamine depleting agents. As would be anticipated, the loss of dopamine secondary to the effect of these drugs can also cause drug-induced parkinsonism. Tetrabenazine also has dopamine receptor blocking activity and may cause drug-induced parkinsonism through both mechanisms.

Treatment

If not disabling, drug-induced parkinsonism does not necessarily require aggressive treatment. Patients with drug-induced parkinsonism usually improve within 3 months of drug discontinuation. Patients who are unable to be discontinued from neuroleptic agents may improve following a reduction in dose. The atypical neuroleptic agents, such as clozapine, olanzapine and quetiapine, are less likely to cause drug-induced parkinsonism and may be useful replacements for those patients who require control of psychosis but yet experience intolerable parkinsonism with traditional neuroleptic agents.

Treating drug-induced parkinsonism with additional agents can be problematic. Anticholinergic agents may improve tremor and rigidity but have an inconsistent effect. Amantadine may be as effective or more so than anticholinergic agents.[26–28] Although levodopa and dopamine agonists are highly effective treatments for idiopathic Parkinson's disease and their use is occasionally justified for patients with severe drug-induced parkinsonism, they must be used with caution in these circumstances because they may exacerbate the psychiatric disorder. If the offending drug has been stopped completely (such as prochlorperazine prescribed for longstanding dizziness), but yet the drug-induced parkinsonism continues, eventually necessitating treatment with levodopa or a dopamine agonist, it is important to try reducing and usually stopping the new drug a few months later.

Pyridoxine has been reported effective in ameliorating both parkinsonism and tardive dyskinesia in uncontrolled observations.[29]

Drug-induced akathisia
Clinical manifestations and epidemiology

Amongst the most agonizing of the neuroleptic-induced movement disorders is akathisia. This term is used to describe a sense of inner restlessness accompanied by an irresistible urge to move. If severe, the inner restlessness may not be alleviated even by extraordinary physical activity. Patients with akathisia find it impossible to remain still. If seated, they may rock in the chair, cross and uncross their legs, fidget with their arms and hands; if standing, they may rock from side to side or pace around the room in a futile attempt to quiet the inner uneasiness (CD 11.1). Early on, akathisia may be described as a sense of inner anxiety, inner tension and dysphoria. As the disorder worsens, the movements begin, mild at first with a stereotyped, purposeful quality. These movements can be voluntarily suppressed but only at the price of a rising sense of discomfort.[30] Because of the nature of the movements and the associated psychological disturbance, akathisia is frequently misdiagnosed as a worsening of the psychiatric disorder leading to an increase in the neuroleptic treatment, and hence a further worsening of the movement disorder.

Akathisia can occur as either an acute or a tardive side-effect of neuroleptic treatment. Its prevalence is unknown; estimates vary from 3 to 50%.[31] Drug-induced akathisia is more frequent with higher doses

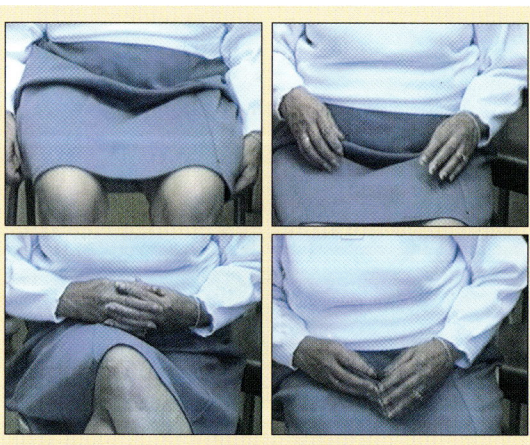

CD 11.1. Neuroleptic induced akathisia.

and with the more potent neuroleptic agents. The onset may be subtle, as the dose of neuroleptic is increased.

Pathophysiology

The pathophysiology of drug-induced akathisia is not understood. The known association with dopamine receptor blockade and the observation that akathisia can occur in Parkinson's disease both suggest that dopamine depletion may be a primary mechanism. Involvement of the mesocortical dopamine system has been proposed.[32] However, improvement in akathisia with a variety of drugs involving other neurochemical systems indicates that the pathophysiology is not solely related to dopamine.

Treatment

Patients with acute neuroleptic-induced akathisia can be treated by a reduction or discontinuation of the neuroleptic agent.[33] In patients with active psychosis, this may not be possible without an exacerbation of the psychiatric disorder. With the possible exception of atenolol,[34] centrally active beta-blocking drugs have been shown to improve akathisia.[35,36] Propranolol is a non-selective, lipophilic beta blocker that was tested in open-label and controlled trials and shown to improve symptoms in 50–100% of patients.[35–38] Other types of centrally active beta-blocking agents have also been reported to be of benefit.

Anticholinergic agents have also been observed to improve akathisia. In particular, patients who have both drug-induced parkinsonism and akathisia tend to improve with this class of drug.[33] Amantadine in doses of 200 mg per day has also been shown to reduce akathisia. Benzodiazepines, especially clonazepam, were quite effective in both open and controlled studies.[39,40] Clonidine, a central, alpha-2 agonist, may also be useful although its usefulness is limited by postural hypotension.[41]

Neuroleptic malignant syndrome

The neuroleptic malignant syndrome is marked by the occurrence of fever, muscle rigidity, movement disorder, autonomic instability and mental status changes.[42,43] The fever may be low-grade or as high as 105°F.[44,45] The rigidity can be extreme, associated with rhabdomyolysis and myoglobinuria, which in turn can lead to acute renal failure in combination with acidosis and hypoxia. Associated movement disorders include parkinsonism, dystonia, tremor, and myoclonus. Autonomic features include cardiac arrhythmias, blood pressure changes, and respiratory instability. Patients may present with intermittent confusion, delirium or frank coma. Laboratory findings include extreme elevations of creatinine phosphokinase, elevated lactic dehydrogenase and other muscle enzymes, leucocytosis and dehydration. Renal failure can lead to profound electrolyte disturbances, and hepatic damage may be reflected in elevations of hepatic enzymes.

The neuroleptic malignant syndrome is an early phenomenon which can be fulminant, either following a single dose of neuroleptic or (more commonly) occurring within the first 2 weeks of starting or increasing the dose of a dopamine receptor antagonist. Fortunately it is quite rare, reported in no more than 1–2% of patients treated with a neuroleptic annually.[43] Friedman found that the incidence was 0.2% among hospitalized psychiatric inpatients.[46] Risk factors for the neuroleptic malignant syndrome include coincidental dehydration, and large doses of the greater potency neuroleptics.

The prognosis for patients with the neuroleptic malignant syndrome is guarded. The disorder has a rapid onset, and generally peaks within 3–4 days. Symptoms usually clear within 1–40 days. Depot neuroleptic agents cause a more prolonged course than the oral formulations. The medical complications of the syndrome affect about 50% of the patients.[44] The mortality from the neuroleptic malignant syndrome is estimated at 20%.[47,48] Early recognition and intervention may prevent the medical complications and reduce mortality.

The differential diagnosis of the neuroleptic malignant syndrome includes infection, heat stroke, malignant hyperthermia and malignant catatonia. Careful assessment for concurrent infection is critical.

Pathophysiology

The neuroleptic malignant syndrome is thought to be primarily related to central dopaminergic mechanisms, since it is typically associated with either beginning (or increasing the dose of) dopamine receptor antagonists or dopamine depleting agents, or else discontinuing levodopa.[48,49] These observations suggest that a precipitous reduction in dopaminergic activity is aetiologically important. The hypothalamus is presumed to be involved in the pathogenesis of the associated hyper-thermia and autonomic lability. Muscle rigidity is thought to be mediated centrally in the basal ganglia, whereas the malignant hyperthermia is believed to be due to peripheral alterations in calcium permeability.[43]

Treatment

Treatment of suspected neuroleptic malignant syndrome involves three steps: first, elimination of infection and any other treatable causes of hyperthermia; second, immediate discontinuation of neuroleptic agents; third, measures to promote cooling, rehydration and preven-tion of complications. If symptoms are moderate or severe, then pharmacological agents are introduced. Dantrolene has peripheral effects on calcium release from the sarcoplasmic reticulum, leading to muscle relaxation. Levodopa or bromocriptine have been reported beneficial. Electroconvulsive treatments may be used to treat coincident psychosis, but carry the potential for serious complications.[50]

Dopamine receptor antagonists: chronic effects (tardive dyskinesia)

Of the drug-induced movement disorders, the most troubling is tardive dyskinesia, the abnormal involun-tary movements which occur following chronic expo-sure to dopamine receptor blocking agents. Neuroleptics are the most frequent cause of tardive dyskinesia although any drug with dopamine receptor antagonist activity can cause the same problem. The definition of tardive dyskinesia used for research purposes includes cumulative neuroleptic exposure of at least 3 months duration with at least moderately severe abnormal movements in one or more body areas or mild movements in two or more body areas, and the absence of other conditions which could produce the involuntary movements.[51] This research definition has many exceptions in clinical practice. For example, tardive dyskinesia has been observed in patients follow-ing very brief exposure to neuroleptic. The movements of tardive dyskinesia may also be masked by the neuroleptic, later emerging when the drug is reduced or discontinued.[52] Withdrawal emergent dyskinesia typically occurs within 2 weeks after a change in neuroleptic dose.[53]

The movements associated with tardive dyskine-sia encompass practically all of the known movement disorders. The movement most characteristically associated with chronic neuroleptic is chorea. However, 'choreatic' neuroleptic-induced movements differ from classic chorea because of the repetitive and predictable nature of the movement. Stacy and Jankovic used the term 'stereotypy' to refer to these repetitive movements, defining stereotypy as a coor-dinated, patterned rhythmic involuntary move-ment.[54] In their series of 100 patients they found that stereotypy was present in 78%, followed by dystonia, akathisia, tremor, chorea and then myoclonus. Many patients had combinations of these different movements. The abnormal move-ments typically start in the head and neck, with orobuccolingual movements being the most frequent at the onset of tardive dyskinesia and continuing, in combination with other movements, throughout the course of the disorder.

Tardive dystonia is less frequent than stereotypy, affecting as many as 4% of the neuroleptic-treated population (CD 11.2).[55] Patients who suffer from tardive dystonia are usually 30–40 years of age, younger than those with stereotypy. As with acute drug-induced dystonia, tardive dystonia may affect one or more body areas. There may be opisthotonus associated with retro-collis that occurs in spasms and worsens with activity. Limb and facial dystonia[56] also occur. The prognosis for recovery from tardive dystonia is grim. Only about 10% of patients spontaneously remit.

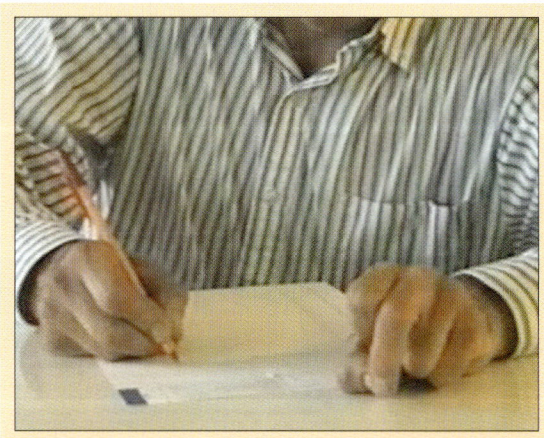

CD 11.2. Tardive dystonia.

Tardive akathisia is clinically similar to acute akathisia, but differs in that it does not improve with a reduction or discontinuation of neuroleptic, and may not improve with the other agents effective for acute akathisia. The onset of symptoms is usually within a year of neuroleptic initiation. Tardive akathisia may occur in combination with the other drug-induced movement disorders described above. Tardive tremor, myoclonus, tics and oculogyric crises[57] have also been described but are rare.

The reported prevalence of tardive dyskinesia varies widely, between 0.5 and 65% of neuroleptic treated patients. This variation in prevalence is likely due to the different populations assessed and the different diagnostic criteria used.[32] Prospective studies of tardive dyskinesia are few. Saltz and associates followed 160 patients older than 55 years for 1–30 months of neuroleptic exposure.[58] They found that 31% developed tardive dyskinesia after cumulative neuroleptic treatment of 43 weeks. In their study, the incidence was not increased in women, neither was it related to the class or dose of neuroleptic. Jeste followed 266 middle-aged and elderly patients on neuroleptic for 3 years and found that the cumulative incidence of tardive dyskinesia increased from 26% after 1 year to 60% after 3 years.[59] Risk factors identified in this study were duration of neuroleptic use, cumulative dose of high-potency neuroleptic, history of alcohol abuse, and tremor. Factors associated with the development of tardive dyskinesia are given in Table 11.3.[59–62]

Chatterjee and colleagues followed 89 schizophrenic patients beginning neuroleptic treatment for the first time and found that 25% developed tardive dyskinesia after 234 weeks of follow-up.[63] Ghadirian and colleagues found in a cross-sectional study that the combination of lithium and neuroleptic was associated with a high prevalence of drug-induced parkinsonism and tremor.[64]

In order to assess the true incidence and prevalence of tardive dyskinesia, the rate of spontaneous dyskinesia in elderly people (around 5–10%) must be subtracted from the reported figures; also, account must be taken of the occurrence of spontaneous movement disorders associated with some subtypes of schizophrenia observed prior to the use of neuroleptic. Chatterjee found that 17% of neuroleptic naïve patients had features of parkinsonism at baseline. These patients were more likely to develop drug-induced parkinsonism, but

● **Table 11.3.** Factors associated with development of tardive dyskinesia [59–62]

Older age[60]
Female gender
Cumulative amount of high–potency neuroleptic[59]
Duration of exposure to neuroleptic[61]
Occurrence of drug-induced parkinsonism
Previous brain injury[62]
Alcoholism

there was no increase in the development of subsequent tardive dyskinesia.[63]

The prognosis for patients with tardive dyskinesia is guarded. Casey and colleagues followed 33 elderly patients with tardive dyskinesia (all of whom who required continuation of low to moderate doses of neuroleptic to control psychotic disorders) for 3–11 years. They found that tardive dyskinesia symptoms remained stable over the course of continued exposure, tending to decrease if neuroleptic dose was increased.[65] If neuroleptic agents can be discontinued, approximately 25–50% of patients improve substantially within the first year.[66] Klawans reported six cases of tardive dyskinesia that resolved 2.5–5 years after neuroleptic discontinuation.[67]

Whether patients susceptible to drug-induced parkinsonism are at increased risk for tardive dyskinesia is not clear. Andrew reviewed this question and concluded that, although there appears to be an increased risk of tardive dyskinesia with the subacute development of extrapyramidal side-effects including parkinsonism, dystonia and akathisia, a causal relationship has not yet been established.[68] The co-existence of drug-induced parkinsonism and tardive dyskinesia increases over time and with increasing doses of neuroleptic; but the presence of drug-induced parkinsonism does not appear to predict the development of tardive dyskinesia.[69]

Pathophysiology

The pathophysiology of tardive dyskinesia is hypothesized to involve the development of dopamine receptor hypersensitivity following chronic pharmacological blockade of dopamine receptors. Andrew suggested that early dopamine hypofunction (manifested by a vulnerability to developing acute dystonic reactions and drug-induced parkinsonism) may increase the risk for subsequent development of dopamine receptor hypersensitivity and tardive dyskinesia. This implies that neuroleptic agents with a reduced tendency to cause subacute side-effects may also have a reduced risk of causing tardive dyskinesia.[68]

Dalgalarrondo and Gattaz compared CT abnormalities among psychotic patients with and without tardive dyskinesia and normal controls.[70] Using a multidimensional scaling and step-wise discriminant analysis, they showed that a reduction in the left caudate volume and enlargement of the left temporal sulci separated the tardive dyskinesia patients from the other two groups. Positron emission tomography (PET) labelling striatal D2 receptors did not demonstrate any differences between tardive dyskinesia and normal controls, although the D2 receptor density in the tardive dyskinesia patients correlated with the severity of the orofacial movements.[71] In animal studies, an increased D2 receptor density has been associated with neuroleptic administration[72,73] and chronic neuroleptic treatment indicates that there may be a hypersensitivity of presynaptic D2 dopamine receptors regulating the release of dopamine.[74]

With the development of a model of basal ganglia circuitry, new theories have focused on the potential role of excitotoxins in the pathophysiology of tardive dyskinesia.[75] In this model, indirect and direct pathways lead from the striatum to the globus pallidus. The indirect pathway is mediated by the D2 receptors, passing via the globus pallidus externa and the subthalamic nucleus. The subthalamic nucleus exerts an excitatory effect on the internal segment of the globus pallidus. The direct pathway has a direct inhibitory effect on the globus pallidus interna. The balance of excitatory and inhibitory influences from the indirect and direct pathways respectively modulates the final inhibitory output from the globus pallidus interna to the thalamus. The loss of integrity of the indirect pathway is thought to play a role in the development of hyperkinetic disorders. Administration of neuroleptic to primates results in an underactivity of the pathway from the subthalamic nucleus to the globus pallidus, leading in turn to an overall increase in excitatory drive from the thalamus to cortical areas.[76] The mechanism whereby neuroleptic agents could cause dysfunction of the indirect pathway is uncertain. It may be through dopaminergic, cholinergic, GABAergic transmitter systems or even an effect on one of the many peptide cotransmitters.

Treatment

The optimal treatment of tardive syndromes is avoidance of all causative drugs, including the antipsychotic agents and anti-emetic drugs with dopamine receptor blocking properties, such as metoclopramide. The need for continuing dopamine receptor blocking medications must be re-evaluated frequently. Prescribing these agents for conditions in which other non-neuroleptic agents may be used (such as for insomnia or mood disorders), is not warranted. In patients with clear indications for neuroleptic agents, evaluating the continued need for these agents is an ongoing process. *Acute* psychotic episodes, for example, may not require *chronic* administration of neuroleptic agents. If the chronic use of these agents is warranted, regular assessments for early signs of tardive dyskinesia are suggested. If tardive dyskinesia appears, discontinuation of the neuroleptic should be strongly considered, but weighed against the continued need for the drug. It may be that switching to an atypical neuroleptic agent, such as clozapine, olanzepine or quetiapine, may improve tardive dyskinesia or reduce the likelihood of progression. These atypical neuroleptic agents have a high affinity for the D4 receptor and are rarely associated with either acute, subacute or chronic neuroleptic side-effects. However, all neuroleptic agents can cause tardive dyskinesia; so the prudent use of these agents will minimize the occurrence of tardive dyskinesia.

Whether concomitant administration of anticholinergic agents increases or decreases the risk of developing tardive dyskinesia is not known. Many practitioners prescribe anticholinergic agents only when indicated to treat drug-induced parkinsonism or oculogyric crisis, when a patient is unable to discontinue neuroleptics without recurrence of psychotic symptoms.

When tardive dyskinesia occurs, treatment depends on the specific form of tardive dyskinesia present. Patients with choreic or stereotypic movements benefit from dopamine-depleting agents, including reserpine (available in the US) or tetrabenazine (available outside the US). Reserpine is a catecholamine-depleting agent with no affinity for dopamine receptors.

Tetrabenazine has both dopamine-depleting activity and mild postsynaptic dopamine receptor antagonism. These agents share certain adverse effects including orthostatic hypotension, depression, sedation, and parkinsonism. The elderly may be particularly prone to the hypotensive effects. Depression can occur in any age group and at any time during therapy. Depression can be quite severe, and if not recognized as a drug side-effect may be misinterpreted as a worsening of the underlying psychiatric disorder. It may take weeks or months to achieve the desired effect from a catecholamine-depleting agent. The upward drug-dose titration is slow. In life threatening cases, it may be necessary to use neuroleptic agents at higher doses to block the receptors until a therapeutic dose is achieved. Other agents that have been used with mixed success for tardive dyskinesia include baclofen, clonazepam, valproic acid, tocopherol and verapamil.[77] A variety of other drugs have been tried, but only with rare anecdotal success.

A general approach to treatment of tardive dyskinesia is shown in Table 11.4.

Drug-induced akathisia and tardive akathisia have been described as the most devastating of the drug-induced movement disorders. Treatment relies on the reduction or discontinuation of neuroleptic. If continued neuroleptic treatment is required or the symptoms of akathisia appear as a tardive phenomenon, several drugs have been shown to offer relief. These include beta-2 adrenergic blocking medications (such as propranolol), anticholinergic agents or benzodiazepines. Dopaminergic agonists (including levodopa, bromocriptine, pergolide or the newer agonists) may be tried if other approaches fail.

Levodopa and dopamine agonist-induced movements

Dopa dyskinesias occur in 30–90% of patients on chronic levodopa therapy.[78,79] In contrast to the cognitive and behavioural complications of dopaminergic therapy, which usually occur after years of treatment, dopa dyskinesias can occur as early as 4 weeks after treatment is started, with up to 50% of patients developing dyskinesias by the end of the first year of therapy.[80,81]

● **Table 11.4.** Drug treatment of tardive dyskinesia

Tardive syndrome	Treatment
Tardive stereotypy	*Reserpine
Tardive chorea	*Tetrabenazine
	Clonazepam
	Baclofen
Tardive akathisia	Tetrabenazine
	Propranolol
	Benzodiazepine (clonazepam)
	Anticholinergic agent
	Atypical neuroleptic agent
Tardive dystonia	Anticholinergic agent
	Baclofen
	Clonazepam
	Tetrabenazine
	Botulinum toxin injections (local treatment only)

*If movements are life threatening, may temporarily increase the neuroleptic agent until reserpine and tetrabenazine are titrated to an effective dose (1–3 months).

A variety of abnormal involuntary movements may be associated with chronic treatment of Parkinson's disease, including chorea, dystonia, myoclonus and asterixis.

Choreic movements may involve face, tongue, hands, limbs and trunk. These movements are rapid and non-stereotyped.[82–84] Ballistic movements may also occur. Involvement of respiratory muscles, manifested by panting, inspiratory spasms and subjective sensations of dyspnoea can occur and are sometimes confused with primary lung disease.[84] The movements tend to become more severe with continued treatment, and may progress to involve more body regions. Not only is chorea a cosmetic problem, it may also interfere with functional activity, impairing eating, swallowing, speech, ambulation, and respiratory status.

In most cases, chorea occurs at the time of maximal drug effect (peak dose), and coincides with the greatest degree of clinical improvement. In this pattern, there is a gradual emergence of chorea following a drug dose, which reaches maximal severity simultaneously with the peak of drug effect (CD 11.3). The chorea wanes as drug effect subsides. Over time, chorea may appear at shorter intervals after the onset of drug effect and may become more prolonged until it may occupy the entire duration of drug efficacy.

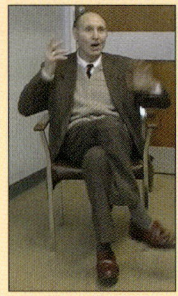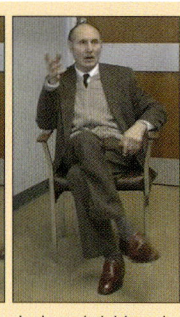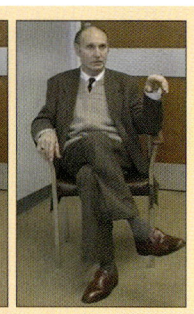

CD 11.3. Levodopa-induced dykinesia.

Diphasic chorea is less frequent and tends to affect younger, akinetic patients. It usually occurs after more prolonged treatment. This pattern of chorea consists of an initial post-dose phase of chorea, followed by a period of improvement without chorea and then the reappearance of the movements as the drug effect wanes.[85]

Dystonic postures in Parkinson's disease are more commonly associated with chronic dopaminergic treatment.[86] There are two types of dystonia in Parkinson's disease patients. Withdrawal dystonia occurs as drug effect disappears, most frequently affecting the patient in the morning before the first dose of medication.[86–89] The second type of dystonia occurs at the same time as drug-induced chorea, usually at peak dose or in a diphasic pattern.[85] Dystonia can occur as the sole manifestation of dopaminergic-induced movement.[90]

There is often a painful dystonic posturing of the feet and toes (see Fig. 2.19) with an equinovarus deformity. The most severe posturing tends to occur on the side most affected by Parkinson's disease.[89,91,92] In addition to foot dystonia, other types of dystonia including orofacial dystonia,[93] and dystonic posturing of limbs, neck and trunk have been reported.[89,94]

Treatment related dystonia tends to occur most frequently in young-onset Parkinson's disease.[81] This is particularly true of diphasic dystonia.[92,94]

Levodopa-induced myoclonus is characterized by brief, lightening-like involuntary jerks which are usually bilateral but may only affect one side. Two types of myoclonus are associated with chronic levodopa use: nocturnal myoclonus and daytime myoclonus. Nocturnal myoclonus is more common and typically occurs during sleep, sometimes awakening the patient. Daytime myoclonus occurs less frequently. Although

associated with prolonged dopaminergic treatment, both types of myoclonus appear to be independent of drug efficacy.[95] The presence of nocturnal myoclonus has been suggested to predict the occurrence of drug-induced mental changes.[96] Leveodopa-induced asterixis may occur in association with a toxic delirium.[97]

Pathophysiology

Factors which appear to be important in the development of drug-induced chorea are the duration of disease, the duration of therapy and the cumulative dose of levodopa.[98,99] A retrospective analysis of the relationship between the timing of the initiation of levodopa and the development of motor response fluctuations and dyskinesia shows that the progression of the underlying diseases may be the major factor in the appearance and severity of the motor complications of levodopa therapy.[100,101] It also appears that the age of Parkinson's disease onset plays an important role. Of those with onset at less than 40 years, most will have abnormal movements by the end of 6 years.[81] This group of young-onset patients tend to develop the more complex patterns of dopa diphasic dyskinesias and often are affected by drug-induced dystonia.[81]

The mechanism underlying drug-induced chorea is not known. However, the pharmacological pathophysiology of choreic disorders in general is believed to involve striatal dopaminergic systems, reflecting a relative over-activity of dopamine. Pharmacodynamic studies have shown that levodopa-induced dyskinesia occurs independently of levodopa-induced improvement in Parkinson's disease symptoms, suggesting that there are different mechanisms mediating the two phenomena.[142,143] Some observations suggest that an abnormal nigrostriatal system may predispose to dopamine-induced chorea. In 1-methyl-4-phenyl-1,2,3,6-tetrahydropyridine (MPTP)-induced parkinsonism, there is a selective degeneration of the substantia nigra.[102,103] Chronic treatment of these patients with levodopa results in movements similar to those found in treated idiopathic Parkinson's disease.[104] In patients with hemiparkinsonism, drug-induced movements occur on the involved side, and in those with thalamotomies, the side contralateral to the surgery is less affected, suggesting a protective influence of thalamotomy for these movements.[84] Although these observations suggest a predisposition to drug-induced movements in those with abnormal dopaminergic pathways, there have been few normal subjects treated chronically with these drugs. Furthermore, tardive dyskinesia does occur in those with normal nigrostriatal pathways. Therefore, whether an altered anatomy is required for the production of levodopa-induced movements remains unknown.

It is unlikely that a single process will explain the diverse clinical manifestations and motor fluctuations that occur. The fact that apomorphine, a direct acting dopamine receptor agonist, and amphetamine, an indirect agonist, can result in movements identical to those occurring with levodopa[105] suggests that the pathophysiology of drug-induced chorea involves the central dopamine receptors.[106]

The role of denervation hypersensitivity in the pathogenesis of chorea is not clear. An elevated density of the D2 dopamine receptors has been demonstrated in untreated Parkinson's disease patients by ligand binding using labelled apomorphine, haloperidol and spiperone.[107] This suggests that in untreated patients, chronic denervation may cause an increase in receptor number. However, in chronically treated patients, the receptor density does not differ from normal controls, suggesting that there is a reversal of the denervation related receptor changes with prolonged levodopa treatment.[108–110]

The current hypothesis is that the movements may be related to agonist-induced hypersensitivity. This hypothesis arose from the observation that in animals chronically pretreated with amphetamine or levodopa, there is a heightened sensitivity to apomorphine and amphetamine induced stereotyped behaviour.[111,112] This suggests that postsynaptic dopaminergic hypersensitivity may develop in chronically treated animals. In support of this theory is the observation that plasma levodopa levels have been found in humans to correlate with dyskinesia which occurs at the time of maximal drug effect,[85] suggesting that in this pattern of chorea, there is a threshold levodopa level above which the movements appear. This would be consistent with the hypothesis of a population of hypersensitive receptors. However, plasma levodopa levels are not correlated with the occurrence of other patterns of dyskinesia.[113] The diphasic movements occur as the plasma level of levodopa is increasing and again as the level is decreasing, suggesting that in this pattern, there is a critical levodopa level at which the movements occur. Therefore, either plasma levodopa levels do not reflect central dopaminergic activity or another mechanism is responsible.

Investigations into the role of dopamine metabolites, specifically 3–O-methyl-dopa, demonstrate that this metabolite is elevated in patients with diphasic dyskinesia and on–off fluctuations.[114–116] It is postulated that 3–O-methyl-dopa competes with levodopa for central transport mechanisms and thus decreases the central availability of levodopa, resulting in motor fluctuations. Others have argued that elevated 3–O-methyl-dopa is unlikely to have a significant effect on response fluctuations[117] and is merely the consequence of the higher doses of levodopa used in treating those with more advanced disease. It may be that additional factors such as dietary protein, or circadian elevations of large chain amino acids, play a role in the more complex forms of movements by interfering with central availability of levodopa.[118]

Drug withdrawal dystonia, which is the most common levodopa-induced dystonia, appears to have a different mechanism from chorea based on pharmacological observations. The parenteral administration of either anticholinergic or dopaminergic agents significantly improves levodopa-induced early morning or off-period foot dystonia,[94] whereas these drugs will often exacerbate chorea. Physostigmine, a centrally acting cholinergic drug, worsens this type of dystonia. Haloperidol, a dopamine receptor antagonist, while worsening parkinsonian symptoms, has little effect on dystonia but significantly improves chorea.[87,94] At this time, the pathogenesis of the early morning dystonia is not known, but pharmacological evidence suggests that the mechanism is distinct from that of chorea.

The mechanism underlying the dystonia occurring simultaneously with chorea may have a common pathogenesis. Little more is known at present.

The mechanism underlying dopaminergic induced myoclonus is postulated to involve alterations in serotoninergic activity. This postulate is based on the observation that methysergide, a serotonin antagonist, has been reported to eliminate levodopa-induced myoclonus.[95]

Treatment

If chorea is the result of a relative overactivity of the striatal dopaminergic system, then reduction of central dopamine activity by reduction in dopaminergic drugs or by dopamine receptor antagonists should be successful in controlling chorea. This strategy, however, usually results in significant and often incapacitating re-emergence of parkinsonian signs.[119]

Fractionation of levodopa dose by giving smaller doses at more frequent intervals can be of benefit primarily in peak-dose dyskinesia,[120] and perhaps in some patients with diphasic dyskinesia.[121] This presumably works by avoiding large fluctuations in plasma levodopa levels. Sustained release levodopa preparations may serve the same function.[122]

Dopamine agonists have been reported to cause less dyskinesia than levodopa. Some have reported that bromocriptine alone can successfully treat the symptoms of Parkinson's disease with a decreased occurrence of dyskinesia.[123] Others have observed that agonist therapy in low doses added to levodopa early in the course of treatment is more effective in treating symptoms and avoiding dyskinesia.[124,125] However, the efficacy of either of these options is limited.

Many clinicians attempt to delay the time of onset of dyskinesia by delaying the use of levodopa. Evidence in support of this is provided by one series, which found a similar mean interval from time of levodopa onset to the time of side-effect, regardless of their age at Parkinson's disease onset.[126] Many investigators now recommend that levodopa therapy be delayed until postural reflex impairment occurs.[99,127,128] In addition, when possible, the use of agents other than levodopa, including anticholinergic drugs and amantadine,[129] alone or in combination, may forestall the initiation of levodopa and therefore delay the occurrence of dyskinesia.

Withdrawal dystonia can be significantly improved in some patients by the use of anticholinergic drugs. Dopamine agonists such as bromocriptine and pergolide mesylate may also be effective.[88,92,130] Baclofen has also been reported to help some patients.[91] In patients not responding to these drugs, lithium carbonate at therapeutic blood levels has been reported to be of use,[131] although the potential for serious adverse effects with this drug must be considered.

All patterns of drug-induced dystonia respond to the discontinuation of dopaminergic therapy during drug holidays. However, drug holidays are least likely to benefit those with early-morning and off-period dystonia. This type of dystonia tends to recur very early after the reintroduction of dopaminergic therapy.[132]

Myoclonus has been effectively treated with methysergide although the side-effects associated with chronic use limit long-term benefit.[95] Periactin, with less associated toxic effects, may decrease myoclonus.

Table 11.5 shows the effects that different kinds of drugs can have on movement disorders.

Other drugs associated with movement disorders

The medical literature is replete with case reports of movement disorders blamed on drug treatment. In some cases causality is clear, in others it is possible, in yet others it seems highly improbable. Nevertheless, it is wise to keep the possibility of pharmacological causation in mind, whatever the clinical syndrome. The brief notes which follow are intended as a 'sample' of the literature of diverse associations between drugs and involuntary movements; the list is far from complete.

Calcium-channel blockers have been used widely for the treatment of hypertension and cardiovascular disease. Flunarizine and cinnarizine have been reported in multiple case histories to cause drug-induced parkinsonism which resolves with discontinuation. Drug-induced basal ganglia disorders are rare with the other types of calcium-channel blockers.[133,134]

A less common side-effect of oestrogen-containing medications, specifically the oral contraceptive agents, is chorea. Oral contraceptive induced chorea tends to occur in women with a previous history of injury to the basal ganglia including Sydenham's chorea and systemic lupus erythematosus.[135] Oestrogen treatment has also been reported to both worsen and improve parkinsonism. While it is difficult to reconcile these contrasting observations, oestrogen clearly has a modulatory effect on central dopamine activity, and that effect may vary depending on the particular dopamine systems and receptors involved.

Dyskinesias have been occasionally reported in patients treated with tricyclic antidepressants.[136]

● **Table 11.5.** Drugs which cause or worsen some movement disorders and improve others

Drug class	Movement disorders caused and/or worsened	Movement disorders improved
Anticholinergics	Chorea	Tremor Dystonia Akathisia
Anticonvulsants	Chorea Dystonia Tremor	Paroxysmal movement disorders
Dopamine agents	Chorea Dystonia	Parkinsonism Dystonia Akathisia
Dopamine-depleting agents (reserpine, tetrabenazine)	Parkinsonism Tremor	Chorea Tics Hemiballismus Dystonia
Oestrogen-containing compounds	Chorea ?Parkinsonism	?Parkinsonism
Antidepressants	Myoclonus Periodic movements of sleep Tics	?Dystonia
Lithium	Parkinsonism Tremor Myoclonus Chorea	?Chorea
Stimulants (methylphenidate, pemoline, amphetamine)	Chorea Tics Stereotyped movements Tremor	?Parkinsonism
Antibiotics	Tremor Myoclonus	?
Calcium-channel blockers	Parkinsonism	?

Likewise, there have been scattered reports of basal ganglia disorders associated with use of serotonin reuptake inhibitors. These reports are rare.[137]

There have been occasional reports of myoclonus occurring in patients treated with chlorambucil.[138]

Sodium valproate is recognized as a cause of tremor. Dyskinesias have been reported in patients on phenytoin and, less commonly, with carbamazepine.[139] Carbamazepine may also cause tics, even at therapeutic levels and without other evidence of toxicity.[140]

Amiodarone has been associated with a postural tremor; but there have also been occasional reports of parkinsonism.[141] Lithium commonly causes a postural tremor but probably does not cause parkinsonism.

References

1. Weiner W J, Lang A E. Drug induced movement disorders. Mount Kisco, NY: Futura Publishing Co., 1992

2. Singh H, Levinson D F, Simpson G M et al. Acute dystonia during fixed-dose neuroleptic treatment. J Clin Neuropharmacol 1990; 10: 389–396

3. Swett C. Drug-induced dystonia. Am J Psychiat 1975; 132: 532–533

4. McCann U D, Penetar D M, Belenkey G. Acute dystonic reaction in normal humans caused by catecholamine depletion. Clin Neuropharmacol 1990; 13: 565–568

5. Groves J E, Mandel M R. The long-acting phenothiazines. Arch Gen Psychiat 1975; 32: 893–900

6. Burke R E, Reches A, Traube M M et al. Tetrabenazine induces acute dystonic reactions. Ann Neurol 1985; 17: 200–202

7. Keepers G A, Casey D E. Prediction of neuroleptic-induced dystonia. J Clin Psychopharmacol 1987; 7: 164–166

8. Keepers G A, Casey D E. Use of neuroleptic-induced extrapyramidal symptoms to predict future vulnerability to side effects. Am J Psychiat 1991; 148: 85–89

9. Armstrong M, Daly A K, Blennerhasset R et al. Antipsychotic drug-induced movement disorders in schizophrenics in relation to CYP2D6 genotype. Br J Psychiat 1997; 170: 23–26

10. Ayd F. A survey of drug-induced extrapyramidal reactions. J Am Med Assoc 1961; 175: 102–108

11. Garver D L, Davis J M, Dekirmenjian H et al. Dystonic reactions following neuroleptics: Time course and proposed mechanisms. Psychopharmacology 1976; 47: 199–201

12. Sayers A C, Burki H R, Ruch W, Asper H. Anticholinergic properties of antipsychotic drugs and their relation to extrapyramidal side effects. Psychopharmacology 1976; 51: 15–22

13. Snyder S, Greenberg D, Yamamura H et al. Antischizophrenic drugs and brain cholinergic receptors. Arch Gen Psychiat 1974; 31: 58–61

14. Coffin V L, Latranyi M B, Chipkin R C. Acute extrapyramidal syndrome in Cebus monkeys: Development mediated by dopamine D2. J Pharmacol Exp Ther 1989; 249: 769–774

15. Comella C, Tanner C M. Anticholinergic drugs in Parkinson's disease. In: Koller W C et al. (eds) Therapy of Parkinson's disease. New York: Marcel Dekker, 1994: 123–141

16. Tonda M E, Guthrie S K. Treatment of acute neuroleptic-induced movement disorders. Pharmacotherapy 1994; 14: 543–560

17. Steck H. Le syndrome extrapyramidal et diencéphalique au cours des traitements au largactil at au serpasil. Ann Méd Psychiat 1954; 2: 737–744

18. Ditfurth v H. Anwendungsmöglichkeiten des Megaphens in der psychiatrischen Klinik und Forschung. Nervenarzt 1955; 2: 54–59

19. Freyhan F A. Psychomotility and parkinsonism in treatment with neuroleptic drugs. Arch Neurol Psychiat 1957; 78: 465–471

20. Miller L G, Jankovic J. Neurologic approach to drug-induced movement disorders: A study of 125 patients. South Med J 1990; 83: 525–532

21. Bollini P, Pampallona S, Orz M J. Antipsychotic drugs: Is more worse? A meta-analysis of the published randomized control trials. Psychologica Med 1994; 24: 307–316

22. Jankovic J. Tardive syndromes and other drug induced movement disorders. Clin Neuropharmacol 1995; 18: 197–214

23. Schwab S G, Scherer J, Wildenauer D B. Presymptomatic testing in families with Wilson's disease (7). Lancet 1994; 343: 1637–1638

24. Melamed U D, Achiron A, Shapira A, Davidoviez S. Persistent and progressive parkinsonism after discontinuation of chronic neuroleptic therapy: An additional tardive syndrome? Clin Neuropharmacol 1991; 14: 273–278

25. Hansen T E, Brown W L, Weigel R M, Casey D E. Risk factors for drug induced parkinsonism in tardive dyskinesia patients. J Clin Psychiat 1988; 49: 139–141

26. Pacifici G M, Nardini M, Ferrani P. Effect of amantadine on drug induced parkinsonism: Relationship between plasma levels and effect. Br J Clin Pharmacol 1976; 3: 883–889

27. Silver H, Geraisy N, Schwartz M. No difference in the effect of biperiden and amantadine on parkinsonism and tardive dyskinesia type involuntary movements: A double blind crossover, placebo-controlled study in medicated chronic schizophrenic patients. J Clin Psychiat 1995; 56: 167–170

28. Kelly T J, Zimmerman R L, Abuzzahab F S, Schiele B C. A double blind study of amantadine HCL versus benztropene mesylate in drug induced parkinsonism. Pharmacology 1974; 12: 65–73

29. Sandyk R, Pardeshi R. Pyridoxine improves drug-induced parkinsonism and psychoses in a schizophrenic patient. Int J Neurosci 1990; 52: 225–232

30. Gibb W R G, Lees A J. The clinical phenomenon of akathisia. J Neurol Neurosurg Psychiat 1986; 49: 861–866

31. Van Putten T. The many faces of akathisia. Compr Psychiat 1975; 16: 43–47

32. Marsden C D, Jenner P. The pathophysiology of extrapyramidal side effects of neuroleptic drugs. Psycholog Med 1980; 10: 55–72

33. Braude W M, Barnes T R C, Gore S M. Clinical characteristics of akathisia. Br J Psychiat 1983; 143: 134–150

34. Reiter S, Adler L, Angrist B et al. Atenolol and propranolol in neuroleptic induced akathisia. J Clin Psychopharmacol 1987; 7: 279–280

35. Adler L A, Angrist B, Peselow E. A controlled assessment of propranolol in the treatment of neuroleptic-induced akathisia. Br J Psychiat 1986; 149: 42–45

36. Adler L A, Angrist B, Weinred H, Rostrosen J. Studies on the time course and efficacy of beta-blockers in neuroleptic-induced akathisia and the akathisia of idiopathic Parkinson's disease. Psychopharmacol Bull 1991; 27: 107–111

37. Lipinski J F, Zubenko G S, Barriera P, Cohen B M. Propranolol in the treatment of neuroleptic induced akathisia. Lancet 1983; ii: 685–686

38. Kramer S M, Gorka R A, DiJohenson C, Sheves P. Propranolol in the treatment of neuroleptic induced akathisia (NIA) in schizophrenics: A double blind, placebo controlled study. Biol Psychiat 1988; 24: 823–827

39. Kutcher S P, MacKenzie S, Galarraga P, Szalai J. Clonazepam treatment of adolescents with neuroleptic induced akathisia. Am J Psychiat 1987; 144: 823–824

40. Kutcher S, Williamson P, MacKenzie S et al. Successful clonazepam treatment of neuroleptic induced akathisia in older adolescents and young adults: A double blind study. J Clin Psychopharmacol 1989; 9: 403–406

41. Zubenko G S, Cohen B M, Lipinski J F, Jonas J M. Use of clonidine in the treatment of akathisia. Psychiat Res 1984; 13: 253–259

42. Buckley P F, Hutchinson M. Neuroleptic malignant syndrome. J Neurol Neurosurg Psychiat 1995; 58: 271–273

43. Factor S A, Singer C. Neuroleptic malignant syndrome. In: Lang A E et al. (eds) Drug-induced movement disorders. Mount Kisco, NY: Futura Publishing Co, 1992: 199–230

44. Addonizio G, Sussman V L, Roth S D. Neuroleptic malignant syndrome: Review and analysis of 115 cases. Biol Psychiat 1987; 22: 1004–1020

45. Rosebush P, Stewart T. A prospective analysis of 24 episodes of neuroleptic malignant syndrome. Am J Psychiat 1989; 146: 717–725

46. Friedman J H, Davis R, Wagner R L. Neuroleptic malignant syndrome: The results of a 6-month prospective study of incidence in a state psychiatric hospital. Clin Neuropharmacol 1988; 11: 373–377

47. Carnoff S N. The neuroleptic malignant syndrome. J Clin Psychol 1980; 41: 79–83

48. Gibb W R G, Lees A J. The neuroleptic malignant syndrome — a review. Q J Med 1985; 220: 421–429

49. Kurlan R, Hamill R, Shoulson I. Neuroleptic malignant syndrome. Clin Neuropharmacol 1984; 7: 109–120

50. Jessee S S, Anderson G F. ECT in neuroleptic malignant syndrome. J Clin Psychiat 1983; 44: 186–188

51. Schooler K, Kane J M. Research diagnosis for tardive dyskinesia. Arch Gen Psychiat 1982; 39: 486–487

52. Woerner M, Kane J M, Lieberman J. The prevalence of tardive dyskinesia. J Clin Psychopharmacol 1991; 1: 34–42

53. Dufresne R L, Wagner R L. Antipsychotic withdrawal akathisia verus antipsychotic induced akathisia: Further evidence for the existence of tardive akathisia. J Clin Psychiat 1988; 49: 435–438

54. Stacy M, Cardosa F, Jankovie J. Tardive stereotype and other movement disorders in tardive dyskinesias. Neurology 1993; 43: 937–941

55. Raja M. Tardive dystonia. Prevalence risk factors and comparison with tardive dyskinesia in a population of 200 acute psychiatric inpatients. Eur Arch Psychiat Clin Neurosci 1995; 245: 145–151

56. Ananth J, Edelmuth E, Dargan B. Meige's syndrome associated with neuroleptic treatment. Am J Psychiat 1988; 145: 513–515

57. Sachdev P. Tardive and chronically recurrent oculogyric crises. Mov Dis 1993; 8: 93–97

58. Salz B L, Woerner M G, Kane J M et al. Prospective study of tardive dyskinesia incidence in the elderly. J Am Med Assoc 1991; 266: 2402–2406

59. Jeste D V, Claigiuri M P, Paulsen J S. Risk of tardive dyskinesia in older patients. A prospective longitudinal study of 266 outpatients. Arch Gen Psychiat 1995; 52: 756–765

60. Bak T H, Bauer M, Schaub R T. Myoclonus in patients treated with clozapine: A case series. J Clin Psychiat 1995; 56: 418–422

61. Sweet H. Le syndrome extrapyramidal et diencephalique au cours des traitements au largactil et au serpasil. Ann Med Psychiat 1995; 52: 478–486

62. Pourcher E, Baruch P, Bouchard R H. Neuroleptic associated tardive dyskinesias in young people with psychosis. Br J Psychiat 1995; 166: 768–772

63. Chatterjee A, Chakos M, Koreen A et al. Prevalence and clinical correlates of extrapyramidal signs and spontaneous dyskinesia in never-medicated schizophrenic patients. Am J Psychiat 1995; 152: 1724–1729

64. Ghadirian A M, Annable L, Belanger M C, Chouinard G. A cross-sectional study of parkinsonism and tardive dyskinesia in lithium treated affective disordered patients. J Clin Psychiat 1996; 57: 22–28

65. Casey D E, Povlsen U J, Meidahl B, Gerlach J. Neuroleptic-induced tardive dyskinesia and parkinsonism: Changes during several years of continuing treatment. Psychopharmacol Bull 1986; 22: 250–253

66. Task force on the late neurological effects of antipsychotic drugs. Tardive dyskinesia: A summary of a task force report of the American Psychiatric Association. Am J Psychiat 1980; 137: 1163–1172

67. Klawans H L, Tanner C M, Barr A. The reversibility of 'permanent' tardive dyskinesia. Clin Neuropharmacol 1984; 7: 153–159

68. Andrew H G. Clinical relationship of extrapyramidal symptoms and tardive dyskinesia. Can J Psychiat 1994; 39(Suppl 2): S76–S80

69. Elliott K J, Lewis S, El-Mallakh R S, Looney S W, Caudill R, Bacani-Oropilla T. The role of parkinsonism and antiparkinsonian therapy in the subsequent development of tardive dyskinesia. Ann Clin Psychiatry 1994; 6: 197–203

70. Dalgalarrondo P, Gattaz W F. Basal ganglia abnormalities in tardive dyskinesia. Possible relationship with duration of neuroleptic treatment. Eur Arch Psychiat Clin Neurosci 1994; 244: 272–277

71. Blin J, Baron J C, Cambon H. Striatal dopamine D2 receptors in tardive dyskinesia: PET study. J Neurol Neurosurg Psychiat 1989; 52: 1248–1252

72. Boyson S J, McGogigle P, Luthin GR et al. Effects of chronic administration of neuroleptic and anticholinergic agents on densities of D2 dopamine and muscarinic cholinergic receptors in rat striatum. J Pharmacol Exp Ther 1988; 244: 987–993

73. Burt D R, Creese I, Snyder S H. Antischizophrenic drugs: Chronic treatment elevates dopamine receptor binding in brain. Science 1977; 196: 326–327

74. Calabresi P, DeMurtas M, Mercuri N B, Bernardi G. Chronic neuroleptic treatment: D2 dopamine receptor supersensitivity and striatal glutaminergic transmission. Ann Neurol 1992; 31: 366–373

75. Alexander G E, Crutcher M D, Delong M R. Basal ganglia-thalamocortical circuits: Parallel substrates for motor, oculomotor, 'prefrontal' and 'limbic' functions. Prog Brain Res 1990; 85: 119–146

76. Feve A, Angelard B, Fenelon G. Neuroleptic-induced tardive dyskinesia in the Cebus monkey. Mov Dis 1990; 7: 32–37

77. Abad V, Ovsiew F. Treatment of persistent myoclonic dystonia with verapamil. Br J Psychiat 1993; 162: 554–556

78. Bergman K J, Mendoza M R, Yahr M D. Parkinson's disease and long term levodopa therapy. Adv Neurol 1986; 45: 463–467

79. Keenan R E. The Eaton collaborative study of levodopa therapy in parkinsonism: A summary. Neurology 1970; 20: 46–59

80. Markham C H, Treciokas L J, Diamond S G. Parkinson's disease and levodopa-a five year follow up and review. West J Med 1974; 121: 188–206

81. Quinn N, Critchley P, Marsden C. Young onset Parkinson's disease. Mov Dis 1987; 2: 73–91

82. Sweet R D, McDowell F H. Five years treatment of Parkinson's disease with levodopa: Therapeutic results and survival of 100 patients. Ann Int Med 1975; 83: 456–463

83. Barbeau A. L-dopa therapy in Parkinson's disease: A critical review of nine years' experience. Can Med Ass J 1969; 101: 59–68

84. Mones R J, Elizan T S, Siegel G J. Analysis of L-dopa induced dyskinesias in 51 patients with Parkinsonism. J Neurol Neurosurg Psychiat 1971; 34: 668–673

85. Meunter M D, Sharpless N S, Tyce G M, Darley F L. Patterns of dystonia ('I-D-I AND 'D-I-D') in response to L-dopa therapy for Parkinson's disease. Mayo Clin Proc 1977; 52: 163–174

86. Melamed E. Early morning dystonia, a late effect of long-term levodopa therapy in Parkinson's disease. Arch Neurol 1979; 36: 308–310

87. Peowe W, Lees A, Stern G. Foot dystonia in Parkinson's disease: Clinical phenomenology and neuropharmacology. Adv Neurol 1986; 45: 357–360

88. Newman R, LeWitt P, Shults C et al. Dystonia: Treatment with bromocriptine. Clin Neuropharm 1985; 8: 328–333

89. Kidron D, Melamed E. Forms of dystonia in patients with Parkinson's disease. Neurology 1987; 37: 1009–1011

90. Parkes J, Bedard P, Marsden C. Chorea and torsion in parkinsonism. Lancet 1976; 1: 155

91. Nausieda P A, Weiner W J, Klawans H L. Dystonia: Foot response of parkinsonism. Arch Neurol 1980; 37: 132–136

92. Ilson J, Fahn S, Cote L. Painful dystonic spasms in Parkinson's disease. Adv Neurol 1984; 40: 395–398

93. Weiner W, Nausieda P. Meige's syndrome during long term dopaminergic therapy in Parkinson's disease. Arch Neurol 1982; 39: 451–452

94. Poewe W H, Lees A J, Stern G M. Dystonia in Parkinson's disease: Clinical and pharmacologic features. Ann Neurol 1988; 23: 73–78

95. Klawans H L, Goetz C G, Bergen D. Levodopa-induced myoclonus. Arch Neurol 1975; 32: 331–334

96. Nausieda P A, Glantz R, Weber S et al. Psychiatric complications of levodopa therapy of Parkinson's disease. Adv Neurol 1984; 40: 271–277

97. Glantz R, Weiner W J, Goetz C G et al. Drug-induced asterixes in Parkinson's disease. Neurology 1982; 32: 553–555

98. Lesser R P, Fahn S, Snider S R et al. The clinical problems in parkinsonism and the complications of long-term levodopa therapy. Neurology 1979; 29: 1253–1260

99. Rajput A H, Stern W, Laverty W H. Chronic low-dose levodopa therapy in Parkinson's disease an argument for delaying levodopa therapy. Neurology 1984; 34: 991–996

100. Horstink M W I M, Zijlmans J C M, Pasman J W et al. Severity of Parkinson's disease is a risk factor for peak-dose dyskinesia. J Neurol Neurosurg Psychiat 1990; 53: 224–226

101. Cederbaum J M, Gandy S E, McDowell F H. Early initiation of levodopa treatment does not promote the development of motor response fluctuations, dyskinesias, or dementia in Parkinson's disease. Neurology 1991; 41: 622–629

102. Davis G C, Williams A C, Markey S P et al. Chronic parkinsonism secondary to intravenous injection of meperidine analogues. Psychiat Res 1979; 1: 249–254

103. Burns R S, Chiueh C C, Markey S P et al. A primate model of parkinsonism: Selective destruction of dopaminergic neurons in the pars compacta of the substantia nigra by N-methyl-4-phenyl-1,2,3,6-tetrahydropyridine. Proc Natl Acad Sci 1983; 80: 4546–4550

104. Langston J W. MPTP-induced parkinsonism: How good a model is it? In: Fahn S (ed) Recent developments in Parkinson's disease. New York: Raven Press, 1986: 119–126

105. Cotzias G C, Papavasiliou P S, Fehling K et al. Similarities between neurologic effects of L-dopa and of apomorphine. N Engl J Med 1970; 282: 31–33

106. Carlsson A. Biochemical implications of dopa-induced actions on the central nervous system, with particular reference to abnormal movements. In: Barbeau A et al (eds) L-dopa and parkinsonism. Pennsylvania: FA Davis Co., 1970: 205–213

107. Lee T, Seeman P, Rajput A, Farley I J, Hornykiewicz O. Receptor basis for dopaminergic supersensitivity in Parkinson's disease. Nature 1987; 273: 59–61

108. Jenner P, Marsden C D. Interpretation of radioactive ligand binding to cerebral dopamine receptors. In: Marsden C D et al (eds) Movement disorders. London: Butterworth Scientific, 1982: 356–368

109. Guttman M, Seeman P. L-dopa reverses the elevated density of D2 receptors in Parkinson's diseased striatum. J Neural Trans 1985; 64: 93–103

110. Guttman M, Seeman P, Reynolds G et al. Dopamine D2 receptor density remains constant in treated Parkinson's disease. Ann Neurol 1986; 19: 487–492

111. Klawans H L, Margolin D I. Amphetamine-induced dopaminergic hypersensitivity in guinea pigs, implications in psychosis and human movement disorders. Arch Gen Psychiat 1975; 32: 725–732

112. Klawans H L, Goetz C G, Nausieda P A, Weiner W J. Levodopa-induced dopamine receptor hypersensitivity. Ann Neurol 1977; 2: 125–129

113. Meunter M D, Tyce G M. L-dopa therapy of Parkinson's disease. Plasma L-dopa concentration, therapeutic response and side effects. Mayo Clin Proc 1971; 46: 231–239

114. Feurestein C L, Serre F, Gavend M, Pellat J, Perret J, Tanche M. O-methyldopa in levodopa-induced dyskinesias: A biochemical investigation. Acta Neurol Scand 1977; 56: 508–524

115. Reches A, Fahn S. O-methyldopa interferes with striatal utilisation of levodopa. Ann Neurol 1981; 10: 94

116. Mena M A, Muradas V, Bazan E et al. Pharmacokinetics of L-dopa in patients with Parkinson's disease. Adv Neurol 1986; 45: 481–486

117. Fabbrini G, Juncos J L, Mouradian M M et al. 3–O-methyldopa and motor fluctuations in Parkinson's disease. Neurology 1987; 37: 856–859

118. Nutt J G, Woodward W R, Hammerstad J P et al. The 'on–off' phenomenon in Parkinson's disease: Relation to levodopa absorption and transport. N Engl J Med 1984; 310: 483–488

119. Klawans H L, Weiner W J. Attempted use of haloperidol in the treatment of L-dopa induced dyskinesias. J Neurol Neurosurg Psychiat 1974; 37: 427–430

120. Jankovic J. Management of motor side effects of chronic levodopa therapy. Clin Neuropharmacol 1982; 5(Suppl. 1): 19–28

121. Lhermitte F, Agid Y, Signoret J. Onset and end-of-dose levodopa-induced dyskinesias: Possible treatment by increasing the daily doses of levodopa. Arch Neurol 1978; 35: 261–263

122. Chase T, Serrati C, Fabbrini G, Bruno G. Fluctuations in response to levodopa therapy: Pathogenetic and therapeutic considerations. Adv Neurol 1986; 45: 477–480

123. Lees A J, Stern G M. Sustained bromocriptine therapy in previously untreated patients with Parkinson's disease. J Neurol Neurosurg Psychiat 1981; 44: 1020–1023

124. Rinne U K. Combined bromocriptine-levodopa therapy early in Parkinson's disease. Neurology 1985; 35: 1196–1198

125. Rinne U K. Early combination of bromocriptine and levodopa in the treatment of Parkinson's disease: A five year follow-up. Neurology 1987; 37: 826–828

126. Tanner C M, Kinori I, Goetz C G et al. Age at onset and clinical outcome in idiopathic Parkinson's disease. Neurology 1985; 35(Suppl. 1): 276

127. Melamed E. Initiation of levodopa therapy in parkinsonian patients should be delayed until the advanced stages of the disease. Arch Neurol 1986; 43: 402–405

128. Fahn S, Bressman S B. Should levodopa therapy for parkinsonism be started early or late? Evidence against early treatment. Can J Neurol Sci 1984; 11: 200–205

129. Timberlake W H, Vance M A. Four year treatment of patients with parkinsonism using amantadine alone or with levodopa. Ann Neurol 1978; 3: 119–128

130. Lieberman A N, Goldstein M. Treatment of advanced Parkinson's disease with dopamine agonists. In: Marsden C D et al (eds) Movement disorders. London: Butterworth Publishing, 1982: 146–165

131. Quinn N, Marsden C D. Lithium for painful dystonia in Parkinson's disease. Lancet 1986; 1: 1377

132. Goetz C G, Tanner C M, Klawans H L. Drug holiday in the management of Parkinson's disease. Clin Neuropharm 1982; 5: 351–364

133. Daniel J R, Mauro V F. Extrapyramidal symptoms associated with calcium channel blockers. Ann Pharmacother 1995; 29: 73–75

134. Garcia-Ruiz P J, Garcia de Yebenes J, Jimenez-Jimenez F J et al. Parkinsonism associated with calcium channel blockers: A prospective follow up study. Clin Neuropharmacol 1992; 15: 19–26

135. Wadlington W B, Erlendson I W, Burr I M. Chorea associated with the use of oral contraceptives. Report of a case and review of the literature. Clinical Paediatrics 1981; 20: 804–806

136. Fann W E, Sullivan J L, Richman B W. Dyskinesias associated with tricyclic antidepressants. Br J Psychiat 1976; 128: 490–493

137. Arya D. Extrapyramidal symptoms with selective serotonin reuptake inhibitors. Br J Psychiat 1994; 165: 728–733

138. Wyllie A R, Bayliff C D, Kovacs M J. Myoclonus due to chlorambucil in two adults with lymphoma. Ann Pharmacother 1997; 31: 171–174

139. Schwartzman M J, Leppik I E. Carbamazepine-induced dyskinesia and ophthalmoplegia. Cleve Clin J Med 1990; 57: 367–372

140. Robertson P L, Garofalo A G, Silverstein F S, Komarynski M A. Carbamazepine-induced tics. Epilepsia 1993; 34: 965–968

141. LeMaire J F, Autret A, Biziere K et al. Amiodarone neuropathy: Further arguments for human drug-induced neurolipidosis. Eur Neurol 1982; 21: 65–68

142. Schuh L A, Bennett J P. Suppression of dyskinesias in advanced Parkinson's disease. Neurology 1993; 43: 1545–1550

143. Mouradian M M, Heuser I J E, Baronti F, et al. Pathogenesis of dyskinesias in Parkinson's disease. Ann Neurol 1989; 25: 523–526

chapter 12

Paediatric movement disorders

Helen Cross, Lucinda Carr and Stewart Boyd

Introduction

This chapter aims to give an overview of the more common paediatric motor disorders. Whilst there is often overlap of conditions seen in paediatric and adult populations, many chronic and degenerative conditions present in childhood. The overall approach is different in paediatrics. In contrast to adults, presentation is usually parent led and they will give the history. Formal neurological examination is often difficult in the younger child so that clinical observation is a vital part of the assessment. Early diagnosis is particularly important, not just in planning future management for the child but for the genetic implications a diagnosis may have for both the child and his parents. The management of a child with a neurological disorder requires a holistic approach, since in addition to the medical problems, educational and social issues will also need addressing. The expertise of a multidisciplinary team is often required.

The history is often the most important guide to the diagnosis and much information can be gained by repeated careful history taking. The particular feature one is trying to determine at the outset is whether the disorder is acute, subacute or chronic, or indeed stable or progressive. Furthermore particular confusion may be caused in trying to determine whether a motor disorder is epileptiform or non-epileptiform in origin. Features in the history that may aid in such a distinction are the predictability of the movement (including any triggering factors), the duration, the repetitive and stereotypic nature of the attacks, and retention of awareness. These aside, some features may be common to epileptiform and non-epileptiform attacks. Furthermore, considerable overlap exists amongst conditions that fall into both groups. Apparent cortical myoclonus and epilepsia partialis continua may occur without electrical correlate. Hyperekplexia is another condition that although entitled 'startle epilepsy' again has no apparent cortical electrical correlate.

Any childhood motor disorder has to be seen within its developmental context. A child typically acquires cognitive and motor skills in a standard progression at recognized ages; these constitute the developmental milestones. These must be evaluated before it can be determined whether motor control is delayed, deviant or regressing (see Table 12.1).

Motor development may be constrained by other developmental problems, such as global delay or visual impairment. It may be also be directly affected by other medical conditions, such as poorly controlled epilepsy, cardiac, respiratory or gastroenterological disease. Thus, in addition to a detailed developmental history, a full medical history should be taken. This should include

● **Table 12.1.** Main developmental milestones. (Adapted from Illingworth 1985 and Frankenburg 1969)[2]

Gross and fine motor	Mean age skill acquired
Grasps objects	3 months
Transfers objects from hand to hand	5 months
Rolls over	5 months
Sits independently	6 months
Crawls	9 months
Neat pincer grip	9 months
Walks around furniture	10 months
Walks independently	13 months
Pedals a tricycle	2.5 years
Hops on one foot	3.5 years
Language	
Babbles	6 months
Uses 'Dada'/'Mama' appropriately	10 months
Utters 2-word sentences	2 years
Social	
Smiles	6 weeks
Wary of strangers	9 months
Uses spoon	12 months
Dresses	3 years
Ties shoelaces	5 years

● **Table 12.2.** Key points in history

Current parental concerns	
Antenatal	Concerns in pregnancy (e.g. infection, bleeding etc)
	Significant maternal illness and drug ingestion
	Quality of fetal movements
	Oligo/polyhydramnios
	Multiple pregnancy
Perinatal	Intrauterine growth retardation and low birth weight
	Prematurity
	Significant neonatal illness (e.g. neurological [seizures]/infection/metabolic/respiratory complications)
Postnatal	Significant illness or trauma (as above)
	Ease of early handling and feeding
	Acquisition of developmental milestones
	Loss of developmental milestones

● **Table 12.3.** Key points of examination

General	Growth parameters (including head circumference)
	Presence of dysmorphic features
	Neurocutaneous stigmata
	Deformity or scoliosis
	Systemic examination to include palpation for organomegaly and examination of genitalia
Neurological	Full examination to include gait:
	Tone/power/sensation and deep tendon reflexes
	Evaluation of persisting primitive reflexes
	Development of postural reflexes
	Fog's test
	Cerebellar signs
	Cranial nerve examination

antenatal, perinatal and postnatal events detailed in Table 12.2. For a more detailed description the reader is referred to any standard paediatric textbook.[1]

The younger child or a child with learning difficulties may have difficulty complying with formal neurological testing, particularly sensory testing. For this reason examination is initially based on observation. Much information can be derived from this, such as muscle power and coordination, the quality of gross and fine movements and the level of the child's interaction and play. Following this a full medical and neurological examination should be attempted (Table 12.3).

The primitive reflexes (Table 12.4) are useful indicators of central nervous system (CNS) maturity and of functional integrity. They should be elicited with the child awake but relaxed. Any asymmetry should be noted. In general these reflexes are strongest in the neonatal period and are fading by 3 months of age. Persistence beyond 6 months is abnormal (except in specific circumstances) and may be an early sign of CNS dysfunction, in particular of cerebral palsy.

● **Table 12.4.** Primitive reflexes

Reflex	Key features
Moro	Elicited by dropping head back when infant supine
	Initial extension and abduction of arms followed by flexion and adduction
	Fingers extend, hips and thighs may flex
Suck	Elicited by placing finger into mouth
Root	Examiner's finger touches corner of mouth, infant's head turns to finger (and may then suck)
Stepping	Infant is supported under axillae and inclined forward to elicit automatic walking
Grasp	The palmar grasp is elicited by placing a finger firmly in the infant's palm
Asymmetric tonic neck reflex	When the infant's head is turned to one side the arm on that side extends and the opposite arm flexes. The asymmetric tonic neck reflex is strongest between 2–4 months and is normally hard to elicit beyond 6 months

Specific conditions

Cerebral palsy

Cerebral palsy has an incidence of 2–2.5/1000 live births. It is an umbrella term covering a number of different pathological and clinical entities but describes any persistent disorder of movement and posture that is caused by non-progressive pathology of the immature brain. Most cases are congenital, with damage occurring in the pre- or perinatal period. Causes may include cortical migration defects, *in utero* vascular events, perinatal asphyxia and perinatal bleeds. Modern studies confirm that perinatal asphyxia was over-represented as a cause of cerebral palsy by earlier epidemiological studies. Significant perinatal asphyxia presents in the neonatal period with clinical features of hypoxic ischaemic encephalopathy such as seizures and organ dysfunction. Around 10% of cases are acquired in early childhood as a result of metabolic or vascular insults, infection or trauma.

A careful history and examination are required to make the diagnosis. Often there are clear risk factors in the history such as premature delivery and low birth weight. Neuroimaging will often demonstrate the underlying pathology. However, unusual features in the history and examination should alert the clinician to the possibility of another diagnosis, such as a degenerative, genetic or metabolic disorder. Further investigations are then indicated and are discussed in later sections of the chapter. Table 12.5 lists some of the warning features.

The motor manifestations of cerebral palsy are not unchanging, despite the underlying pathology. Motor milestones are generally delayed or deviant. Early manifestations may include abnormalities of muscle tone, feeding difficulties and irritability. As the child matures muscle contractures and bony deformities may ensue, requiring the involvement of an orthopaedic surgeon. In addition non-motor features are often associated with the condition. These are particularly seen in the more severe forms of cerebral palsy (Table 12.6). For this reason multidisciplinary expertise is often required for comprehensive management and is likely to involve education and social services.

Classification of cerebral palsy

Cerebral palsy is classified according to the geographical pattern of involvement and the neurological features. Spastic forms predominate and account for around 65% of cerebral palsies. These reflect pyramidal tract damage. Dyskinetic and ataxic forms are less common.

Spastic diplegia

Spastic diplegia remains the commonest form, with an incidence of 0.9/1000 live births. The majority result from periventricular lesions, particularly cystic

● **Table 12.5.** Warnings to question diagnosis

Cerebral palsy is unexplained

Positive family history

Episodes of encephalopathy or regression

Pure neurological signs, e.g. nystagmus, myoclonus, cerebellar ataxia

Dysmorphic features

● **Table 12.6.** Non-motor features associated with cerebral palsy

Learning difficulties

Disorders of vision (especially squint) and hearing

Feeding difficulties and dysarthria

Epilepsy

Sensory loss

Behavioural problems

leukomalacia occurring in the preterm infant. Involvement is greatest in the lower limbs. The increased tone leads to delayed sitting and standing, and delayed or absent independent walking. The gait is abnormal, often crouched with toe walking. Physical interventions are aimed at promoting mobility and preventing contractures by maintaining muscle length. These are likely to include the early introduction of physiotherapy, with the judicious use of orthotics, casting and more recently botulinum toxin injections. Surgical intervention is often required later in childhood. The hips should be monitored since they are at increased risk of dislocation, particularly in the non-ambulant child. The upper limbs and sometimes the bulbar musculature are involved in the motor disorder, albeit to a lesser extent than the lower limbs. Other associations include squint, visual impairment and posthaemorrhagic hydrocephalus. Where hydrocephalus is significant, ataxia is often noted. Epilepsy and learning difficulties are found in only a minority of children.

Hemiplegic cerebral palsy

Hemiplegic cerebral palsy is seen in around 0.8/1000 live births. Around 85% of cases are congenital, with the damage occurring prenatally in the majority. Vascular and subcortical cystic lesions may be seen. Motor involvement is unilateral, with variable upper and lower limb involvement. Early hand preference, with failure to develop prehension, is a common early manifestation. Around 50% of children show delayed walking. In contrast to adult hemiplegia, speech is likely to develop normally irrespective of the side of the lesion, unless the hemiplegia is acquired in late childhood (>6 years). Sensory disturbance often accompanies the motor deficit. Facial weakness, visual field defects, epilepsy and learning difficulties are found in the minority.

Four limb cerebral palsy

Four limb cerebral palsy (tetraplegia/quadriplegia/total body involvement) is the most severe form with involvement of all four limbs. It occurs in around 0.2/1000 live births. The infant often has abnormal early behaviour, particularly abnormal tone and feeding difficulties. Visual impairment, pseudobulbar palsy and orthopaedic problems are common. The majority also have severe learning difficulties, with epilepsy and microcephaly. Many remain totally dependant for their care.

Worster–Drought syndrome

Worster–Drought syndrome (bulbar variant) is uncommon. Involvement is predominantly of the bulbar musculature, with a pseudobulbar palsy. There is minor involvement of the limbs and often a degree of learning difficulties. Presentation is usually with severe feeding problems and speech delay.

Dyskinetic cerebral palsy

Dyskinetic cerebral palsy (dystonic or choreoathetoid) comprises around 15% of cases of cerebral palsy. Children in this group have the highest incidence of perinatal factors, including perinatal asphyxia. Kernicterus was once a common cause of dyskinetic cerebral palsy but with modern management of rhesus incompatibility and neonatal hyperbilirubinaemia it is now rare. Damage typically involves the basal ganglia resulting in extrapyramidal signs, namely variations in muscle tone, abnormal postures and involuntary movements. Primitive reflexes are likely to persist and there is often a degree of spasticity. The infant is often hypotonic initially with dystonia or abnormal movements evolving later. Dysarthria and hearing loss are common associations and intelligence is generally reasonably preserved.

Ataxic cerebral palsy

Ataxic cerebral palsy is uncommon (around 5% of cases). It comprises cerebellar features with axial hypotonia, truncal oscillations and intention tremor. Scanning speech may be a feature. There should be caution in making this diagnosis; genetic and metabolic causes, hydrocephalus, posterior fossa tumours and progressive ataxias should all be considered.

Genetic and dysmorphic syndromes

Developmental delay may be a presenting or integral part of a dysmorphic, genetic syndrome ultimately manifesting in part as a movement disorder (Table 12.7). Angelman's syndrome, previously the 'Happy Puppet' syndrome, is characterized by severe learning difficulties (with little or no acquisition of language), jerky ataxia of the upper limbs and a happy disposition. Typical facial features include prominant lower jaw, wide mouth and tongue thrusting, with blond hair and blue eyes the result of partial albinism. The genetic deletion is seen on chromosome material derived from the mother at 15q11.2–12. Cortical myoclonus accounts for most of the involuntary movements and makes the gait unsteady. Up to 86% of affected children also have myoclonic seizures. Such myoclonus has been demonstrated to respond to piracetam, although the seizures themselves may show a favourable response to benzodiazepines. The movement disorder may also be compounded by the predisposition to nonconvulsive

● **Table 12.7.** Genetic/dysmorphic syndromes		
Cause	**Clinical features**	**Investigations**
Angelman's syndrome	Dysmorphic	Genetics – FISH (15q)
	Happy disposition	EEG
	Jerky ataxia	
	Severe learning difficulty (SLD)	
	Epilepsy	
Rett syndrome	Hand stereotypies	Clinical
	Hyperventilation	EEG
	SLD	
	Scoliosis	
	Microcephaly	
Joubert's syndrome	Hyperapnoea	Neuroimaging
	Ataxia	
	SLD	

status. The electroencephalogram (EEG) may aid in diagnosis of Angelman's syndrome showing runs of slow 3Hz activity, especially posteriorly, occasionally associated with sharp waves (Fig. 12.1).

Rett syndrome is a condition only as yet reported in girls. There is a history of normal development over the first year of life followed by developmental plateau and delay with regression particularly in hand function, although some studies suggest early development in the majority is not strictly normal. Familial cases are reported but rare, with genetic and environmental factors implicated in the aetiology but not fully elucidated. The movement disorder is manifest by stereotyped repetitive hand movements associated with an apparent loss of hand function. Furthermore, although motor milestones are usually reached within normal time limits, the gait becomes increasingly stiff and apraxic. Episodes of hyperventilation occur in many patients. The diagnosis is made on the basis of clinical criteria, although the EEG may help particularly in the early stages by the demonstration of central sylvian discharges, possibly enhanced by finger tapping (Fig. 12.2).

ANGELMAN'S SYNDROME

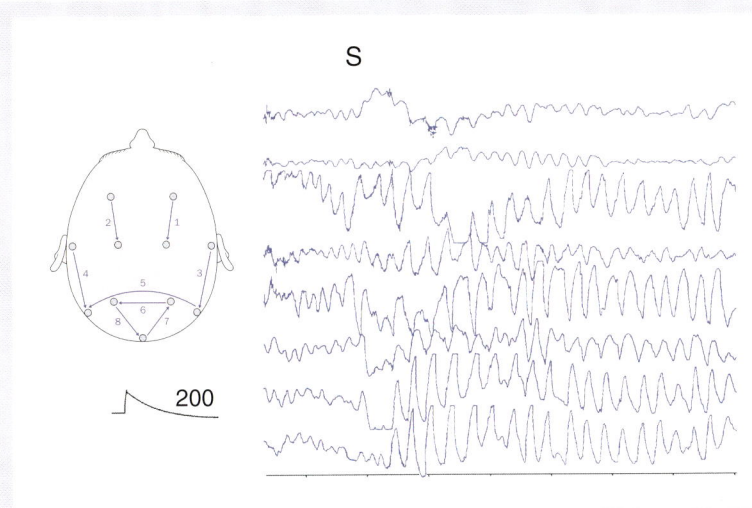

Figure 12.1. EEG features of a child with Angelman's syndrome at the age of 2 years 6 months. Note the large amplitude, rhythmic delta and theta activity. Spikes are usually inconspicuous, but can be seen over the right posterior temporoparietal region, enhanced following eye closure (S). (Calibration in microvolts, time marker in seconds.)

RETT SYNDROME

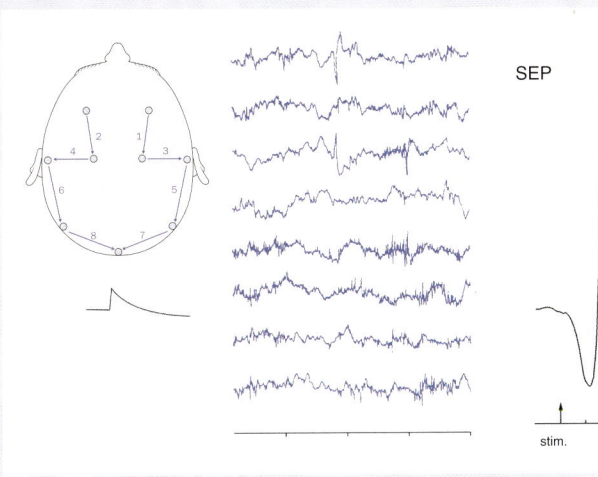

Figure 12.2. (a) EEG findings in a 4-year-old girl with Rett syndrome. Note the right central spike which could be facilitated by tapping the hands. There is a poverty of normal rhythmic activities. (Calibration in microvolts, time marker in seconds.) (b) Median nerve somatosensory evoked potential showing enlarged components (after 50 ms).

Joubert's syndrome is an autosomal recessive condition that may manifest with respiratory anomalies as early as the neonatal period. Ataxia, abnormal eye movements and severe learning difficulties then manifest in later infancy and childhood. Such problems may be attributable to the agenesis of the cerebellar vermis (Fig. 12.3) and associated developmental defects of the brainstem.

Ataxia

Table 12.8 lists the key causes and aids to diagnosis of ataxia in childhood. In childhood, particularly in the first 5 years of life, it can be difficult to determine true primary cerebellar ataxia from other causes of movement disorder that lead to unsteadiness and therefore pseudoataxia. For example, a peripheral neuropathy, as seen in acute conditions such as Guillain–Barré, or more chronic neurodegenerative conditions such as metachromatic leucodystrophy, may lead to a deterioration in gait,

manifesting with a wide base and therefore as apparent ataxia. Close observation, however, will reveal the characteristic hyperextension of the knees on walking and loss or diminished deep tendon jerks may be confirmative. Subtle myoclonus may lead to pseudotremor, and a pseudoataxic gait as seen in late infantile Batten's disease. Non-convulsive status (Fig. 12.4), particularly

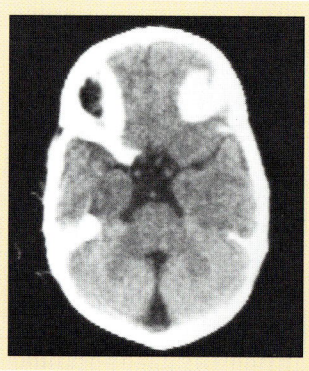

Figure 12.3. CT scan showing agenesis of the cerebellar vermis in Joubert's syndrome.

NON-CONVULSIVE STATUS EPILEPTICUS

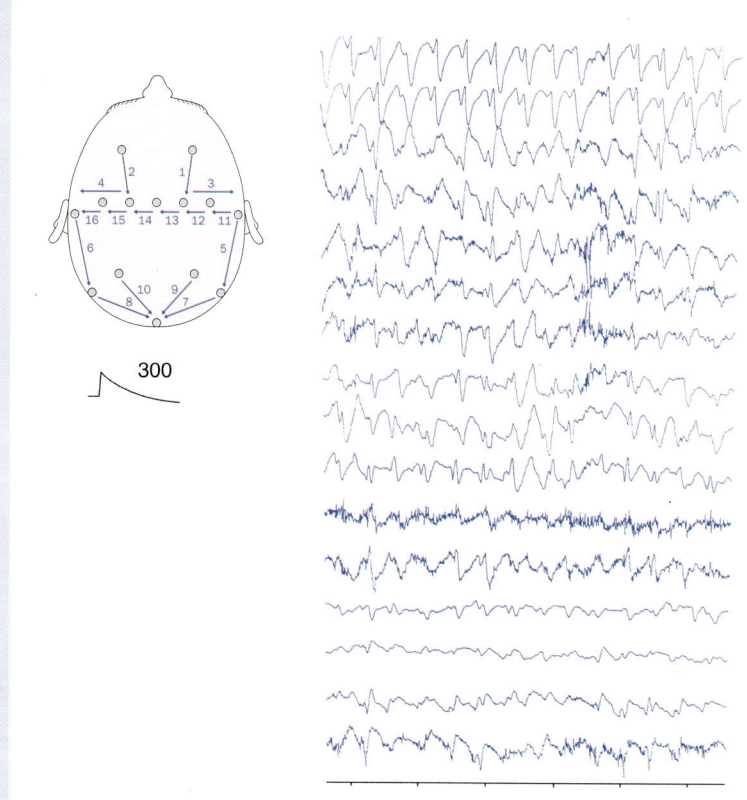

Figure 12.4. EEG features of non-convulsive status epilepticus. Note the spike wave complexes seen most clearly over the frontocentral regions. (Calibration in microvolts, time marker in seconds.)

● **Table 12.8.** Ataxia in childhood

	Cause	Clinical features	Investigations
Congenital	Cerebral palsy	Motor delay Intention tremor	Plasma amino acids Urine organic acids Neuroimaging
	Metabolic: Refsum's disease	Night blindness Ataxia Peripheral neuropathy	Plasma phytanic acid
	Abetalipoproteinaemia	Ataxia Loss of deep tendon jerks Pigmentary retinal degeneration	Acanthocytosis β-lipoproteins Electroretinogram (ERG)
	Organic acidaemias Ornithine carbonyl transferase deficiency	Intermittent ataxia	Urine for organic acids Ammonia/urinary orotic acid
	Cerebellar malformations	Ataxia	Neuroimaging
Acquired:	Pseudoataxia: Peripheral neuropathy	Loss of deep tendon jerks Hyperextended knees	Nerve conduction studies
	Non-convulsive status	Fluctuating responsiveness	EEG
	Late infantile neuroronal ceroid lipofusunosis	Age 2–4 years Myoclonus Developmental regression	EEG, Visual-evoked response Rectal biopsy
Acute	Toxic: Anticonvulsant Piperazine Antihistamines		History Drug levels
	Structural: Tumour	Ataxia Vomiting Headache	Neuroimaging
	Parainfectious: Mycoplasma Varicella	Respiratory tract infection Characteristic rash	Neuroimaging
	Benign paroxysmal vertigo		Neuroimaging, history
Chronic	Ataxia telangiectasia	Progressive ataxia or dystonia Neurocutaneous telangiectasia Eye movement abnormality	α-feto-protein DNA fragility
	Friedreich's ataxia	Progressive ataxia Absent deep tendon jerks, pyramidal limb signs	Nerve conduction studies DNA (expansion of GAA repeat within X25, chromosome 9)

in the difficult symptomatic polymorphic epilepsies, may lead to an extremely subtle change in apparent awareness, as well as subtle myoclonus and carers may only be aware of the apparent onset of unsteadiness. This may also demonstrate a fluctuating intermittent course.

Once the presence of true ataxia has been established, the history remains the most important aspect to determining the cause, in particular whether the problem is of recent onset or is longstanding (Fig. 12.5). Ataxia present from infancy most often manifests in the first instance as a delay in motor milestones, ataxia only becoming apparent after some time into walking. True congenital ataxic cerebral palsy is rare although recognized, and it is extremely important to exclude an

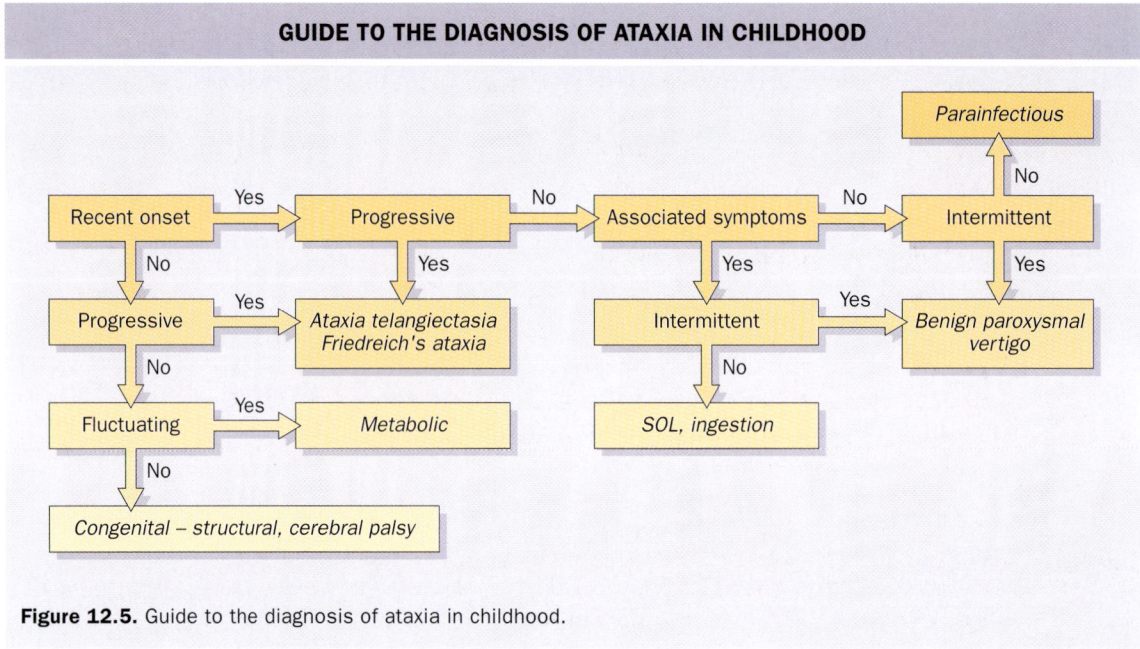

GUIDE TO THE DIAGNOSIS OF ATAXIA IN CHILDHOOD

Figure 12.5. Guide to the diagnosis of ataxia in childhood.

underlying metabolic disorder by appropriate investigation. Clues to a metabolic diagnosis may lie in the family history, or an episodic nature to the degree of movement disorder. Structural abnormalities of the cerebellum ordinarily manifest with a long-standing history from early infancy although may present with apparent acquired problems later in childhood.

If there is definite evidence of a period of normal development, so the ataxia appears acquired, then it is important to determine the speed of onset, history of intoxication, or concurrent symptomatology (for example, a space-occupying lesion of the posterior fossa will have associated symptoms of raised intracranial pressure). Recent history of a respiratory tract infection in the absence of a structural lesion, or a recent history of chickenpox, may suggest a parainfectious cerebellar syndrome with good prognosis. A further syndrome in childhood with apparent intermittent ataxia is benign paroxysmal vertigo. This usually manifests in the first 5 years of life with the child intermittently seeking attention due to probable dizziness. Horizontal nystagmus may often be seen during the attacks, and the child retains awareness. The attacks are short-lived, usually minutes, and have a good prognosis, becoming less frequent with age. Intervention is usually not required, and is anyway usually unhelpful.

Ataxia telangiectasia is aptly described by its title, characterized by progressive truncal ataxia and oculocutaneous telangiectasia (Fig. 12.6). The progressive nature of the condition in its early stages may be masked as the rate is often slower than acquisition of motor skills, although the majority present within the first 5 years of life with motor delay. Eye movement abnormalities (dyspraxia of rapid saccadic eye movements in the vertical and horizontal fields) are usually present by the age of 3 years. Extrapyramidal movements may later develop, though dystonia has been reported as a presenting feature. Many children with the disorder demonstrate an increased frequency of infections, with reduced IgA noted in

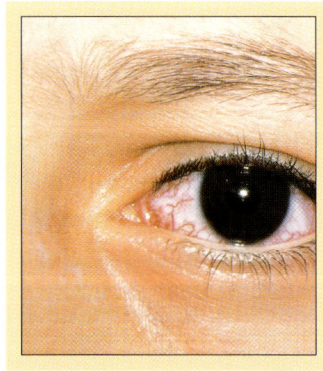

Figure 12.6.
Conjunctival telangiectasia as seen in ataxia telangiectasia.

around 75% of patients. Raised serum α-fetoprotein and enhanced DNA fragility confirm the clinical diagnosis. Friedreich's ataxia may present to the paediatric neurologist, although the onset of symptoms may be insidious. Atypical forms may present with cardiomyopathy in childhood. Early diagnosis of these chronic progressive conditions is important in order to outline prognosis to the parents, as well as to explain the genetic implications for the rest of the family.

The following sections will briefly discuss the 'extrapyramidal' movement disorders, namely chorea, athetosis, dystonia and tics. All are characterized by abnormalities in the regulation of muscle tone and/or in the coordination of movement. They have been described in detail in preceding chapters, however in children these disorders rarely present in such pure forms, for example choreoathetosis is seen in dyskinetic cerebral palsy (see above) and in juvenile Huntington's disease there is often marked rigidity and akinesia.

Chorea

Characterized by 'dancing' involuntary movements, these are rapid irregular jerks. If unilateral they are described as hemichorea or hemiballismus. The main paediatric causes of chorea are listed in Table 12.9 with their key features.

● **Table 12.9.** Chorea in childhood

	Cause	Clinical features	Investigations
Congenital	Cerebral palsy	Initial hypotonia Motor delay Involuntary movements	Neuroimaging Exclude metabolic disorders
Genetic	Huntington's disease	Rigidity and/or chorea Dysarthria Dementia	DNA for CAG repeats of Huntington gene
	Benign hereditary chorea	Non-progressive chorea Onset <5 years No dementia	
	Neuroacanthocytosis	Added extrapyramidal Features: 　Cognitive dysfunction 　Depressed tendon jerks	Fresh blood for acanthocytes Nerve conduction studies
	Organic acidaemias: 　*Methylmalonic* 　*Proprionic*	Recurrent coma Failure to thrive	Acidosis Urinary organic acids
Acquired	Sydenham's chorea	Emotional lability Facial dyskinesias Carditis	ECG (Streptococcal antibody titres)
	Vascular	Post bypass Post stroke	
	Systemic lupus erythematosus	Systemic symptoms Systemic sign Cutaneous	Antibodies: 　*Antinuclear* 　*Double stranded DNA*
	Thyrotoxicosis	Systemic signs	Thyroid function
	Toxic	Anticonvulsants Neuroleptics Amphetamines	

A number are genetically determined: Huntington's disease rarely presents under the age of 20 years. In over 90% of those that do present below this age, the gene is paternally transmitted and in the majority the parent is also clinically affected by the time of presentation. Clinically, these early cases are more likely to resemble the Westphal variant, showing rigidity and akinesia. Seizures are also more frequent and dementia more severe in this group. Clinical suspicion is confirmed by demonstrating expanded trinucleotide CAG repeats in the HD locus on chromosome 4p. International guidelines have been published regarding the more difficult issues of prenatal and presymptomatic testing.[3] Despite parental pressure, presymptomatic testing in childhood is strongly discouraged.

Of acquired causes, Sydenham's chorea, although uncommon, is still seen as a late feature of rheumatic fever following streptococcal A infection. Presentation is between 7 and 12 years in two-thirds of patients. Onset is usually insidious with fidgety behaviour gradually replaced by more obvious involuntary movements. These may be asymmetrical and true hemichorea is sometimes seen. Proximal myoclonic jerks are associated with complex distal movements and this leads to the 'dancing' appearance. Typically facial movements are also prominent and dysarthria is common. Emotional lability is a further feature. Carditis occurs in around 30% of patients and should be excluded. Complete recovery is usually seen within 2–3 months but recurrences may occur, particularly during pregnancy. Haloperidol is classically used in treatment.

Other transient causes of chorea may result from drug ingestion, particularly amphetamines and phenytoin. It is also seen in children following bypass procedures for cardiac surgery. Chorea or hemichorea is seen in <5% of patients with systemic lupus erythematosus but may precede systemic manifestations by many months or years.

Dystonia

The dystonic syndromes are characterized by involuntary muscle contractions leading to abnormal postures and sometimes pain. It is most important to distinguish primary from secondary (symptomatic) dystonia.

Primary, idiopathic torsion dystonia (ITD) has been discussed in Chapter 6. It often presents in adolescence with variable clinical features; distribution may be focal, segmental or generalized. The majority of cases are dominantly inherited but show variable penetrance and there is considerable genetic heterogeneity. In large Jewish kindreds with ITD the gene has been isolated on chromosome 9q allowing carrier detection and prenatal diagnosis.

Dopa-responsive dystonia is clinically distinct from ITD. Symptoms are usually present from childhood, but may be misdiagnosed as cerebral palsy or a functional motor disorder. In the classical Segawa syndrome the child presents with postural dystonia, predominantly affecting the lower limbs. Symptoms show marked diurnal fluctuations, worsening through the day and improved by sleep. The signs are dramatically improved by small doses of levodopa, without adverse side-effects. The disease is caused by mutations of the GTP-cyclohydrolase 1 gene located on chromosome 14q. Dopa-responsive dystonia should be considered in any child with an unexplained diplegia who has dystonic features.

Non-epileptiform paroxysmal movements are also seen in children. The classical manifestations of the paroxysmal kinesogenic and non-kinesogenic dystonia/choreoathetosis syndromes (as classified by Lance)[4] are similar to adults and will not be discussed further. However, paroxysmal dystonia and paroxysmal torticollis has been described in infants, which is transient and may represent a separate disorder. Spasmodic posturing of the head and neck is also a feature of Sandifer's syndrome. In this condition movements typically increase around mealtimes. This is a rare manifestation of gastro-oesophageal reflux and the movements are cured by fundoplication. Finally, paroxysmal movements are seen in hyperekplexia. Excessive stiffening occurs, usually in response to a stimulus. This is so sudden and severe that it causes falls and often injury, whilst the individual remains fully aware. It may present as early as the first year of life with episodes of apparent 'apnoea', found to be secondary to the stiffening, and may be so profound as to be associated with heart block and sudden death. It is an autosomal dominant condition caused by a point mutation in the alpha 1 subunit of the glycine receptor. It responds poorly to most anticonvulsants although success has been demonstrated with the benzodiazepines.

Dystonia presenting in childhood is generally secondary (symptomatic). Cerebral palsy is an important cause, although rarely causes pure dystonia. There are a number of neurodegenerative and metabolic conditions that should be actively excluded, particularly Wilson's disease which may present in childhood and is treatable. Presentation in the younger child is often hepatic, with chronic or fulminant hepatic failure, however more insidious neurological presentation is recognized. Typically, schoolwork slowly deteriorates before variable motor signs ensue. These may include tremor, cerebellar signs, dystonia and rigidity. Dysarthria and scanning speech are common.

Lesch–Nyhan disease is an X-linked disorder of purine metabolism, where deficiency of the enzyme hypoxanthine guanine phosphoribosyl transferase results in defective regulation of uric acid synthesis. Production of uric acid is increased and hyperuricaemia develops. Clinical manifestations are of progressive motor and cognitive deterioration with early hypotonia followed by opisthotonic spasms and athetosis before spasticity develops. Seizures occur in around 50%. Compulsive self-mutilation develops between 2 and 4 years of age. This is distressing for both the child and carers and often requires physical restraint. Gout, renal calculi and ultimately renal failure are late features of the disease. Allopurinol lowers the uric acid level but does not improve the neurological features. Partial deficits of the enzyme result in clinical variants of the disease.

Pelizaeus–Merzbacher disease is also confined to boys. There is profound delay in central myelination classically due to mutations of the proteolipid protein gene on the X chromosome. Presentation is usually in the first year of life with the onset of rotatory or nystagmoid eye movements and often stridor. Disease progression is variable but hypotonia is generally followed by mixed spastic, dystonic and cerebellar signs accompanied by optic atrophy and ultimately decorticate behaviour. Death occurs in the second or third decade. A more severe and rapid course is seen in the congenital or connatal form. This may be autosomal recessive and has been described in girls.

Hallervorden–Spatz disease is a recessively inherited progressive dystonia that typically presents in early childhood. Choreoathetosis is seen in around 50% of patients and there are often pyramidal tract signs.

There is no confirmatory diagnostic test but classical magnetic resonance imaging (MRI) features are recognized, including the 'eye of the tiger' sign in the basal ganglia (secondary to ferrocalcific pigment accumulation in the pallidum and substantia nigra). The outcome is uniformly poor.

Table 12.10 lists some of the important causes of dystonia in childhood. Whilst dystonia is generally a major feature of these disorders it is rarely 'pure' and there are often other superadded motor features.

Tics

Tics are very common in childhood, particularly simple motor tics involving the face or upper limbs. It is well recognized but uncommon for children to progress to multifocal motor tics with vocalization as seen in Tourette's syndrome. In children with simple tics there is usually a family history, that may or may not be apparent to the individual family, and intervention is rarely required. When profound they can be extremely difficult to distinguish from myoclonus. When such difficulty is encountered, the two may be distinguished by determining that tics may be suppressed by the individual when they are aware of their occurrence. Ritualistic repetitive behaviour may at times be confused with a motor disorder, especially when such behaviours involve subtle stereotyped movements.

Myoclonus

Myoclonus (Table 12.11) by definition is a single movement of one or more muscle groups, arising as a result of a higher neuronal discharge. This in the majority is cortical, although at times it is difficult to demonstrate such on EEG, and indeed at other times it may be evident that it is arising from a lower level, namely the spine. As in other movement disorders it is important to establish whether the myoclonus is of recent onset or is longstanding, and whether intermittent or persistent.

Acute onset

A condition seen most commonly in the younger age group is that of the 'dancing eyes' syndrome, or 'opsoclonus myoclonus'. This is aptly described by either terminology; opsoclonus referring to the marked eye movement disorder and the myoclonus to the associ-

● **Table 12.10.** Dystonia in childhood

	Cause	Clinical features	Investigations
Congenital	Cerebral palsy	Initial hypotonia Motor delay	Neuroimaging Exclude metabolic disorders
Genetic: **Primary**	Idiopathic	Isolated dystonia No other neurological signs	DNA sequencing of 9q
	Dopa-responsive	Symptoms fluctuate Predominate in lower limbs	DNA sequencing of GTP-cyclohydrolase
	Paroxysmal	Kinesogenic/non-kinesogenic	
Secondary	Wilson's disease	Progressive dementia with tremor/dystonia/dysarthria Kayser-Fleisher ring	Low serum Cu and caeruloplasmin Raised urinary Cu MRI/CT
	Lesch–Nyhan disease	Progressive dystonia/spasticity Cognitive regression Self-mutilation	Serum and urinary Uric acid HGPRT assay (blood/skin)
	Mitochondrial disease (Leigh's syndrome)	Early regression Mixed motor signs	Blood/CSF lactate MRI scan Mitochondrial DNA
	Pelizaeus–Merzbacher	Nystagmus Stridor Progressive mixed motor signs	MRI scan PLP gene
	Gangliosidoses (GM1/GM2)	Regression Mixed motor signs Macular cherry red spot (GM2)	Leucocyte enzymes β-galactosidase (GM1) Hexosaminidase A (GM2)
	Homocystinuria	Learning difficulties Ectopia lentis Thromboembolic events	Plasma/urine amino acids
	Hallervorden–Spatz disease	Progressive dystonia	Acanthocytes ERG MRI scan
	Ataxia telangectasia		See Table 12.8
	Juvenile Huntington's disease		See Table 12.9
	Glutaric aciduria (1)	Megalencephaly Encephalopathy Dystonia	Urinary organic acids
Acquired	Anticonvulsants/ phenothiazines Basal ganglia damage Infection		Drug levels Neuroimaging

ated movement disorder. The movements vary over time but are not related to attempted movement. There may be a history of a preceding upper respiratory tract infection, although 10% are a presenting feature of neuroblastoma and this must be excluded in all cases. Treatment is with high-dose steroids, to which a response is often rapid although treatment may need to be protracted. Furthermore, a significant number

● **Table 12.11.** Myoclonus in childhood

	Cause	Clinical features	Investigations
Acute	Dancing eyes syndrome	Opsoclonus Myoclonus	Clinical EEG Exclude neuroblastoma
Chronic	Myoclonic epilepsy: Idiopathic (e.g. juvenile myoclonic epilepsy	Age 10–15 years GTC seizures plus morning myoclonus Normal cognition	Clinical EEG
	Symptomatic (e.g. early infantile encephalopathy myoclonic [EIME], Otahara, polymorphic epilepsy)	Age of onset Mixed seizure disorder Developmental regression/plateau	Clinical EEG
	Progressive (e.g. Lafora body, myoclonic epilepsy with ragged red fibres	Age 10–15 years Cognitive regression	Skin biopsy Muscle biopsy
Neuro-degenerative	Late infantile Batten's disease	Age 2–4 years Myoclonic seizures Developmental regression	EEG, VER Rectal biopsy
	Subacute sclerosing panencephalitis	Behaviour change Cognitive regression Periodic jerks	EEG CSF measles titre

although demonstrating a prompt response with regard to the acute movement disorder may show long-term motor, verbal or intellectual deficits. Postanoxic myoclonus, although relatively common in adults, is rarely seen in childhood.

Chronic

Myoclonus is commonly associated with epilepsy. Early-onset myoclonus may form part of a malignant seizure disorder, associated with a poor prognosis for seizure control. Early myoclonic encephalopathy (Otahara's syndrome) and early infantile myoclonic encephalopathy appear to differ only in their age of onset, the latter being in the neonatal period. Both demonstrate a 'burst suppression' pattern on EEG (Fig. 12.7). Myoclonic epilepsy with a (generally) slightly later onset is seen as part of a mixed seizure disorder associated with a variable degree of learning difficulties; myoclonus possibly presenting as a cause of 'drop' attacks. Later in childhood,

myoclonus is seen as a part of idiopathic generalized epilepsy, namely juvenile myoclonic epilepsy. Such children may present with other seizure types, such as absence seizures or generalized tonic clonic seizures, particularly on waking, and morning myoclonus may only be determined from direct questioning in the history. The diagnosis may easily be distinguished from the progressive forms of myoclonic epilepsy, associated with poor response to anticonvulsants and progressive cognitive decline. Although a large number remain of unknown aetiology, investigation must exclude such disorders as Lafora body disease and the mitochondrial cytopathies.

Neurodegenerative

Some relatively early onset neurodegenerative disorders have myoclonus as a major presenting feature. Late infantile neuronal ceroid lipofuscinosis (late infantile Batten's disease) may present to the paediatrician with epilepsy at around 3 years with myoclonus as a major component, at times with almost continuous subtle jerks causing 'pseudoataxia'. Developmental 'plateau' may go unrecognized until direct questioning, with regression evident with time. Neurophysiological testing may be revealing, with the EEG demonstrating spikes and polyspikes enhanced by photic stimulation (Fig. 12.8), and a reduced or absent ERG with enlarged early components of the VEP being virtually pathognomonic. Diagnosis may be confirmed on blood and skin biopsy.

EARLY INFANTILE MYOCLONIC ENCEPHALOPATHY

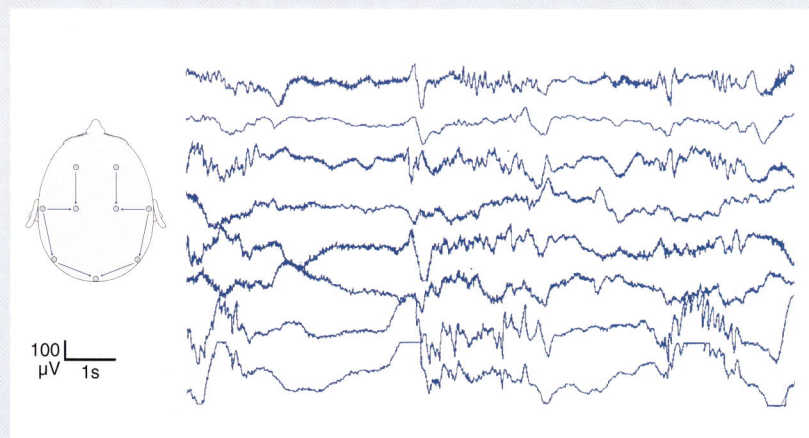

Figure 12.7. EEG of a 1-month-old baby with continuing seizures from birth. Note the abnormal discontinuous nature of the EEG, in addition to the abnormal EEG components.

LATE INFANTILE NEURONAL CEROID LIPOFUSCINOSIS

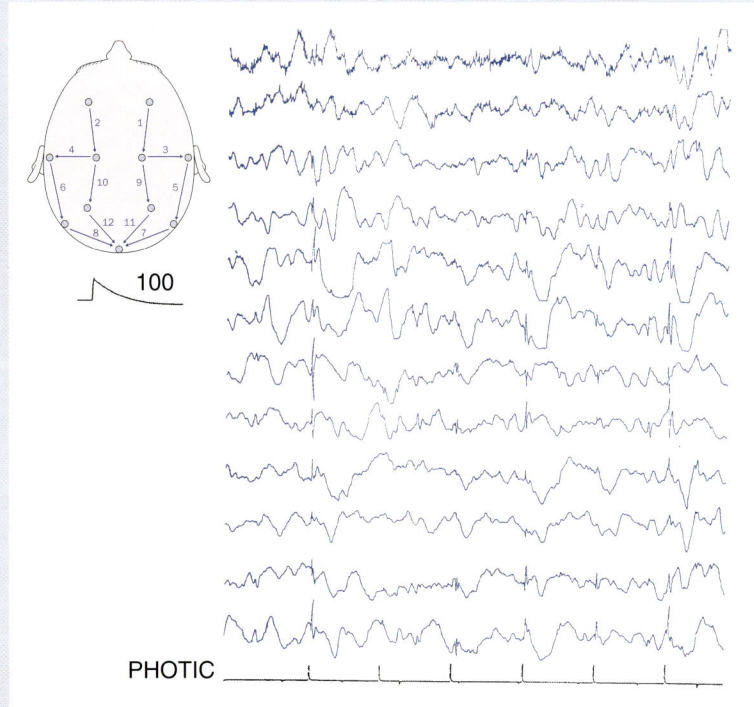

Figure 12.8. EEG findings in a boy aged 3 years 8 months with a history of jerks from age 3 years and developmental regression from 3 years 5 months. Note the spikes with a posterior emphasis evoked by photic stimulation at 1/s, consistent with late infantile neuronal ceroid lipofuscinosis (Batten's disease). (Calibration in microvolts, time marker in seconds.)

Subacute sclerosing panencephalitis (SSPE) is a neurodegenerative condition that is a late consequence of measles infection. It is now rare, as a result of the introduction of measles vaccination, but not extinct, and may be seen in atypical presentation. Most commonly onset is between 5 and 15 years and is usually insidious with a change in behaviour and cognitive performance, that may only retrospectively be recognized as significant. Characteristic periodic involuntary movements are subsequently apparent. These movements or 'jerks' have a sudden onset similar to myoclonus, but they do not have the same abrupt end, ceasing gradually. They are usually symmetrical and bilateral, but may be unilateral or asymmetrical. Characteristic periodic complexes are seen on EEG in association with muscle contraction on EMG that may suggest the diagnosis (Fig. 12.9), confirmed by measles titre within the CSF. Later in the disease signs of extrapyramidal and/or pyramidal dysfunction are evident, with continued dementia, and ultimately coma and death.

Sleep phenomena

Movements during sleep are common in children, and often present to the paediatrician with a possible diagnosis of epilepsy. They may present as early as the neonatal period when benign neonatal sleep myoclonus may present as a major management problem. Careful history taking and observation reveal brief, albeit frequent, jerks to only be present during sleep, sleep taking up a large proportion of time in a small baby. When difficulty arises in diagnosis, confirmation will be provided by a normal EEG during such movements. The jerks will become less frequent with age and rarely persist much longer than 6 months.

Periodic movements of sleep are common in the older child, and may only come to light when the parent sleeps in close contact with the child.

Epilepsy may also manifest as a nocturnal movement disorder. Benign epilepsy with centrotemporal spikes usually presents with episodes from sleep, between the ages of 5–10 years. These episodes may simply be temporary short-lived paralysis of an upper limb, with facial involvement. The diagnosis may be difficult in the absence of witnessed convulsive movements. An EEG again may then be helpful in the diagnosis, with discharges seen over the centrotemporal areas, particularly in sleep.

SUBACUTE SCLEROSING PANENCEPHALITIS

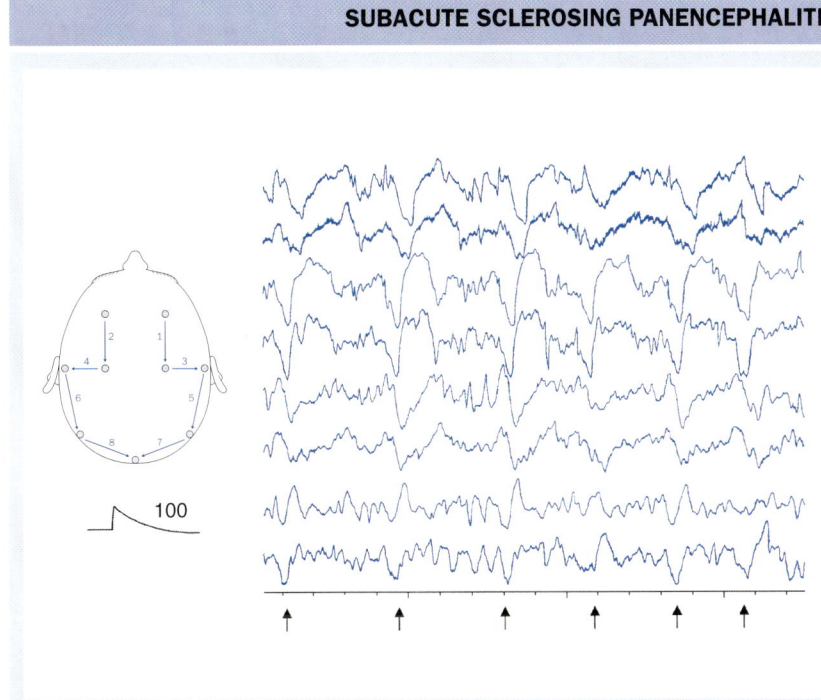

Figure 12.9. EEG features of subacute sclerosing panencephalitis (SSPE). Note the periodic complexes recurring approximately every 3 seconds. Any type of EEG activity, including normal alpha rhythm, may be seen between the complexes. (Calibration in microvolts, time marker in seconds.)

100

Conclusion

This chapter has reviewed the movement disorders presenting in childhood, in particular outlining the difficulties in determining their presence and underlying aetiology. Although there is much overlap with disorders seen in adults, some conditions are unique to this age group. Furthermore, the whole approach to the diagnosis and management of movement disorders in young children differs to that in adults as each presentation has to be recognized in the context of the developing nervous system, and therefore early neurodegenerative disease may be masked. For this reason, a paediatrician should always be involved in the management of such children. In addition, the diagnosis of any disorder will have far-reaching psychosocial consequences, not only within the family with regard to genetic counselling and management of the individual, but also with education and schooling. This highlights the role of the multidisciplinary team, particularly in the chronic non-progressive movement disorders such as cerebral palsy.

References

1. Hull D, Johnston D I. Essential paediatrics. Edinburgh: Churchill Livingstone, 1981: 1–13

2. Illingworth R S. The development of the infant and young child, normal and abnormal. Edinburgh: Churchill Livingstone, 1987

3. World Federation of Neurology Research Group on Huntington's Disease. Presymptomatic testing for HD: a worldwide survey. J Med Genet 1993; 30: 1020–1022

4. Lance J W. Familial paroxysmal dystonic choreoathetosis and its differentiation from related syndromes. Ann Neurol 1977; 2: 285–292

5. Aicardi J. Diseases of the nervous system in childhood. Clin Devel Med Nos 115/118. London: Mac Keith Press, 1992

chapter 13

Psychogenic movement disorders

Guy Sawle

As in all of medicine, and neurology in particular, it is dangerous to diagnose movement disorders as psychogenic (Fig. 13.1). New organic disorders are constantly being reported. Genetic and other insights into aetiology demand that we struggle constantly to understand the relationship of one phenotype to another. Put simply, we dare not diagnose a psychogenic movement disorder on the basis of 'I've never seen it before', however fantastic the movements (or lack of them) may appear; it may be a new disorder, or a new presentation of a familiar one. There are many examples in the literature of disorders once thought to be entirely functional (such as cervical dystonia and blepharospasm) which have a clearly organic basis.

But it would be equally fanciful to suggest that every patient who presents with a disorder of movement has an organic disease. There are, undoubtedly, some patients with psychogenic disorders and there are a small number of patients with organic disease who 'elaborate' their symptoms. So how can we distinguish between the two (CD 13.1)?

General points

The first rule is simple. If in doubt, assume the condition is real. Far fewer mistakes are made and far fewer fingers are burned in this way. Secondly, if all other doctors who have seen the patient think the disorder is fake, then there is still a very good chance that it is real. Thirdly, if at first sight you think the condition is a fake, you are likely to be wrong and the condition is probably real. Lastly, if after careful consideration you come to the conclusion that the bulk of what you see is fake, it is still dangerous to assume that it did not begin with a less dramatic disorder which may still be present and which is real.

In some patients it is easy to be sure that a movement disorder has a psychological basis; in others it may be better to include with any such diagnosis an estimate of certainty, ranging from a documented psychogenic disorder to a possibly psychogenic disorder.[1]

Categories of diagnostic certainty

A 'documented psychogenic movement disorder' is one where the symptoms have already been shown to be completely relieved by 'psychological means', or where there is clear evidence of malingering. Psychological treatments may include treatment of an underlying psychiatric condition, or some kind of

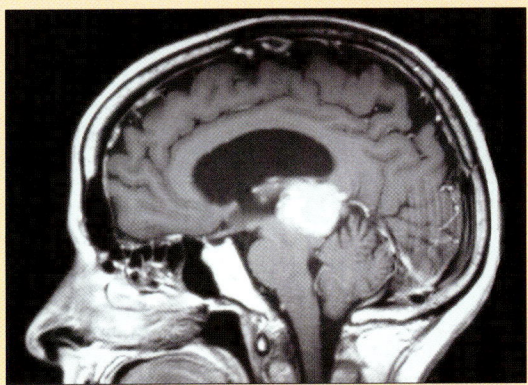

Figure 13.1. Pineal tumour with hydrocephalus. This patient had a long history of severe anxiety and depression. The presenting system was a bizarre, unclassifiable, distractible and inconsistent gait.

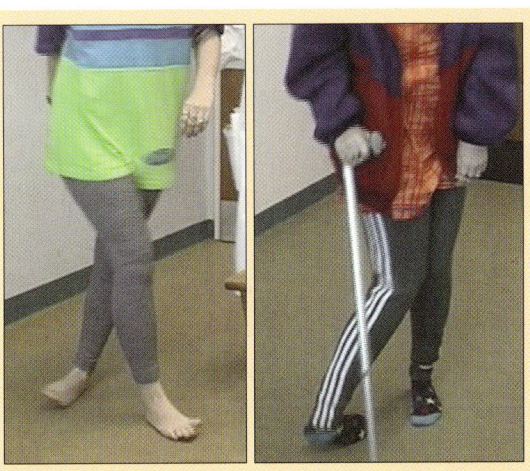

CD 13.1. Functional scissoring gait in a patient with organic leg dystonia.

placebo. Patients may prove to be malingering if they behave completely normally when they think they are not being observed.

A 'clinically established psychogenic movement disorder' is one for which the clinical features are inconsistent over time, or else they are unlike any known movement disorders, and in which at least one additional feature is present, such as definitely fake neurological signs, multiple somatizations, obvious psychiatric disturbance, or excessive and deliberate slowness of movement.

The next lower degree of certainty applies to patients in whom the movement disorder is probable, such as those in whom either the movement disorder looks genuine but it disappears (unexpectedly) on distraction, or there are accompanying definitely fake signs, or there are multiple somatizations. This category also applies to patients in whom the movement disorder does not look real, but in whom there are no supportive signs such as fake signs, distractibility or multiple somatizations.

Lastly, patients with possibly psychogenic movement disorders have signs which look like an organic disorder, but they also have obvious emotional disturbance. Clearly this end of the spectrum could be interpreted to include many patients with definite organic disease in whom psychological factors also play a part.

Dealing with intermittent disorders

The whole process of deciding between psychological and organic movement disorders is made even more complicated when the symptoms are intermittent. Fortunately, many such patients can be encouraged to have 'an attack' when seeing the doctor, and then the same process as above (except for termination by distraction, which could be simply the genuine end of an attack) apply (CD 13.2). Other patients report frequent attacks at home and yet never have such an attack in the consulting room. I have found it helpful to ask patients if they have (or know somebody with) a video camera. The result is then usually a 3 or 4 hour long video tape, but a few minutes spent with one's hand on the forward-preview knob may be sufficient to identify a series of widely varying attacks, sufficient to confirm the diagnosis of psychogenic attacks.

Relevant psychiatric diagnoses

A particular problem in the management of such patients is that psychiatrists are usually reluctant to make a firm 'psychiatric' diagnosis. So a patient in whom the neurologist suspects a psychogenic disorder, if sent to a psychiatrist, is unlikely to return with a definite psychiatric diagnosis. Psychiatrists are understandably wary of diagnosing any kind of physical disease as psychogenic. There are, however, several categories recognized under DSM IIIR[2] which apply to some movement disorder patients.

Somatoform disorder

This is where the physical symptoms are caused by psychological factors, but are not under voluntary control. There are two kinds: conversion disorder and somatization disorder.

Conversion disorder

In this case, psychological factors are manifest as physical symptoms.

Somatization disorder

This term is used to denote a chronic condition characterized by a history of numerous, recurrent physical complaints that begin in early life (before the age of 30 years) and persist for many years.[3] Such patients have usually complained of pain in a variety of body sites, and had other gastroenterological, sexual and pseudoneurological symptoms. Somatization disorder is ten times more common in women than men, with

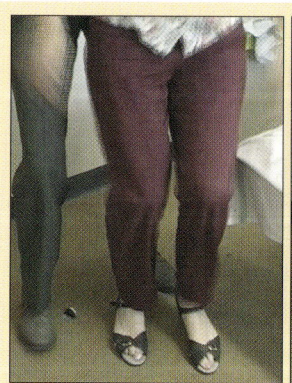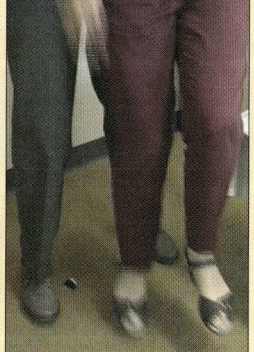

CD 13.2. Unusual jumping attack.

a population lifetime prevalence of 0.1–0.2%, though subthreshold disorders may be 100 times as common. Patients with somatization disorders have a heightened awareness of, and pay increased attention to, a wide variety of bodily sensations, many of which are common in the general population but which most people choose to ignore.

Factitious disorder

This refers to patients in whom the symptoms are deliberately put on in order to satisfy some kind of psychological need. It includes Münchausen's syndrome, and the so-called Münchausen-by-proxy (in which usually a parent fakes or deliberately precipitates symptoms in a child).

Malingering

This is the situation where a psychiatrically sound patient fakes illness in order to avoid work, criminal prosecution, or other similarly unattractive alternatives.

Clues on examination

The commonest fake symptoms in psychogenic movement disorders are tremors and peculiarities of gait. Other patients may exhibit a wide range of different abnormal movements; but this is a trap for the unwary, because some organic disorders are characterized by mixtures of, for example, ataxia and myoclonus, or parkinsonism, dystonia and chorea; so a detailed knowledge of what is normal across a wide variety of genuine conditions is needed before jumping to conclusions about unusual combinations of signs.

There are a number of clinical features which are closely associated with hysteria. These include 'la belle indifference' and secondary gain. It is my experience that these phrases are rarely used in circumstances *except* when discussing hysteria. It is important to remember, however, that both of these signs (and many other features typically seen in psychogenic illness) also occur in a significant number of patients with structural organic disease.[4] Also, patients with organic movement disorders may have psychogenic features added, so correctly identifying the latter is not necessarily enough to exclude the former.[5]

It is usually the clinical features of the condition which make one consider the possibility of psychogenic aetiology. Typically some aspect of the clinical presentation fails to ring true and then one begins to search for other signs. Much the same occurs in psychiatric practice, of course, where the experienced psychiatrist develops a feel for the symptoms and signs which are usual in psychiatric disease. Every now and then a psychiatrist spots an incongruous sign or behaviour that leads ultimately to the diagnosis of a 'neurological' disease.

Psychogenic tremor

Tremor comprises up to 50% of psychogenic movement disorders.[6] Typical clinical features are shown in Table 13.1. When asked to perform a rhythmic task with an unaffected limb, the tremor frequency may alter, becoming synchronized with the newly started movement (CD 13.3). Where recordings of tremor frequency are possible, psychogenic tremors usually demonstrate fluctuations in frequency; a feature not normally seen in organic disorders. Patients with large amplitude tremors may show reduction in amplitude when approaching the target during the finger–nose test (CD 13.4).

Noise-induced psychogenic tremor has been described in a patient with the post-traumatic stress disorder following a marine disaster in which many of the patient's colleagues drowned.[7] The tremor settled when the patient was distracted, even though he could

Table 13.1. Clinical features of psychogenic tremor.[13]

Abrupt onset
Static course
Spontaneous remissions
Unclassifiable tremors
Clinical inconsistencies
Changing tremor characteristics
Unresponsiveness to antitremor drugs
Tremor increases with attention
Tremor lessens with distraction
Responsiveness to placebo
Absence of other neurological signs
Remission with psychotherapy

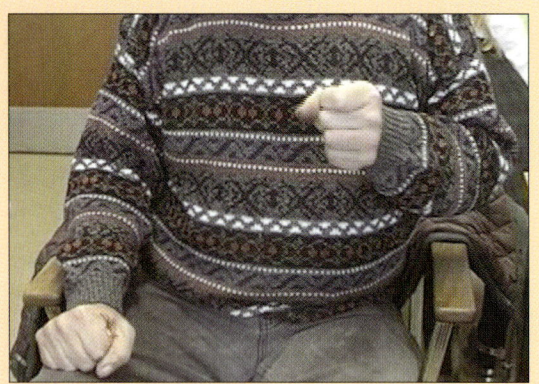

CD 13.3. Alteration of tremor speed by contralateral voluntary movement.

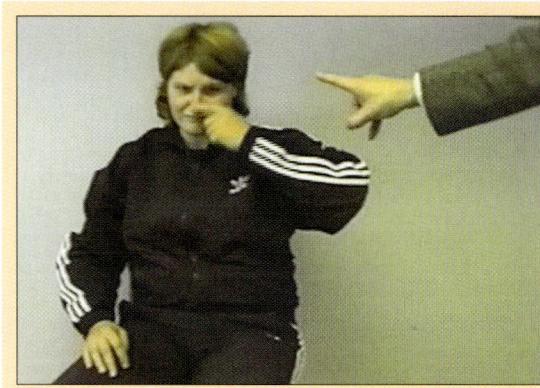

CD 13.4. Reduction in tremor amplitude on approaching a target.

not consciously suppress the movements. In this particular patient, the tremor persisted for several days after hearing a loud noise.

Psychogenic dystonia

In one large series, 2.6% of patients presenting to a specialist dystonia research centre were considered to have documented or clinically established psychogenic dystonia.[8]

Psychogenic dystonia may begin with fixed dystonic postures, whereas the majority of patients with organic dystonia start with action dystonia. Also, onset in the leg is common in psychogenic dystonia, whereas onset in the leg in *adult* onset organic dystonia is unusual. As a result of this disparity, up to a third of adult patients with leg-onset dystonia may have a psychological, rather than a physical, cause for their symptoms (Table 13.2).

Paroxysmal dystonia is a common presentation in psychogenic patients, as a result of which as many as a quarter of patients who present with (non-secondary) paroxysmal dystonia may have psychogenic illness.

Psychogenic dystonia may be severe enough to result in the development of contractures. As with other psychogenic movements, psychogenic dystonia can occur in patients who also have organic dystonia.

Psychogenic parkinsonism

Whilst it is an extremely rare cause of parkinsonism, there are occasional patients in whom the symptoms have a psychogenic basis. In a review of 14 such patients a pattern of common signs emerged.[9] In three of the four patients who underwent fluorodopa PET scans tracer uptake was normal. But a fourth patient had an abnormal scan, suggesting that psychogenic factors were not the full explanation in that case. He was presumed to have psychogenic worsening of underlying idiopathic Parkinson's disease, because his symptoms and signs improved on psychotherapy and haloperidol (which would be expected to worsen symptoms in organic parkinsonism).[9] Patients with psychogenic parkinsonism may be excessively slow, without the decrementing amplitude and speed seen in Parkinson's disease (CD 13.5). Features described above as characteristic of psychogenic tremor may be relevant in these rare patients also (Table 13.3).

Psychogenic myoclonus and chorea

Clinically, similar considerations apply in the diagnosis of 'jerking' disorders as psychogenic. Clinical incongruity is usual and patients often improve with distraction.[10] A patient with chorea due to systemic lupus erythematosus improved on steroids, but then

● **Table 13.2.** Common clinical features of psychogenic dystonia. (Based partly on refs 8 and 14.)

Beginning with fixed dystonia
Adult-onset in the leg (though this happens in genuine dystonia also)
Paroxysmal attacks (also occur in genuine conditions)

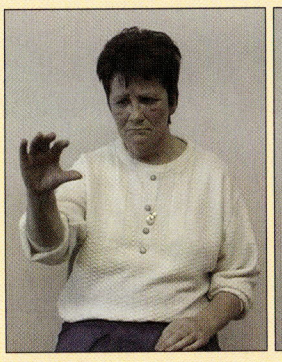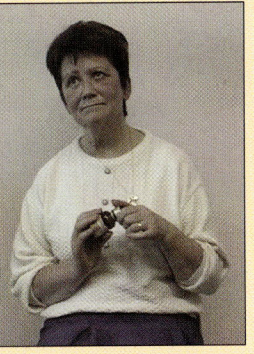

CD 13.5. Extreme and inconsistent slowness of hand movement; psychogenic slowness in a patient with genuine Parkinson's disease.

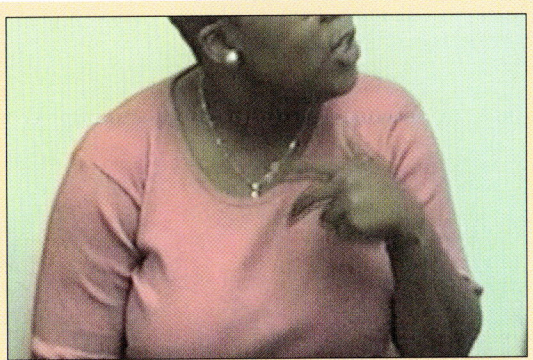

CD 13.6. 'Chorea' movement time-locked to speech.

● **Table 13.3.** Clinical features of psychogenic parkinsonism. (Based partly on ref. 9.)

Abrupt onset (may follow trauma)

Early maximal disability; then static

Rest, postural and action tremor improving with distraction

Feeling of voluntary resistance when testing rigidity, but without cogwheeling

Extreme slowness of movement, without the characteristic decrement of amplitude and rate

Atypical gait

Bizarre response to testing postural reflexes

Normal fluorodopa PET scan

Improvement with neuroleptic or other drugs (not recommended as a diagnostic test)

NEUROPHYSIOLOGICAL RECORDINGS IN PSYCHOGENIC MYOCLONUS

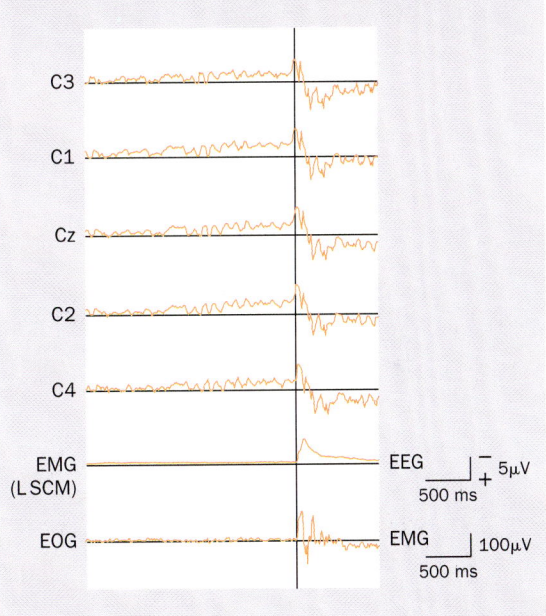

Figure 13.2. Averaged EEG trace, time-locked to the myoclonic jerks recorded by EMG. Slow negative EEG shift precedes the EMG onset by more than 1 second[11].

relapsed as her social circumstances changed. In the relapse, her 'choreic' movements were wide amplitude gesticulations of the arm. When she became animated in conversation her 'chorea' became repetitive and time-locked to the cadence of her speech (CD 13.6).

In patients with spontaneous jerks, good electrophysiological evidence in favour of psychogenic myoclonus is the presence of a slow negative wave, the Bereitschaftspotential (Fig. 13.2), in the EEG back-averaged from the jerks.[11] A similar approach may be used in patients who present with stimulus-sensitive jerks. When these are voluntary, there is generally a variable time interval between the stimulus and the jerk, and the delay between the two lies in the range seen in healthy subjects responding to an external stimulus.[12] The muscles recruited in the jerks vary with repetition and there is habituation with repetition.

Managing psychogenic movement disorders

Managing patients with psychogenic movement disorders is difficult. In some cases, simple reassurance together with a placebo or physiotherapy (to enable the patient to recover without losing face) is sufficient. Other patients, in whom there is an active underlying psychological or psychiatric problem, may not be able to improve until that problem is dealt with and psychiatric help may be necessary. Drug treatment of concurrent depression, psychotherapy and even hypnotherapy can all be helpful.

Not all patients with psychogenic movement disorders (or other neurological symptoms) warm to the idea that their symptoms have a psychogenic basis. Even when the explanation given is that the symptoms are real, but generated on an involuntary basis as an outward manifestation of an otherwise hidden psychological problem, still this may prove unpalatable news and some such patients react aggressively with complaints and at least threats of litigation (on the basis of failing to diagnose a physical disease which they believe must be present).

There is, of course, a circuitous argument in assessing the efficacy of any kind of treatment for these conditions, since many patients with a 'documented psychogenic movement disorder' are categorized in this way on the basis of their symptoms having been completely relieved by psychological means. It is possible that we underestimate the number of patients whose symptoms and signs have a psychological cause. But history is littered with examples of the opposite mistake and anyone who forgets this in clinical practice does so at their own peril.

References

1. Fahn S. Psychogenic movement disorders. In: Marsden C D, Fahn S (eds) Movement disorders 3. Oxford: Butterworth Heinemann, 1994: 359–372

2. American Psychiatric Association. Diagnostic and statistic manual of mental disorders (3rd ed) Washington DC: American Psychiatric Association, 1987

3. Bass G, Murphy M. Somatization disorder in a British teaching hospital. Br J Clin Pract 1991; 45: 237–244

4. Gould R, Miller B L, Goldberg M A, Benson D F. The validity of hysterical signs and symptoms. J Nerv Ment Dis 1986; 174: 593–597

5. Ranawaya R, Riley D, Lang A. Psychogenic dyskinesias in patients with organic movement disorders. Mov Dis 1990; 5: 127–133

6. Factor S A, Podskalny G D, Molho E S. Psychogenic movement disorders: frequency, clinical profile, and characteristics. J Neurol Neurosurg Psychiat 1995; 59: 406–412

7. Walters A S, Hening W A. Noise-induced psychogenic tremor associated with post-traumatic stress disorder. Mov Dis 1992; 7: 333–338

8. Fahn S, Williams D T. Psychogenic dystonia. Adv Neurol 1988; 50: 431–455

9. Lang A E, Koller W C, Fahn S. Psychogenic parkinsonism. Arch Neurol 1995; 52: 802–810

10. Monday K, Jankovic J. Psychogenic myoclonus. Neurology 1993; 43: 349–352

11. Terada K, Ikeda A, Van Ness P C et al. Presence of Bereitschaftspotential preceding psychogenic myoclonus: Clinical application of jerk-locked back averaging. J Neurol Neurosurg Psychiat 1995; 58: 745–747

12. Thompson P D, Colebatch J G, Brown P et al. Voluntary stimulus-sensitive jerks and jumps mimicking myoclonus or pathological startle syndromes. Mov Dis 1992; 7: 257–262

13. Moon S L, Koller W C. Psychogenic tremor. In: Findley L J, Koller W C (eds) Handbook of tremor disorders. New York: Marcel Dekker, Inc., 1995: 491–494

14. Lang A E. Psychogenic dystonia: a review of 18 cases. Can J Neurol Sci 1995; 22: 136–143

chapter 14

Other dyskinesias

Guy Sawle

However carefully we devise a scheme of classification, there will always be 'left over' conditions which do not easily fit into other categories. As our understanding of movement disorder genesis and relationships evolves, there will doubtless be a re-ordering of many conditions. Some will migrate out of this chapter to others; some may remain, and doubtless new conditions will be added. For now, these are the conditions it would seem wrong to omit, yet which do not obviously belong in any of the previous chapters.

Belly dancer's dyskinesia

This description was first used in the literature in 1990, in a paper describing five patients with focal involuntary movements affecting the abdominal wall.[1] One had diaphragmatic flutter, but the others all had writhing movements and contractions of the abdominal muscles (CD 14.1).

Once witnessed, this condition is easily recognized the second time around. The movements vary somewhat, but are unlike any other movement disorder such as dystonia, myoclonus or tics. The onset is usually gradual. In one-third or more of patients the movements

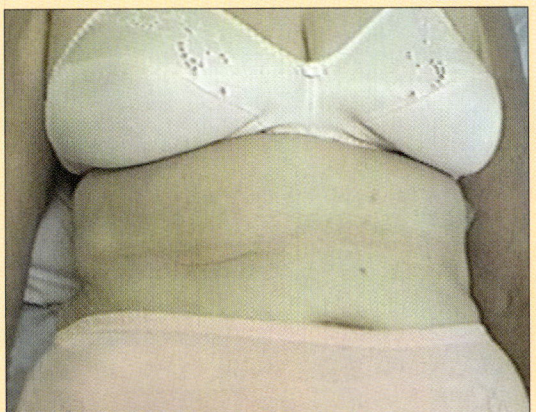

CD 14.1. Belly dancer's dyskinesia.

begin after local trauma or surgical procedures, such as appendicectomy or laparoscopy. The movements are not associated with neuroleptic or other medication. They cannot be voluntarily suppressed.

Investigations such as spinal and abdominal imaging fail to explain the movements. They are usually refractive to treatment, and long lasting if not permanent.

Other unusual focal dyskinesias

A range of other curious focal segmental involuntary movements have been described, including movements of the ears, back, shoulder girdle and upper extremity.[2] The movements are broadly similar to those of belly dancer's dyskinesia. They are stereotyped, consisting of local or segmental movements lasting for up to a few seconds and recurring in a sometimes rhythmical fashion, or else they comprise an apparently continuous writhing movement. The movements do not spread to involve other body parts.

Onset is usually gradual. There may be a history of prior trauma, though not necessarily to the body part in question, so the significance of such a trauma history is uncertain. A variety of accompanying sensory symptoms are reported, varying from minimal discomfort to quite severe pain. In those patients who report bad pain, the movements and pain do not necessarily vary in tandem.

The involuntary movements are often improved by stress, concentration and movement of other body parts. They are lessened during relaxation, sleep, and contraction of the affected muscles.

As with belly dancer's dyskinesia, investigations and treatment are usually unrewarding.

Stiff person syndrome

The stiff person syndrome (formerly the stiff man syndrome when first described by Moersch and

Woltman in 1956)[3] comprises axial and proximal limb muscle rigidity with painful muscle spasms of varying intensity. The symptoms usually begin insidiously over weeks or months, ultimately culminating in extreme axial rigidity, typically with an exaggerated lumbar lordosis (CD 14.2a). All neck and trunk movements become severely restricted.

Many patients also report superimposed muscle spasms, which may be triggered off by a variety of stimuli, including touch, stretch, deliberate movement, noise or emotion. The spasms can lead to falls, making walking effectively impossible. The spasms can even result in fractures of long bones or of the pelvis (Fig. 14.1). The rigidity and spasms are less severe or absent during sleep, general anaesthesia, myoneural blockade and peripheral nerve blockade.

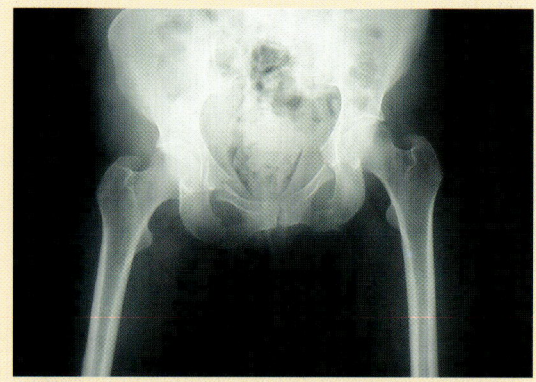

Figure 14.1. Photograph of pelvic fracture in patient with stiff person syndrome. (Same patient as CD 14.2)

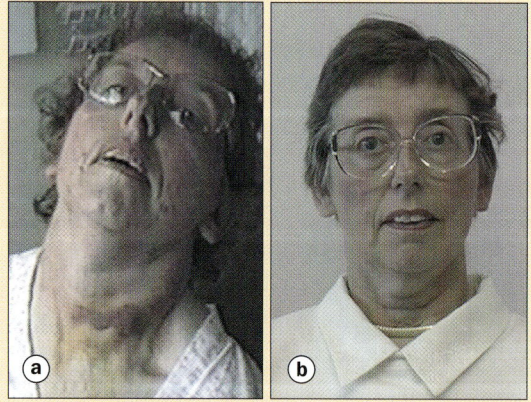

CD 14.2. (a) Stiff person syndrome: before treatment. (b) On treatment.

In most patients the condition runs a lengthy course and the prognosis may be affected by associated underlying conditions. Sudden death has been reported in patients whose attacks of muscle spasms were associated with paroxysmal autonomic dysfunction including transient hyperpyrexia, tachycardia and hypertension.[4]

There are well established links with type-I diabetes mellitus and, less commonly, a range of other autoimmune conditions such as vitiligo, pernicious anaemia and thyroid disease. Some patients have an underlying malignancy.

Physical examination, except for the muscular rigidity, abnormal posture, and spasms, is usually normal.

Investigation

Many patients (around 60%) have autoantibodies against glutamic acid decarboxylase in their serum and cerebrospinal fluid (CSF).[5] Some may have oligoclonal bands.

EMG reveals continuous normal motor unit potentials in the affected muscles, which the patients are unable to abolish through relaxation. Agonist and antagonist muscles may be affected concurrently. If spasms are induced by touching nearby muscles, they are manifest as a marked increase in motor unit activity.

Muscle biopsy does not show any diagnostic features. Imaging of the brain and spinal cord is usually normal.

Treatment

The muscle spasms are usually lessened by diazepam;[6] other benzodiazepines such as clonazepam may also be effective. Baclofen is also usually effective. Both drugs cause sedation as a dose-limiting side-effect, and this may be lessened by using the two drugs, in lower doses, in combination (CD 14.2b). Anticonvulsants have also been tried; there have been anecdotal reports of response to valproic acid.[7]

There have also been reports of beneficial response to steroids, though high doses are necessary and patients may relapse when the drugs are stopped.[8]

Plasmapheresis has been variably reported as either effective[9] or ineffective. Botulinum toxin injections may help,[10] though the widespread muscle involvement in most patients preclude this as a practical treatment in most cases.

Progressive encephalomyelitis with rigidity

This condition is much rarer than the stiff person syndrome. It has a much worse prognosis, with relentless progression. Patients may die in a few weeks[11] or survive up to around 3 years. In some cases there is an underlying malignancy, in which case the pathological features are those of a paraneoplastic encephalomyelitis. In cases without recognized malignancy, there is widespread encephalomyelitis with lymphoid infiltration and neuronal loss in the brainstem and spinal cord.[12]

The clinical features include evidence of cranial nerve involvement (such as nystagmus, loss of eye movements, dysarthria) and long tract signs. The rigidity is very severe, worse than is generally encountered in parkinsonian syndromes. Severe and painful muscle spasms occur too, and are typically accompanied by profuse sweating.

As with the stiff man syndrome treatment is usually with baclofen and diazepam. In one patient who had frequent episodes of severe generalized muscle spasms with piloerection and hyperventilation and in whom a cervical cord biopsy showed perivascular cuffing and a mononuclear infiltration, treatment with intravenous high-dose methylprednisolone was associated with considerable clinical improvement.[13]

Painful legs and moving toes

The principal clinical features of this condition are painful legs and moving toes! The phrase was coined by Spillane and colleagues who described six affected patients in 1971.[14] In most cases the pain starts days or even years before the movements.[15] It is usually constant and described as burning, crushing, or throbbing and there may be accompanying changes in cutaneous sensitivity as seen in causalgia.

The movements are either unilateral or bilateral and comprise a range of flexion, extension, abduction and adduction movements of the toes at a rate of 1–2 Hz.[15] They defy imitation. Some patients are able to suppress them briefly. Occasional patients have the same movements without any pain.[16]

There are a broad range of associated neurological lesions. Some patients have an axonal peripheral neuropathy, whilst others have evidence of spinal nerve root damage or else have had lower leg fractures or varicose vein surgery.[15]

The origin of the syndrome is unknown; suggestions have included activation of spinal motor neurons by afferents via the posterior root[17] and an irritative central or spinal disorder associated with a peripheral lesion.[18] A spectrum of disorders between causalgia (pain alone), through painful legs and moving toes, to moving toes *without* pain, has been suggested, each due to alterations in suprasegmental central sensorimotor circuits.[15] Yet in a patient with similar clinical features associated with nerve entrapment in the tarsal tunnel, the movements were abolished by nerve blockade distal to the point of nerve compression, suggesting a peripheral ectopic generator in the region.[19]

Occasional patients improve if the underlying cause can be found and is remediable. Some patients gain useful pain relief from lumbar sympathetic blockade. Others are treated with a range of agents including benzodiazepines, baclofen, carbamazepine and tricyclic antidepressants. Response to these agents is generally poor and the condition usually long-lasting. A combination of transcutaneous electrical nerve stimulation and vibratory stimulation was helpful in one patient.[20]

Broadly similar upper limb disorders have also been reported, as painful arm and moving fingers (in a patient with a brachial plexus lesion),[21] and painful hand and moving fingers (following trauma and amputation).[22]

Hemifacial spasm

Unilateral involuntary contractions of facial muscles are generally due to hemifacial spasm. The disorder is the facial nerve 'equivalent' of trigeminal neuralgia.

The movements occur in bursts lasting a few seconds at a time. They may be triggered by speaking or eating. Both upper and lower facial muscles are affected, but it is usually the twitching movement around the eye which patients find most annoying (CD 14.3). The condition can usually be easily distinguished from blepharospasm because the latter condition is nearly always bilateral.

The cause of hemifacial spasms is most commonly compression of the facial nerve close to the root entry zone, though rarely compression further out along the course of the nerve may be the cause,[23,24] and there have been anecdotal reports of lesions within the brainstem (a multiple sclerosis plaque, for example).[25] The usual cause of root entry zone compression is compression by a tortuous but otherwise normal vessel, typically the anterior or posterior inferior cerebellar artery or the vertebral artery.[26] A broad range of other mass lesions at the same site have been described.

Investigation should include imaging of the root entry zone. With modern magnetic resonance methods it may be possible to image the vessels in this region without risk of vascular disruption (Fig. 14.2). On the rare occasions when a mass lesion (such as a meningioma) is revealed, this must be treated on its own merits. In other cases where a compressing vessel has been demonstrated, some physicians (and many surgeons) favour a 'curative' surgical procedure to decompress the root entry zone. This operation is generally successful and usually safe,[27,28] but like all such procedures it does carry some risk and many physicians prefer treatment with botulinum toxin (see section on botulinum toxin in Chapter 6).

Other forms of drug therapy are usually unhelpful, though there have been anecdotal reports of response to pizotifen,[29] gabapentin,[30] and felbamate.[31]

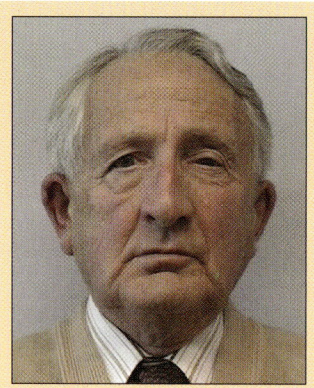

CD 14.3. Hemifacial spasm.

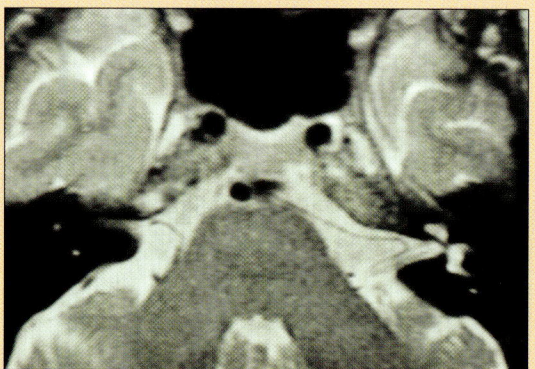

Figure 14.2. MR image to show left (right of image) posterior inferior cerebellar artery loop compressing facial nerve. (Courtesy of Dr T. Jaspan.)

References

1. Iliceto G, Thompson P D, Day B L et al. Diaphragmatic flutter, the moving umbilicus syndrome and 'belly dancer's' dyskinesia. Mov Dis 1990; 51: 15–22

2. Caviness J N, Gabellini A, Kneebone C S et al. Unusual focal dyskinesias: the ears, the shoulders, the back and the abdomen. Mov Dis 1994; 9: 531–538

3. Moersch F P, Woltman H W. Progressive fluctuating muscular rigidity and spasm (stiff-man syndrome): report of a case and some observations in 13 other cases. Mayo Clin Proc 1956; 31: 421–427

4. Mitsumoto H, Schwartzman M J, Estes M L et al. Sudden death and paroxysmal autonomic dysfunction in stiff-man syndrome. J Neurol 1991; 238: 91–96

5. Blum P, Jankovic J. Stiff-person syndrome: an autoimmune disease. Mov Dis 1991; 6: 12–20

6. Howard F M. A new and effective drug in the treatment of stiff-man syndrome. Mayo Clin Proc 1963; 38: 203–212

7. Spehlmann R, Norcross K, Rasmus S C, Schlageter N L. Improvement of stiff-man syndrome and sodium valproate. Neurology 1981; 31: 1162–1163

8. Piccolo G, Cosi V, Zandrini C, Moglia A. Steroid-responsive and dependent stiff-man syndrome: a clinical and electrophysiological study of two cases. Ital J Neurol Sci 1988; 9: 559–566

9. Brashear H R, Phillips II L H. Autoantibodies to GABAergic neurons and response to plasmapheresis in stiff-man syndrome. Neurology 1991; 41: 1588–1592

10. Davis D, Jabbari B. Significant improvement of stiff-person syndrome after paraspinal injection of botulinum toxin A. Mov Dis 1993; 8: 371–373

11. Whiteley A M, Swash M, Urich H. Progressive encephalomyelitis with rigidity. Its relation to 'subacute myoclonic spinal neuronitis' and to the 'stiff man syndrome'. Brain 1976; 99: 27–42

12. Howell D A, Lees A J, Toghill P J. Spinal internuncial neurones in progressive encephalomyelitis with rigidity. J Neurol Neurosurg Psychiat 1979; 42: 773–785

13. McCombe P A, Chalk J B, Searle J W et al. Progressive encephalomyelitis with rigidity: a case report with magnetic resonance imaging findings. J Neurol Neurosurg Psychiat 1989; 52: 1429–1431

14. Spillane J D, Nathan P W, Kelly R E, Marsden C D. Painful legs and moving toes. Brain 1971; 94: 541–556

15. Dressler D, Thompson P D, Gledhill R F, Marsden C D. The syndrome of painful legs and moving toes. Mov Dis 1994; 9: 13–21

16. Walters A S, Hening W A, Shah S K, Chokroverty S. Painless legs and moving toes: a syndrome related to painful legs and moving toes? Mov Dis 1993; 8: 377–379

17. Nathan P W. Painful legs and moving toes: evidence on the site of the lesion. J Neurol Neurosurg Psychiat 1978; 41: 934–939

18. Schott G D. Painful legs and moving toes: the role of trauma. J Neurol Neurosurg Psychiat 1981; 44: 344–346

19. Pla M E R, Dillingham D R, Spellman N T et al. Painful legs and moving toes associated with tarsal tunnel syndrome and accessory soleus muscle. Mov Dis 1996; 11: 82–86

20. Guieu R, Tardy-Gervet M F, Blin O, Pouget J. Pain relief achieved by transcutaneous electrical nerve stimulation and/or vibratory stimulation in a case of painful legs and moving toes. Pain 1990; 42: 43–48

21. Verhagen W, Horstink M, Notermans S. Painful arm and moving fingers. J Neurol Neurosurg Psychiat 1985; 48: 384–385

22. Funukawa I, Mano Y, Takayanagi T. Painful hand and moving fingers. J Neurol 1987; 234: 342–343

23. Pego Reigosa R, Pulpeiro Rios J R. Hemifacial spasm. J Neurol Neurosurg Psychiat 1998; 64: 687

24. Ryu H, Yamamoto S, Sugiyama K et al. Hemifacial spasm caused by vascular decompression of the distal portion of the facial nerve. J Neurosurg 1998; 88: 605–609

25. Digre K, Corbett J J. Hemifacial spasm: differential diagnosis, mechanism, and treatment. Adv Neurol 1988; 49: 151–176

26. Magnan J, Caces F, Locatelli P, Chays A. Hemifacial spasm: endoscopic vascular decompression. Otolaryngology — Head Neck Surg 1997; 117: 308–314

27. Illingworth R D, Porter D G, Jakubowski J. Hemifacial spasm: a prospective long term follow up of 83 cases treated by microvascular decompression at two neurosurgical centres in the United Kingdom. J Neurol Neurosurg Psychiat 1996; 60: 72–77

28. Ji C S, Ui H C, You C K et al. Prospective study of microvascular decompression in hemifacial spasm. Neurosurgery 1997; 40: 730–735

29. Gross M L P. Hemifacial spasm: treatment with pizotifen. J Neurol Neurosurg Psychiat 1996; 61: 118

30. Patel J N. Gabapentin for the treatment of hemifacial spasm. Clin Neuropharmacol 1996; 19: 185–188

31. Mellick G A. Hemifacial spasm: successful treatment with felbamate. J Pain Symp Man 1995; 10: 392–395

Index

CD-ROM Instructions

1. Insert the CD into your computer's CD-ROM drive.
2. Refer to the appropriate system:

For Windows® 95 / 98 or Windows NT®:

Simply double click your CD-ROM drive icon. Then double click the ISIS.EXE program icon to run the program. The program will not run without an appropriate QuickTime installation. If an appropriate version of QuickTime is not found on your computer you will be given the opportunity to install QuickTime 2.1 onto your hard drive.

For Macintosh:

Please ensure that the sound is turned up to a comfortable listening level. Double click on the ISIS.EXE program icon to run the program.

General Requirements:

Great care has been taken to incorporate videos of high detail in order to represent accurately a number of movement disorders. Therefore, it is recommended that your system run at a minimum of 200 MHz and that your monitor be set to a minimum of 640x480 (16 bit/thousands of colour). A minimum 4X speed CD-ROM drive is also required.

It is recommended that screensavers be turned off while viewing the program. This product runs from the desktop and installation onto your hard drive is not required.

This product is non-refundable if the seal on the CD wallet is broken.

Isis Medical Media does not offer technical support.